Pregnancy-Related Anxiety

This book provides a collective examination of the theoretical, empirical, and clinical perspectives of pregnancy-related anxiety. Pregnancy-related anxiety is a distinct form of anxiety that is experienced by pregnant women and is characterized by pregnancy-specific fears and worries. This form of anxiety has been associated with a range of negative obstetric, neonatal, and maternal outcomes. There has been increased research interest in this form of anxiety, particularly over the last 15 years.

The content is organized in three parts. Part I provides a thorough understanding of pregnancy-related anxiety, ranging from its historical development, evidence of its distinctiveness to the antecedents, and outcomes of this anxiety for the mother and child. Part II examines key clinical issues around diagnosis and treatment specifically, current diagnosis/screening for this anxiety, and approaches for intervention and treatment. Part III considers emerging areas of research such as pertinent issues around culture and acculturation, which are key issues in an increasingly multicultural world. Moreover, the effects of pregnancy-related anxiety on the woman's broader psychosocial functioning are considered with specific chapters on body image and sexual abuse, two key areas of concern.

A seminal resource, this book provides a broad examination of the topic from multiple frameworks and perspectives, which sets this book apart from other books in print. This book intends to inform and stimulate future research studies, as well as increase awareness and understanding of pregnancy-related anxiety. It is a must-read for researchers, educators, clinicians, and higher education students who care about delivering better support and services to pregnant women, particularly those who are vulnerable and distressed.

Rachel Dryer is an Associate Professor at Australian Catholic University, Australia.

Robyn Brunton is a Lecturer at Charles Sturt University, Australia.

Routledge Research in Women's Mental Health

This series offers an international forum for original and innovative research being conducted across the field of Mental Health. Titles in the series are empirically or theoretically informed and explore a range of dynamic and timely issues and emerging topics with particular relevance to women's mental health. The series is aimed at upper-level and post-graduate students, researchers, and research students, as well as academics and scholars.

Recent titles in the series include:

Understanding Complex Trauma and Post-Traumatic Growth in Survivors of Sex Trafficking
Foregrounding Women's Voices for Effective Care and Prevention
Heather Evans

Pregnancy-Related Anxiety
Theory, Research, and Practice
Edited by Rachel Dryer and Robyn Brunton

For more information about this series, please visit www.routledge.com/Routledge-Research-in-Womens-Mental-Health/book-series/RRWMH

Pregnancy-Related Anxiety
Theory, Research, and Practice

Edited by Rachel Dryer and
Robyn Brunton

Routledge
Taylor & Francis Group

LONDON AND NEW YORK

First published 2022
by Routledge
2 Park Square, Milton Park, Abingdon, Oxon OX14 4RN

and by Routledge
605 Third Avenue, New York, NY 10158

Routledge is an imprint of the Taylor & Francis Group, an informa business

© 2022 selection and editorial matter, Rachel Dryer and Robyn Brunton; individual chapters, the contributors

The right of Rachel Dryer and Robyn Brunton to be identified as the authors of the editorial material, and of the authors for their individual chapters, has been asserted in accordance with sections 77 and 78 of the Copyright, Designs and Patents Act 1988.

British Library Cataloguing-in-Publication Data
A catalogue record for this book is available from the British Library

Library of Congress Cataloging-in-Publication Data
A catalog record for this book has been requested

ISBN: 978-0-367-85630-4 (hbk)
ISBN: 978-1-032-12500-8 (pbk)
ISBN: 978-1-003-01400-3 (ebk)

DOI: 10.4324/9781003014003

Typeset in Galliard
by Apex CoVantage, LLC

This book is dedicated to every woman who has experienced anxiety during pregnancy. Pregnancy should be a time that is joyous and filled with the anticipation of a new baby. Sadly, for many women, pregnancy is experienced with fearful thoughts and feelings of dread. We hope that this book will contribute to increased awareness and understanding about pregnancy-related anxiety among clinical/postgraduate students, researchers, and professional staff in medical and allied health disciplines, so that women are better supported during this joyful, yet vulnerable time.

Contents

Figures

Tables

Contributors

Hamideh Bayrampour, PhD, MSc, is Assistant Professor in the Department of Family Practice, an associate member in the School of Population and Public Health, and a faculty member in Reproductive and Developmental Sciences program at the University of British Columbia, Canada. Dr. Bayrampour's research interests are in the areas of maternal mental health and pregnancy outcomes with particular interest in maternal anxiety and its assessment during the perinatal period. Dr. Bayrampour has research expertise in conducting systematic reviews, quantitative and qualitative research, mixed methods studies, and concept and trajectory analyses.

Katherine S. Bright, PhD, is Registered Nurse and Triage Coordinator at the Women's Mental Health Clinic at Alberta Health Services and Postdoctoral Fellow in the Cumming School of Medicine (Department of Community Health Sciences) at the University of Calgary in Canada. Her research interests are in virtual and digital delivery of mental health interventions for women during the perinatal period.

Jessica Brunner, BA, is a research coordinator and graduate student at the University of Rochester. Her interests are in maternal and child public health.

Robyn Brunton, PhD (Psychology) (Charles Sturt University, School of Psychology, Bathurst NSW 2795, Australia) has research interest in the area of women's psychosocial health with a particular interest in perinatal mental health and how childhood adversity impacts women and their children in later life. She teaches both undergraduate and postgraduate students and is Fellow of the UK Academy of Higher Education (Advance HE).

Helen Cheyne is Midwife and Professor of Maternal and Child Health Research and Deputy Director of the Chief Scientist Office Nursing, Midwifery and Allied Health Professions Research Unit (NMAHP RU) based at the University of Stirling. Her research interests are in perinatal mental health problems, women's experiences of maternity care, models of maternity care, and implementation science.

Allison Cunning, BA, a research associate at the University of Rochester and is now a graduate student at University of South Florida. Her interests are in child and maternal health and eating disorders.

Elysia Poggi Davis is Professor of Psychology at the University of Denver. Her program of research evaluates the way that biological and behavioral processes during the prenatal and postnatal periods are incorporated into the developmental program and the influence this has on physical and mental health across the lifespan. Professor Davis has led a research program that has been continuously funded by the National Institutes of Health for the past 17 years, including current support from grants P50 MH096889 and R01 MH109662, and she has published over 100 journal articles and book chapters.

Rachel Dryer, PhD, is a registered psychologist and an Associate Professor in the School of Behavioural & Health Sciences (Faculty of Health Science) of the Australian Catholic University in Australia. Her recent research interests are in health psychology, particularly women's mental health, body image, and disordered eating behavior. She teaches psychological testing and assessment to undergraduate and postgraduate students.

Christine Dunkel Schetter, PhD, is Professor of Psychology and Psychiatry at UCLA with training in social and health psychology. She is also Director of a training program in Biobehavioral Issues in Mental and Physical Health and Co-Chair of the Health Psychology PhD program. Her program of research in maternal child health focuses on biopsychosocial processes in pregnancy and prediction of birth, maternal, and child outcomes.

Sarah E. Garcia, PhD, is a clinical psychologist and Assistant Research Professor in the Department of Psychology at the University of Denver. Her research interests are in developmental psychopathology, including the intergenerational transmission of anxiety and depression.

Laura M. Glynn, PhD, is Professor of Psychology and Associate Dean for Research in Crean College of Health and Behavioral Sciences at Chapman University. Her program of research focuses on how the pre- and postnatal periods shape lifespan developmental trajectories of both mother and child.

Betty Goguikian Ratcliff, PhD, is a clinical psychologist and psychotherapist, senior lecturer, and researcher in the Faculty of Psychology and Educational Sciences at the University of Geneva, Switzerland. Her field of academic expertise is the intercultural clinical psychology. She is head of the research unit on intercultural and interpersonal clinical psychology, which aims to better understand the psychosocial vulnerability and protection mechanisms underlying the mental health outcomes of individuals in different contexts of migration.

Ella-Marie P. Hennessey, MA, is a graduate student in the University of Denver's Clinical Psychology PhD program. She is interested in the development of stress physiology in early childhood and the influence of prenatal factors upon child development more broadly.

Anja C. Huizink, PhD, is physiologist and neuropsychologist and a full professor at the Department of Clinical, Neuro and Developmental Psychology of the Vrije Universiteit Amsterdam, the Netherlands. Her research interests are in stress and anxiety across the lifespan, particularly in developmental transitional phases, such as pregnancy and adolescence, and in substance use and abuse among youth and emerging adults.

Melissa Julian, MA, is a predoctoral student in clinical psychology at George Washington University. Her research focuses on factors that contribute to resilience in the context of perinatal mood and anxiety disorders. Her published papers include work on resilience in pregnant women and a scale to measure resilience resources. Her clinical and research interests are in acceptance and mindfulness-based interventions in perinatal and other medical populations.

Ntemena Kapula, BA, a research associate at the University of Rochester, and at present a graduate student at University of California, San Francisco. Her research interests are in maternal and child health.

Jane Kohlhoff, PhD, is Associate Professor in the School of Psychiatry (Faculty of Medicine & Health) at the University of New South Wales, Australia, and Research Fellow at an Australian early parenting organization, Karitane. She conducts clinically oriented research in the areas of perinatal, infant, and early childhood mental health, and has particular interests in the interplay between early parenting, attachment, and child outcomes.

Bronwyn Leigh is a clinical psychologist and Director of the Centre for Perinatal Psychology and the Perinatal Training Centre. Bronwyn is deeply interested in the psychological aspects of becoming a parent, the emotional development of infants, and parent-infant relationships. She has coauthored a self-help workbook, contributed to research, and provided media interviews in the perinatal field.

Margaret Maxwell is Sociologist and Professor of Health Services and Mental Health Research, and Director of the Chief Scientist Office Nursing, Midwifery and Allied Health Professions Research Unit (NMAHP RU) based at the University of Stirling. Her research interests are in common mental health problems (depression and anxiety), suicide prevention, comorbid mental and physical illness, and implementation science.

Hannah Murphy, BA, is a research associate and graduate student at the University of Rochester. Her interests are in maternal and child health.

Thomas G O'Connor, PhD, is the Wynne Distinguished Professor at the University of Rochester, with appointments in Psychiatry, Psychology, Neuroscience, and Obstetrics and Gynecology. His clinical research considers the mechanisms by which early exposures shape child health outcomes.

Sarah E. D. Perzow, PhD, is a clinical psychologist and postdoctoral fellow at the University of Denver. Her research interests are in developmental psychopathology, particularly prevention, intervention, and stress and coping. She is currently a study therapist and researcher for The Care Project.

Carolyn Ponting, MA (Department of Psychology, University of California) is an advanced predoctoral student in clinical psychology at UCLA. She is interested in the acceptability and efficacy of psychological interventions for prenatal anxiety, especially among ethnic and racial minority women. She will continue her training as a bilingual clinical intervention scientist focused on the prenatal period at the University of California, San Francisco, where she will complete a clinical internship and postdoctoral fellowship and obtain her PhD in 2022.

Emma Robertson-Blackmore, PhD, Assistant Professor of Psychiatry at the University of Rochester, is now with the University of Florida and Florida Health Care Plans. Her interests are in perinatal mental health.

Shahirose Sadrudin Premji, BSc, BScN, MScN, PhD, FAAN, is a registered nurse and Director and Full Professor in the School of Nursing at York University in Toronto, Ontario, Canada. Her program of research on perinatal mental health brings new knowledge and innovation in improving mental health and well-being of women and their children from local to global.

Anna Sharapova, PhD, is a clinical psychologist and psychotherapist. She is member of the research unit on intercultural and interpersonal clinical psychology at the Faculty of Psychology and Educational Sciences in Geneva University. Her research interests are in perinatal mental health, particularly migrant women's psychological well-being during the perinatal period.

Andrea Sinesi, PhD, is a research psychologist in the Nursing, Midwifery and Allied Health Professions Research Unit (NMAHP RU) at the University of Stirling in the UK. His current research interests are in the areas of perinatal mental health and psychometrics, with a focus on improving the identification and care of women experiencing poor mental health during pregnancy and in the postnatal period.

Foreword

It is my genuine pleasure to write the foreword to this important book. Perinatal mental illness has always been with us. It makes my skin crawl to contemplate the generations of women, and men, who have suffered anxiety and depression in this context. What sets perinatal mental illness apart is the context. There is an almost universal acceptance that pregnancy is happy, positive, life-affirming, and desirable. Parenting should be filled with heart-aching love, laughter, and joy and the needs of the child, born and unborn, hold primacy over all other needs and desires, particularly for a mother. That a mother, or father, might experience anxious or depressive thoughts strikes a discordant note in every society's air-brushed, commercial view of this most precious of human experiences. It doesn't fit with an accepted narrative.

The responsibility of academia is to challenge perceived norms and assumptions, even when that is uncomfortable. Recognition that women are always autonomous beings, including when they are pregnant, or mothers, is essential. Asking the question, through screening and dialogue, is the only way to begin a conversation. There is a need to explore the cultural, social, and personal history, economic and social experiences that shape the person who then experiences, and reacts to, the reproductive journey. Then, we must challenge ourselves and ask whether our questions and interventions make that journey better, or worse. We need data, both qualitative and quantitative.

From my own lived experience, through my wife's severe perinatal mental illness nearly 30 years ago, I know that these matters are profound. Two ordinary people, a happy marriage, two beautiful boys, torn apart by crippling anxiety, suicidal ideation, a marriage breakdown, and then years of recovery. We are survivors, but many others have suffered and some, too many, have lost their lives. We can do better, to the benefit of individuals, families, and society as a whole. Serious academic interrogation should underpin any programs, or interventions and, the chapters in this book, *Pregnancy-related Anxiety: Theory, Research and Practice*, reflect the thoughtful, intellectual rigor, and commitment of the authors to this integral, human subject.

by Dr Vijay Roach, MBBS MRCOG FRANZCOG
President of the Royal Australian and New Zealand
College of Obstetricians and Gynecologists

Acknowledgments

This book has only been made possible because of the generous help of many people. The editors wish to first express their sincere gratitude to all the chapter authors for their generous involvement and fine contribution to the book. Second, we would like to sincerely thank the following colleagues who freely gave up their time and shared their knowledge to read and provide constructive comments on the chapters during the review process.

Anne Buist, Austin Health, University of Melbourne, Melbourne, Australia

Jan K. Buitelaar, Radboud University, Nijmegen, The Netherlands

Chui yi Chan, Caritas Institute of Higher Education, Hong Kong

Sheri Cassity, Foothills Medical Center, Calgary, Alberta, Canada

Christine Dunkel-Schetter, University of California, Los Angeles (UCLA), California, USA

Laura M. Glynn, Chapman University, Orange, California, USA

Hilde Grimstad, Norwegian University of Science and Technology, Norway

Rachael Hickinbotham, North Shore Private Hospital, Royal North Shore Hospital and the Mater Hospital, North Sydney, New South Wales, Australia

Calvin Hobel, Cedars Sinai Health Center, Los Angeles, California, USA

Eeva-Leena Kataja, University of Turku, Finland

Rachel Lev-Weisel, University of Haifa, Mount Carmel, Haifa, Israel

Roberta Mancuso, Regis University, Denver, Colorado, USA

Cathy McMahon, Macquarie University, North Ryde, New South Wales, Australia

Stephen Matthey, University of New South Wales; South West Sydney Local Health District, Sydney, Australia

Karen Matvienko-Sikar, University College Cork, Ireland

Sandra Nakic Rados, Catholic University of Croatia, Croatia

Shahirose Sadrudin Premji, York University, Toronto, Ontario, Canada

Vijay Roach, North Shore Private Hospital, Royal North Shore Hospital and the Mater Hospital, North Sydney, New South Wales, Australia

Emma Robertson-Blackmore, University of Florida and Florida Health Care Plans, Daytona Beach, Florida, USA
Rachel Rodgers, Northeastern University, Boston, Massachusetts, USA
Panagiota "Penny" Tryphonopoulos, Western University, London, Ontario, Canada
Hedwig van Bakel, Tilburg University, Tilburg, The Netherlands

In addition, we would also like to thank our universities (Australian Catholic University and Charles Sturt University) for their support. We also sincerely thank our Editor, Katie Peace, for all her support to realize this book. And lastly, on a personal note, we would like to thank our respective families for their constant love, support, and encouragement.

Abbreviations

ACOG	American College of Obstetricians and Gynecologists
AHDC	anxiety concerning health and defects in the child scale
AIDS	acquired immunodeficiency syndrome
ALSPAC	Avon longitudinal study of parents and children
ANRQ	Antenatal Risk Questionnaire
ART	assisted reproductive technology
AUROC	Area Under the Receiver Operating Characteristic Curve
BAI	Beck anxiety inventory
BDI	Beck depression inventory
BELIEF	birth emotions and looking to improve expectant fear
BIPS	body image in pregnancy scale
BMI	body mass index
CALM	coping with anxiety through living mindfully
CBQ-VB	Children's Behavior Questionnaire – Very Brief
CBT	cognitive behavior therapy
CES-D	Center for Epidemiological Studies – Depression
COPE	Centre of Perinatal Excellence
CRH	corticotropic-releasing hormone
CWS	Cambridge Worry Scale
DASS	depression, anxiety and stress scales
DoHaD	developmental origins of (mental) health and disease
DSM-IV	Diagnostic and Statistical Manual version 4
DSM-V	Diagnostic and Statistical Manual version 5
EPDS	Edinburgh Postnatal Depression Scale
GAD	Generalized Anxiety Disorder
GAD-2	Generalized Anxiety Disorder Scale – 2 items
GAD-7	Generalized Anxiety Disorder Scale – 7 items
GHQ	General Health Questionnaire
GP	General Practitioner
HADS	Hospital Anxiety And Depression Scale
HADS-A	Hospital Anxiety and Depression Scale, Anxiety Subscale
HIV	human immunodeficiency virus
HPA	hypothalamic-pituitary axis

ICD-10	International Classification of Diseases version 10
IVF	in vitro fertilization
K-10	Kessler Psychological Distress Scale
NICE	National Institute for Health and Care Excellence
NOSI	Nijmeegse Ouderlijke Stress Index
PAS	pregnancy-related anxiety scale
pCRH	placental corticotropic-releasing hormone
PHQ-4	Patient Health Questionnaire 4
POMS	profile of mood symptoms
POQ	Pregnancy Outcome Questionnaire
PRAQ	Pregnancy-Related Anxiety Questionnaire
PRAQ-R	Pregnancy-Related Anxiety Questionnaire – Revised
PRAQ-R2	Pregnancy-Related Anxiety Questionnaire – Revised (2)
PRAS	pregnancy-related anxiety scale
PRT	pregnancy-related thoughts
PSAS	pregnancy-specific anxiety scale
PSEQ-SF	Prenatal Self-Evaluation Questionnaire – Short Form
PSS	perceived stress scale
PSWQ	Penn State Worry Questionnaire
PTSD	post-traumatic stress disorder
RCT	randomized control trial
SAAS	Stirling Antenatal Anxiety Scale
SAS	self-rating anxiety scale
SCID	Structured Clinical Interview for DSM-IV
SCS	self-compassion scale
STAI	State-Trait Anxiety Inventory
STAIX	State Anger Inventory
UK	United Kingdom
USA	United States of America
WHO	World Health Organization

Introduction

Rachel Dryer and Robyn Brunton

Pregnancy is a significant period of transition for women. While there is the joyful anticipation of new life and a new role as a "mother," there is also a heightened sense of responsibility and uncertainty about the future. Therefore, it is not surprising that expectant mothers are vulnerable to developing psychological distress during this period (Bayrampour et al., 2015; Parfitt & Ayers, 2014). Pregnancy-related anxiety (also referred to as pregnancy anxiety and pregnancy-specific anxiety) is a distinct, multidimensional form of anxiety that is experienced by expectant mothers and characterized by pregnancy-specific fears and worries about the well-being of the unborn child, one's own health and well-being, childbirth, and body image (Bayrampour et al., 2016; Brunton et al., 2019). Unlike other forms of anxiety where the individual can avoid the places, people, and/or events that trigger their anxiety-related symptoms in order to experience a temporary sense of relief, engaging in avoidance behaviors is a lot more difficult for women with this form of anxiety. The significant physical, physiological, social, and psychological changes associated with pregnancy often serve as ever present reminders of the woman's fearful thoughts, worries, and feelings of dread.

Over the last decade or so, there has been a significant increase in research conducted on pregnancy-related anxiety in terms of how best to conceptualize and measure this form of anxiety, the antecedents/predictors of pregnancy-related anxiety, as well as the associated negative outcomes for both mother and child. However, despite this increased attention from researchers, we have not yet reached the stage where expectant mothers are routinely screened for pregnancy-related anxiety and there have been very few investigations conducted on the efficacy and effectiveness of common psychological approaches/interventions for addressing this anxiety construct, let alone interventions that have been developed to specifically address it. We also observed, while conducting our own research in this area, the lack of scholarly books dedicated to this topic.

This book is divided into three parts. In Part I of the book (*Understanding pregnancy-related anxiety*), we provide the reader with a thorough understanding of what pregnancy-related anxiety is and what it isn't. Chapter 1 (Dunkel Schetter and Ponting) provides an examination of the theoretical and empirical grounded definition of this form of anxiety as well as an overview of some of the key issues of contention and areas of research that are examined in more

DOI: 10.4324/9781003014003-1

detail in later chapters in the book. This is followed by Chapter 2 (Huizink) that examines the distinctiveness of pregnancy-related anxiety from general anxiety and depression and Chapter 3 (O'Connor et al.) that provides a review of the research on pregnancy-related anxiety in relation to other affective disorders in pregnancy. The last three chapters in this part provides a discussion of the antecedents (Chapter 4 – Bayrampour), birth outcomes (Chapter 5 – Dunkel Schetter et al.), and outcomes for the infant/child (Chapter 6 – Garcia et al.).

Part II of the book (*Implications for practice*) focuses on issues relevant to clinical practice, which includes a critical examination of the current diagnostic practices and their limitations (Chapter 7 – Kohlhoff), a critical review of the current scales to measure pregnancy-related anxiety and their psychometric properties (Chapter 8 – Sinesi et al.), and a critical examination of current psychological and psychosocial interventions for anxiety during pregnancy (Chapter 9 – Leigh and Brunton).

Part III of the book (*Future directions*) examines the core gaps in the current research on pregnancy-related anxiety. The first two chapters in this section examine cross-cultural perspectives of pregnancy-related anxiety (Chapter 10 – Bright and Premji) and issues of acculturation on antenatal anxiety in migrant women (Chapter 11 – Sharapova and Goguikian Ratcliff). The last two chapters examine the psychosocial functioning of pregnant women in relation to past childhood sexual abuse (Chapter 12 – Brunton) and body dissatisfaction (Chapter 13 – Dryer).

We hope that by providing a comprehensive coverage of research on pregnancy-related anxiety by key and prominent researchers in this field of study will contribute to greater awareness and understanding about this form of anxiety among professionals, clinicians, and postgraduate students in medical and allied health disciplines. We also hope that pulling together the current and emerging literature on pregnancy-related anxiety in one book will stimulate current and emerging researchers to address the gaps in the literature identified by the various contributing authors in the book.

References

Bayrampour, H., Ali, E., McNeil, D. A., Benzies, K., MacQueen, G., & Tough, S. (2016). Pregnancy-related anxiety: A concept analysis. *International Journal of Nursing Studies*, 55, 115–130. https://doi.org/10.1016/j.ijnurstu.2015.10.023

Bayrampour, H., McDonald, S., & Tough, S. (2015). Risk factors of transient and persistent anxiety during pregnancy. *Midwifery*, 31(6), 582–589. https://doi.org/10.1016/j.midw.2015.02.009

Brunton, R. J., Dryer, R., Saliba, A., & Kohlhoff, J. (2019). The initial development of the pregnancy-related anxiety scale. *Women Birth*, 32(1), 118–130. https://doi.org/10.1016/j.wombi.2018.05.004

Parfitt, Y., & Ayers, S. (2014). Transition to parenthood and mental health in first-time parents. *Infant Mental Health Journal*, 35(3), 263–273. https://doi.org/10.1002/imhj.21443

Part I

Understanding
pregnancy-related anxiety

1 What is pregnancy-related anxiety?

Christine Dunkel Schetter and Carolyn Ponting

What is pregnancy-related anxiety?

The term *pregnancy-related anxiety* is now common in the literature on pregnancy. It appears in nursing, psychological, psychiatric, and obstetrics publications among others. Yet it does not have one agreed-upon definition. Slightly different terms in the literature refer to overlapping yet distinct concepts. For example, *pregnancy anxiety, pregnancy-specific anxiety, pregnancy distress, and pregnancy concerns* are all terms that are used. Moreover, these terms are not always well defined. Researchers have too often designed assessment tools and then created a title for the instrument, not always accurately reflecting the content assessed. In our own research, we prefer the term *pregnancy anxiety*. Therefore, in this chapter, we will use the term pregnancy anxiety when describing the development of our scales and related studies. In all other aspects, the term *pregnancy-related anxiety* will be used for consistency in terminology throughout this book. Pregnancy-related anxiety is most often conceptualized as an affective state consisting of any combination of concerns about one's pregnancy, baby, self, hospital and health care, childbirth, and future parenting (Dunkel Schetter, 2011).

The difficulty in coming to agreement on the definition of pregnancy-related anxiety is readily apparent in several systematic reviews published since 2011 on anxiety and stress during pregnancy (Evans et al., 2015; Nast et al., 2013; Sinesi et al., 2019). Some of the reviews focus on clinical screening for anxiety symptoms and clinical disorders during pregnancy (Meades & Ayers, 2011). Others focus more broadly and include at least some measures of pregnancy-related anxiety. For example, Sinesi et al. (2019) reviewed anxiety scales used in pregnancy and reported on 22 relevant studies, 11 of which use instruments that measured "general worries" experienced during pregnancy, whereas 3 studies involved instruments measuring pregnancy-specific worries, distress, or anxiety. Similarly, Evans et al. (2015) conducted a systematic review of anxiety instruments in pregnancy in which 4 of 17 scales were on pregnancy-related anxiety, while 3 more were on pregnancy distress that is broader. Similarly, Nast et al. (2013) systematically reviewed instruments measuring psychosocial stress in pregnancy, finding 11 anxiety scales and 6 scales measuring pregnancy-specific stress. In that review, some of the scales classified under anxiety were actually on pregnancy-related

DOI: 10.4324/9781003014003-3

anxiety, but others were more general, exemplifying the ongoing confusion about the concepts involved.

In sum, there are a plethora of measures of anxiety and stress used in pregnancy research, as well as a number of instruments developed to assess pregnancy-related anxiety and pregnancy stress. The large number of instruments and their assessment of various interrelated concepts together contribute to the absence of an agreed-upon definition of pregnancy-specific anxiety (Brunton et al., 2015) and to lack of agreement on the adoption of common assessment tools.

History of research on pregnancy-related anxiety

The earliest published work on pregnancy-related anxiety or distress was conducted by Pleshette, Asch, and Chase who in 1956 reported that half to two-thirds of women feared pain and injury during delivery, losing their baby, or fetal abnormality. Later, Light and Fenster (1974) created one of the first inventories on pregnancy-related anxiety with 62 items on maternal concerns during pregnancy, including those about the baby, birth, self, family, medical care, and finances. At about the same time, Burstein et al. (1974) also developed a dichotomous (true/false) 25-item pregnancy anxiety scale (PAS) that captured psychosomatic concerns regarding a woman's pregnancy and concerns about hers and the baby's health, including the postpartum period. In later work (Glazer, 1980), researchers found that 94% of a sample of 100 women in a Midwestern region of the United States were concerned about whether the baby would be healthy and normal, 93% about the baby's condition at birth, 91% about her appearance as an expecting mother, and 89% about unexpected events during birth. Standley et al. (1979) and Lederman (1984) were also pioneers in this area of research conducting interviews to assess a woman's acceptance of her pregnancy, parenting confidence, and concerns over her relationship with the baby's father.

Since then, others around the world have developed concepts, measures, and programmatic research on pregnancy-related anxiety. Research teams in the United Kingdom, Belgium, Australia, and various parts of the United States continue to push this work forward. Notably, Van den Berg, Huizink, and colleagues have a large program of work on pregnancy-related anxiety, based on the Pregnancy-Related Anxiety Questionnaire (PRAQ) that is translated into many languages, including Spanish and German (Huizink et al., 2004, 2016; Sikkema et al., 2001; Van den Bergh, 1992).

What is pregnancy-related anxiety and what isn't it?

Bayrampour et al. (2016) have added to our understanding of pregnancy-related anxiety by differentiating it from other forms of distress. Reviewing qualitative and quantitative data from 38 studies, these researchers conducted a concept analysis based on the premise that pregnancy-related anxiety is a distinct concept from general anxiety and depression. Their systematic approach to clarifying the concept resulted in the following definition: "nervousness and fear about the baby's health, the mother's health and appearance, experience with the health care system, social and financial issues in the context of pregnancy, childbirth and parenting that are accompanied by excessive worry and somatic symptoms" (p. 121). This definition is similar to how we have defined these phenomena in our work, as "fears about the health and well-being of one's baby, the impending childbirth, of hospital and health care experiences (including one's own health and survival in pregnancy), birth and postpartum, and of parenting or the maternal role" (Dunkel Schetter, 2011, pp. 534–535; Guardino & Dunkel Schetter, 2014).

Worries or concerns about one's pregnancy occurring during a specific pregnancy are a central component of pregnancy-related anxiety. It is important to distinguish this component from worries about becoming pregnant and from symptoms of generalized anxiety. Pregnancy anxiety is distinct from the concepts and measures of general state and trait anxiety, and from current or past anxiety disorder diagnoses. That is, pregnancy-specific anxiety is more than just general anxiety assessed *during pregnancy*. Huizink and colleagues (2004) demonstrated that generalized anxiety and depressive symptoms contributed just 17% of the variance in pregnancy-related anxiety, a finding replicated across early, mid, and late pregnancy by a study in Australia with a much larger sample size ($n = 1209$) (Brunton et al., 2019).

Pregnancy-related anxiety may vary over the course of pregnancy, as may the specific worries a woman experiences. For example, there is maternal worry early in pregnancy associated with unplanned pregnancies (Grussu et al., 2005). In addition, we know that women are often anxious during their first trimester about possible pregnancy loss and as they acclimate to pregnancy-specific physical symptoms and anticipate further changes (Rubertsson et al., 2014). In addition, women who experience high-risk conditions during pregnancy are likely to have concerns about the well-being of their baby (McCoyd et al., 2020). Toward the end of pregnancy, women worry more about impending labor and delivery (Madhavanprabhakaran et al., 2015; Mudra et al., 2020). They also may worry about their own health and even surviving childbirth, especially if they lack confidence in prenatal and maternity care in their health care setting (Davis, 2019; Engle et al., 1990; Backes et al., 2020). Finally, pregnant women worry about being a good mother, and about meeting any cultural expectations associated with pregnancy and motherhood. For example, some cultural groups expect women to be happy and emotionally steady during pregnancy for the baby's sake (Kieffer et al., 2002). Thus, a range of pregnancy-related concerns may arise over the course of pregnancy under the umbrella term of pregnancy-related anxiety.

When researchers describe pregnancy concerns, they appear to be referencing many of these pregnancy-related worries, however, not all concerns that occur in the context of pregnancy should be considered pregnancy-related anxiety. Women who are worried about paying rent or buying food during pregnancy are likely to have worried about these issues before becoming pregnant and will continue to worry about them after pregnancy. These chronic worries are not usually specific to pregnancy, although they may be exacerbated due to prenatal nutrition concerns, but the issues are captured more effectively by other measures in the literature (e.g., Tallis et al., 1994). Social and financial sources of concern reflect stress-related concepts that are clearly distinguishable from anxiety in general or pregnancy-related anxiety. For example, concepts such as financial strain and relationship stress have separate measures and literatures (Dunkel Schetter et al., 2013; Pierce, 1994; Ross et al., 2019). Thus, these need not be confounded with assessments of pregnancy-related anxiety. In contrast, worrying specifically about whether the baby is getting sufficient nutrients and is growing normally is specific to a pregnancy and is what many existing pregnancy-related anxiety measures or scales are designed to measure.

Pregnancy-related anxiety is also differentiable from measures of stress in pregnancy such as the occurrence of stressors captured by negative life event inventories (Mirabzadeh et al., 2013), and from measures of chronic stress that are ongoing stressful conditions of any type (Dunkel Schetter et al., 2016). While acute negative life events and chronic stress may share some of the properties and mechanisms linking them to outcomes such as biological stress responses (Glover, 2014), they do not encompass or define pregnancy anxiety precisely (Meijer et al., 2014).

Figure 1.1 lays out the overlap and distinctions between pregnancy-related anxiety, pregnancy stress, and general prenatal anxiety. Our argument is that all of these concepts pertain to distress during pregnancy, but that general prenatal anxiety, prenatal stress, and pregnancy-related anxiety are distinguishable conceptually and operationally or within the content of assessment tools.

In Figure 1.1, what is labeled "Prenatal General Anxiety" is inclusive of state anxiety, trait anxiety, and clinical symptoms and diagnoses of anxiety disorders. "Prenatal Stress" in Figure 1.1 refers to both stressful conditions (or exposures) such as living in poor neighborhoods, experiencing loss of a loved one, and perceptions or appraisals of stress – but not biological stress markers that have been conceptualized as stress responses (e.g., Lobel, 1994). Most importantly, "Pregnancy-related Anxiety" in the figure is shown as distinct from these

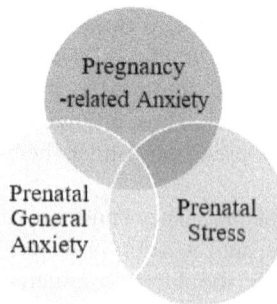

Figure 1.1 Conceptual model of distress during pregnancy

other concepts. As depicted, there is some common variance among these three concepts. Each of these states can be experienced independently or in combination with the other two; each has distinct causes and implications for pregnant women and their offspring. Although pregnancy-related anxiety is distinguishable from other stressors or clinical diagnoses experienced during pregnancy, some pregnancy-related anxiety measures include more than just pregnancy-related anxiety, and therefore confound it with these related concepts. If the goal is to conceptualize and measure pregnancy-related anxiety precisely for basic research and screening, then this lack of precision is not a best practice.

The evolution of our laboratory's understanding of pregnancy anxiety

The definition of pregnancy anxiety in our work evolved after we did several studies that focused on stress and affective states in pregnancy broadly. We created pregnancy anxiety scales that borrowed from Lederman (1984) whose work inspired us. Surprisingly, using very preliminary measures, we found and replicated results demonstrating effects of pregnancy anxiety on length of gestation, and the strength of these effects was often stronger than other standardized measures of stress or anxiety. In a first pilot study, five dichotomous items predicted length of gestation in 90 women (Wadhwa et al., 1993). In a second larger study, a more developed ten-item pregnancy anxiety scale predicted length of gestation in a well-controlled analysis of 230 Latin American and White women (Rini et al., 1999). In a third study, we used a different, much briefer pregnancy-specific anxiety measure consisting of four adjectives and referring to anxiety "regarding your pregnancy" (Roesch et al., 2004). Using advanced multivariate quantitative methods in a sample of 688 diverse women, we found that pregnancy-specific anxiety predicted length of gestation better than standard scale measures of state anxiety or perceived stress. At that point, our program of work expanded to develop the concept and theory surrounding pregnancy anxiety further (Dunkel Schetter, 1998), and we published both scales (Rini et al., 1999; Guardino & Dunkel Schetter, 2014).

In sum, researchers were working on measures of pregnancy-related anxiety as early as 1974, but the onset of systematic work in this area dates to the early 1990s (Chen et al., 1989; Van den Bergh, 1990). At the same time, no one was especially concerned with precisely defining what was being studied. The phenomenon captured attention more than the desire to develop theory. In some cases, a justifiable research goal may have been to study stress or general anxiety symptoms in pregnancy, not pregnancy-related anxiety. However, the history of inadequate conceptualization in this area of research has been a hindrance to progress as noted by several authors (Bayrampour et al., 2016; Dunkel Schetter, 2011; Dunkel Schetter & Glynn, 2011; Field, 2017). As the work has evolved, a narrower definition of pregnancy-related anxiety as a distinct concept has emerged.

Why study pregnancy-related anxiety?

Despite confusion over the definition, some existing measures of pregnancy-related anxiety predict birth outcomes. Reviews conclude that pregnancy-related anxiety predicts shorter length of gestation and sometimes low birth weight across samples of women with diverse nationalities and racial/ethnic identities (Dunkel Schetter & Tanner, 2012; Field, 2017). Another body of research indicates that pregnancy-related anxiety predicts child outcomes, including temperament and cognitive development from infancy through adolescence (Blair et al., 2011; Buss et al., 2011; Ding et al., 2014). Research has also begun to link pregnancy-related worries with offspring mental health. For example, an analysis of three prenatal cohorts combined (n = 19,896) found that a latent factor labeled pregnancy-specific worries composed of pregnancy-specific anxiety and two other related measures was associated with greater general psychopathology in youth at 4–8 years of age, controlling for effects of family socioeconomic status, women's postpartum affective symptoms, and preterm birth of the offspring (Szekely et al., 2021).

While predictive validity is evident from studies showing pregnancy-related anxiety consistently and independently predicts birth, infant, and child outcomes, there are inconsistencies in results from measure to measure, with some instruments more consistently replicating findings for specific outcomes than others. This may be due to lower reliability of some measures, the content of the measures (i.e., their construct validity), or other factors. Nonetheless, this unique contextually based form of anxiety is associated with many adverse maternal and child outcomes (Brunton et al., 2019).

A schematic of our model of pregnancy anxiety appears in Figure 1.2 based on an earlier formulation (Dunkel Schetter, 2011). The framework depicts predictors, mediators, outcomes, and the possible role of moderators, although moderation has rarely been studied. Existing research on pregnancy-related anxiety fits into this overall framework, and the framework suggests avenues for future work.

Are the effects of pregnancy-related anxiety different from other forms of prenatal distress?

Existing evidence suggests that pregnancy-related anxiety is more consistently linked to preterm birth than state or trait anxiety (Dunkel Schetter, 2011). However, there are more studies on state anxiety and it too is consistently associated with adverse neurodevelopmental outcomes in offspring (Glover, 2014). Furthermore, pregnancy-related anxiety predicts birth and postpartum outcomes after controlling for prenatal anxiety disorders (i.e., Generalized Anxiety Disorder – GAD), suggesting an independent effect of pregnancy-related anxiety on maternal physiology and functioning beyond what is accounted for by clinical disorders (Blackmore et al., 2016).

Regarding other types of prenatal distress, there is a much larger literature on depressive symptoms in pregnancy than that on anxiety. This is partly due to an

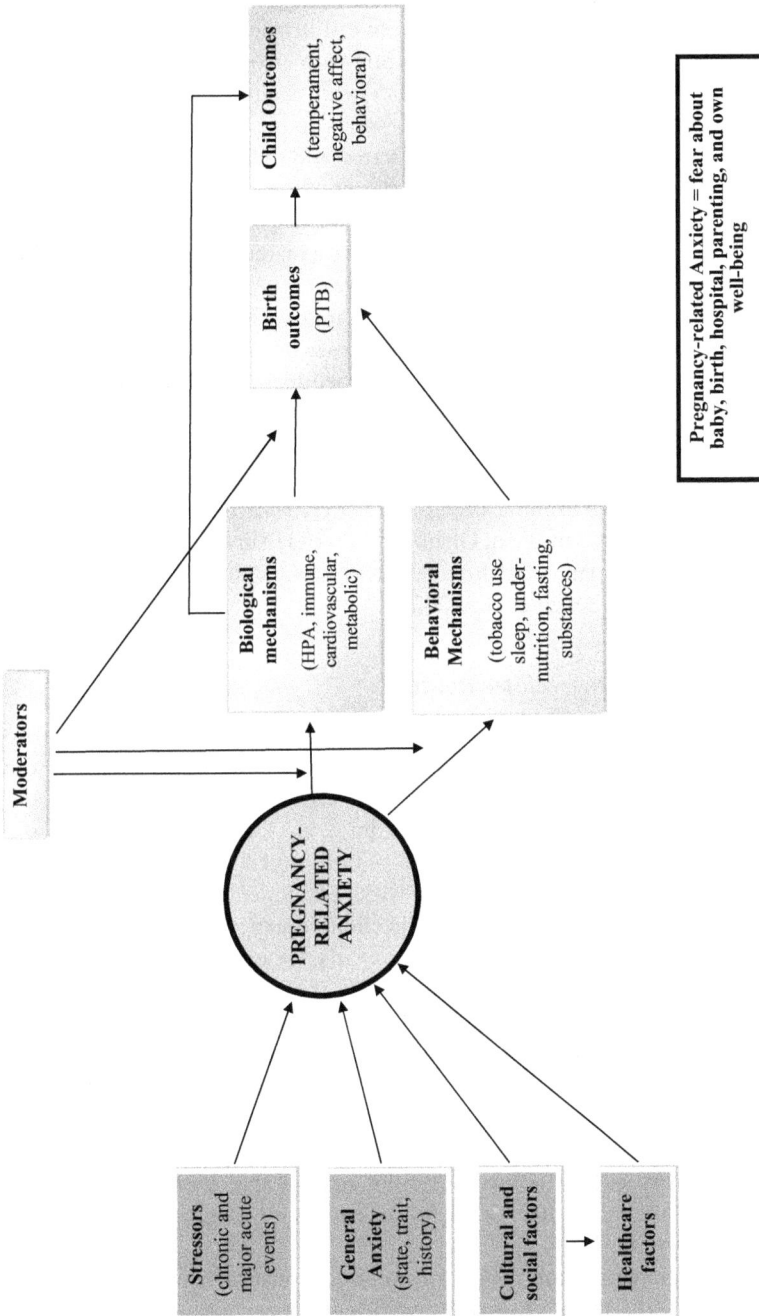

Figure 1.2 Pregnancy-related anxiety processes

emphasis on postpartum depression and its harmful effects on mothers, infants, and their families (Grote et al., 2010; Yim et al., 2015). We know that anxiety and depression are comorbid, but they are quite distinct both in general and during pregnancy. At face value, a mother presenting with anxiety about whether she or her baby will be harmed during labor and delivery is quite different from another presenting with depressed mood or hopelessness about a pregnancy that she feels ill-equipped to manage. These emotional states, and their predisposing and maintaining factors can be distinguished, and may cooccur.

Of note, there is some evidence that prenatal depression, state anxiety, and pregnancy-related anxiety have different effects on maternal behavior, physiology, and birth outcomes. At least one systematic review (Accortt et al., 2015) finds depressive symptoms in pregnancy are associated with low birth weight, possibly due to poor or inadequate diet and sedentary behavior, whereas pregnancy-related anxiety is linked specifically to the neuroendocrine pathways implicated in preterm birth. Child outcomes may also be differentially influenced by prenatal anxiety versus prenatal depression, although few researchers have tested this or reviewed any findings on this issue. Much of the evidence for adverse effects on offspring via fetal programming implicates anxiety (not depression) such as the program of research by Sandman, Glynn, and Davis (Blair et al., 2011; Buss et al., 2010; Davis & Sandman, 2012), and that of Glover and colleagues (Huizink et al., 2003; Van Den Bergh et al., 2005).

Predictors of pregnancy-related anxiety

Dunkel Schetter (2011) presented a comprehensive model of pregnancy-related anxiety and its antecedents, effects, and mechanisms. This model specified some of the factors that predict higher pregnancy-related anxiety such as a preexisting anxiety disorder or history of anxiety (Mudra et al., 2020), major life stressors, medical risks and how they are communicated to women, and cultural influences. Growing evidence indicates that women with certain demographic, medical, and other maternal background factors are likeliest to experience high pregnancy-related anxiety. In the United States and Canada, for example, women are most likely to experience pregnancy-related anxiety if they are having a first birth, are unmarried, were treated for infertility, experienced a prior miscarriage, are at high risk due to medical conditions, are low income, of Latina heritage, or had a prior anxiety disorder (Arch, 2013; Dunkel Schetter et al., 2016; Guardino & Dunkel Schetter, 2014; Tsartsara & Johnson, 2006). Most studies show younger women experience more pregnancy-related anxiety, but women of advanced maternal age are sometimes more anxious than younger women (see Guardino & Dunkel Schetter, 2014 for an overview), suggesting a curvilinear pattern with maternal age.

Other demographic factors also show non-linear relationships with pregnancy-related anxiety. Education is associated with higher pregnancy-related anxiety in some studies, lower levels in others, and sometimes shows no effect. Likely these mixed findings indicate that very low and very high education can produce more anxiety for different reasons, whereas the middle education group is lower in anxiety. For example, highly educated women may seek excessive information about pregnancy, whereas women with less access to formal education may lack basic information, with both extremes fostering anxiety.

Evidence for mechanisms linking pregnancy-related anxiety to outcomes

Two general mechanistic pathways linking pregnancy-related anxiety to birth and child outcomes – biological and behavioral – are shown in Figure 1.2. There is growing evidence for biological mechanisms linking pregnancy-related anxiety to the onset of labor and the timing of delivery (Beijers et al., 2014). Stress hormones and the hypothalamic pituitary axis (HPA) have received the most attention. In pregnancy, levels of placental corticotropic-releasing hormone (pCRH) increase exponentially, reaching high levels in maternal and fetal compartments during late pregnancy and peak concentrations at term and in labor (Hillhouse & Grammatopoulos, 2002; Lindsay & Nieman, 2005; McLean et al., 1995). Studies have shown that premature rises and accelerations in pCRH levels pose higher risk for shortened length of gestation (Sandman, 2015; Wadhwa et al., 1996, 2004). Other studies have shown associations of pregnancy-related anxiety with HPA processes implicated in adverse outcomes such as preterm birth (Hobel, 2004; Kane et al., 2014; Wadhwa et al., 2004).

Very few studies have conducted full mediational analyses with pregnancy-related anxiety predicting a birth or child outcome via biological mediation. Among the first was Mancuso et al. (2004) in a study of 282 pregnant women who reported that higher pCRH levels and higher prenatal anxiety at 28–30 weeks gestation predicted earlier delivery, with analyses supporting pCRH mediation. Pregnancy-related anxiety before 28 weeks did not predict time of delivery in this study, nor did standardized measures of perceived stress and state anxiety at two times in pregnancy. Importantly, perceived stress and state anxiety were also unassociated with pCRH, the proposed biological mechanism linking pregnancy-related anxiety to timing of birth, increasing confidence that pregnancy-related anxiety predicts distinct outcomes through distinct pathways. In a later study, Ramos et al. (2019) replicated and extended those findings in a sample of 337 pregnant women. Pregnancy-related anxiety at 19 and 31 weeks and pCRH at 31 weeks predicted length of gestation. Mediational analyses showed that pregnancy anxiety at 19 weeks and increases from 19 to 31 weeks predicted pCRH at 31 weeks, which in turn predicted timing of delivery in the sample as a whole and especially among Latinas.

Additionally, maternal immune function has been implicated in the relationship between pregnancy-related anxiety and preterm delivery by increased risk for intrauterine bacterial infections (Beijers et al., 2014). Very little research on pregnancy-related anxiety and immune processes has been done to date. One study indicated that pregnancy-specific distress has been linked to inflammatory markers that mediated effects on length of gestation (e.g., Coussons-Read et al.,

2012). More investigations of inflammatory processes as mediators of pregnancy anxiety related effects on outcomes are needed.

In addition to linking pregnancy-related anxiety and birth outcomes via biological mechanisms, there is some evidence for behavioral mechanisms. Substance use (both tobacco and alcohol) are higher in women with high pregnancy anxiety (Dunkel Schetter, 2011; Dunkel Schetter & Lobel, 2012). For example, Arch (2013) found that pregnancy-related anxiety emerged as a strong predictor of alcohol consumption during pregnancy. Pregnancy-related anxiety has also been associated with poor sleep, decreased physical activity, and unhealthy eating (Beijers et al., 2014), as well as excessive weight gain during pregnancy (Westerneng et al., 2017). Adverse health behaviors such as poor diet and their consequences (e.g., excess weight gain) are implicated in fetal development and pregnancy complications (Colón-Ramos et al., 2015; Shin et al., 2015). However, mediational studies that examine these behavioral variables in relation to birth or child outcomes are virtually non-existent. One exception is a study by Lobel et al. (2008) showing that pregnancy-specific stress (a related concept to pregnancy-related anxiety) was associated with smoking, caffeine consumption, and unhealthy eating and lower exercise and vitamin use in pregnancy, but only smoking was associated with shorter gestational age. These potential behavioral mechanisms also warrant future study.

Geographic and cultural factors

Research on pregnancy-related anxiety spans the globe but infrequently addresses the role of geographic or cultural factors. How people in different countries, with diverse ethnic, racial, and cultural backgrounds experience pregnancy-related anxiety is an area rich with opportunity. It is likely that different health care systems, beliefs systems about pregnancy and regarding the transition to motherhood, and cultural norms surrounding birthing practices contribute to differences in rates of pregnancy-related anxiety and responses to it, as well as effects on maternal and child outcomes. In our work, we have examined how pregnancy-related anxiety manifests in women of Latin American heritage and found within-group differences among Latinas based on their level of acculturation and foreign-born status. Specifically, in a sample of 95 women followed from pregnancy to 4 years postpartum, Spanish-speaking women reported more pregnancy-related anxiety than their English-speaking Latina or non-Latina white counterparts (Mahrer et al., 2020). These results were driven by increased fears among the Spanish-speaking women about their own health, the safety of their childbirth, and interactions with the medical system compared to more acculturated Latinas, who were presumably more familiar with US prenatal health care. Of note, Spanish-speaking Latinas in this sample showed stronger associations between pregnancy-related anxiety and offspring negative affect 4 years later compared to more acculturated Latinas or non-Latina White women. Thus, pregnancy-related anxiety may be an especially salient risk factor for adverse intergenerational effects among Latinas.

Finally, qualitative research in our lab with Latinas suggests that cultural factors (e.g., *marianismo*, value of self-sacrifice among Latinas), contextual factors (e.g., perceptions of anti-immigrant sociopolitical climate), and attitudinal factors (e.g., belief that women should feel lucky to be pregnant) may help explain the greater potency of pregnancy-related anxiety in this group (Ramos, 2020).

We have also looked at racial and ethnic differences in pregnancy-related anxiety among White, Latina, and Black women controlling for maternal education and income. Although we found that Latinas generally reported greater anxiety than their non-Latina White counterparts (Campos et al., 2008; Ramos et al., 2019), comparisons of non-Latina White and Black women show no differences (Dominguez et al., 2008). Studies in China (Zhou et al., 2020) and Tanzania (Rwakarema et al., 2015) have shed light on the rates of pregnancy-related anxiety outside of Western cultures, and show that culture and local policy (e.g., availability of prenatal decision-making, two-child policies) influence this affective state. We are encouraged by what we are learning, yet there is still much to understand regarding differences in the expression, and consequences of pregnancy-related anxiety among women of different races, ethnicities, and cultures and within various geographic contexts.

Future directions

Until we are able to further develop the theory and agree upon measurement of the concept, pregnancy-related anxiety will be difficult to screen for broadly and to achieve reduction in adverse outcomes for mothers and children. In future research, pregnancy-related anxiety measures must be based on a well-defined construct upon which scholars agree. Measures need to be validated using strong psychometric standards and compared for convergent, discriminant, and predictive validity with other measures, as is now appearing in some publications (e.g., Brunton et al., 2018; Reck et al., 2013). Understanding what outcomes pregnancy-related anxiety predicts distinctly from perinatal depression or general distress – and why – is critical to building research in this area.

There is also a need to further examine the predictors of pregnancy-related anxiety in order to develop a global understanding of this phenomenon, including variations due to socioeconomic and sociocultural contexts that increase pregnancy-related anxiety and its effects. For example, qualitative work has shown that among women in Malawi (Stewart et al., 2015) and Zambia (Mwape et al., 2012), HIV-related health concerns were common during pregnancy, while in rural parts of Turkey winters with severely cold temperatures and resulting difficulties getting to a hospital were most common (Boyacioğlu & Türkmen, 2008). Understanding pregnancy-related anxiety and improving our theories will require research that carefully attends to culture. Variation in worries, risk factors, and perinatal health systems in different regions of the world and in different cultures are likely to need different or adapted interventions (e.g., Ponting et al., 2020). The study of pregnancy-related anxiety has primarily occurred in North America,

Europe, and in parts of the Middle East, and accordingly we have much to learn about other parts of the world. Community voices in this work are valuable in designing and testing interventions that are effective.

Assuming we can precisely define and reliably and validly measure pregnancy-related anxiety, and given the growing evidence of its effects at birth and on offspring, then what should we do? Screening to identify women experiencing pregnancy-related anxiety and those at risk for it has the potential to permit us to reduce and prevent adverse psychological, birth, and offspring outcomes. Screening for depression during the prenatal period is now done universally and has been well received (El-Den et al., 2015). This is improving the public health of pregnant women. Yet notably absent are agreed-upon screening tools with strong predictive validity and known cutoffs to use widely to assess risk for pregnancy-related anxiety.

When valid screening tools for pregnancy-related anxiety become available, targeted interventions to reduce the specific form of anxiety will be essential. Currently, psychological interventions that target fears about pregnancy or birth are sparse. A recent systematic review of non-pharmacological interventions for fears of childbirth found that only four randomized controlled trials showed significant reductions in pregnancy-specific worries (Stoll et al., 2018). Of note, the majority of interventions reviewed in Stoll et al. (2018) tested childbirth education curriculums or mind-body therapies such as yoga. In other words, psychological interventions were noticeably absent. Promising psychological interventions to reduce anxiety about pregnancy include mindfulness (Guardino et al., 2014), stress management (Urizar et al., 2019), cognitive behavioral therapy (Kaboli et al., 2017), and combinations of these. An important area of research is the extent to which psychological and even complementary and alternative therapies (Newham et al., 2014) are acceptable to pregnant women. Finally, once there is a more established evidence base for efficacious interventions for pregnancy-related anxiety, trials should be designed with state-of-the-art intervention methods, including efforts to model and test mechanisms of symptom change. Thus, we have much to do.

Conclusion

A growing body of research now spanning three decades has identified a new and distinct concept specific to pregnancy, most commonly referred to as pregnancy anxiety or pregnancy-related anxiety. At this point, pregnancy-related anxiety has been measured, and reliably predicts birth and child outcomes. We also know a bit about which women are most likely to experience high pregnancy-related anxiety and of the biological and behavioral pathways to these adverse outcomes. In the future, it behooves those working in this area to be precise in the definitions, and to collaborate to determine best measurement approaches for specific applications. These collective efforts can go beyond theorizing about a distinct affective state during pregnancy or studying its correlates to contribute to translational efforts to reduce pregnancy-related anxiety among women, in effect improving birth outcomes.

References

Accortt, E. E., Cheadle, A. C. D., & Dunkel Schetter, C. (2015). Prenatal depression and adverse birth outcomes: An updated systematic review. *Maternal and Child Health Journal*, (19), 1306–1337. https://doi.org/1 0.1007/s10995-014-1637-2

Arch, J. J. (2013). Pregnancy-specific anxiety: Which women are highest and what are the alcohol-related risks? *Comprehensive Psychiatry*, *54*(3), 217–228. https://doi. org/10.1016/j.comppsych.2012.07.010

Backes, E. P., Scrimshaw, S. C., & National Academies of Sciences, Engineering, and Medicine. (2020). Maternal and newborn outcomes by birth setting. In *Birth settings in America: Outcomes, quality, access, and choice*. National Academies Press (US).

Bayrampour, H., Ali, E., McNeil, D. A., Benzies, K., MacQueen, G., & Tough, S. (2016). Pregnancy-related anxiety: A concept analysis. *International Journal of Nursing Studies*, *55*, 115–130. https://doi.org/10.1016/j.ijnurstu.2015.10.023

Beijers, R., Buitelaar, J. K., & de Weerth, C. (2014). Mechanisms underlying the effects of prenatal psychosocial stress on child outcomes: Beyond the HPA axis. *European Child & Adolescent Psychiatry*, *23*(10), 943–956. https://doi.org/10.1007/s00787-014-0566-3

Blackmore, E. R., Gustafsson, H., Gilchrist, M., Wyman, C., & O'Connor, T. G. (2016). Pregnancy-related anxiety: Evidence of distinct clinical significance from a prospective longitudinal study. *Journal of Affective Disorders*, *197*, 251–258. https://doi.org/10.1016/j.jad.2016.03.008

Blair, M. M., Glynn, L. M., Sandman, C. A., & Davis, E. P. (2011). Prenatal maternal anxiety and early childhood temperament. *Stress*, *14*(6), 644–651. https://doi.org/10.3109/10253890.2011.594121

Boyacioğlu, A. Ö., & Türkmen, A. (2008). Social and cultural dimensions of pregnancy and childbirth in eastern Turkey. *Culture, Health & Sexuality*, *10*(3), 277–285. https://doi.org/10.1080/13691050701673925

Brunton, R., Dryer, R., Saliba, A., & Kohlhoff, J. (2019). Re-examining pregnancy-related anxiety: A replication study. *Women and Birth*, *32*(1), e131–e137. https://doi.org/10.1016/j.wombi.2018.04.013

Brunton, R. J., Dryer, R., Krägeloh, C., Saliba, A., Kohlhoff, J., & Medvedev, O. (2018). The pregnancy-related anxiety scale: A validity examination using Rasch analysis. *Journal of Affective Disorders*, *236*, 127–135. https://doi.org/10.1016/j.jad.2018.04.116

Brunton, R. J., Dryer, R., Saliba, A., & Kohlhoff, J. (2015). Pregnancy anxiety: A systematic review of current scales. *Journal of Affective Disorders*, *176*, 24–34. https://doi.org/10.1016/j.jad.2015.01.039

Burstein, I., Kinch, R. A., & Stern, L. (1974). Anxiety, pregnancy, labor, and the neonate. *American Journal of Obstetrics and Gynecology*, *118*(2), 195–199. http://dx.doi.org/10.1016/0002-9378(74)90549-3

Buss, C., Davis, E. P., Hobel, C. J., & Sandman, C. A. (2011). Maternal pregnancy-specific anxiety is associated with child executive function at 6–9 years age. *Stress*, *14*(6), 665–676. https://doi.org/10.3109/10253890.2011.623250

Buss, C., Davis, E. P., Muftuler, L. T., Head, K., & Sandman, C. A. (2010). High pregnancy anxiety during mid-gestation is associated with decreased gray matter density in 6–9-year-old children. *Psychoneuroendocrinology*, *35*(1), 141–153. https://doi.org/10.1016/j.psyneuen.2009.07.010

Campos, B., Schetter, C. D., Abdou, C. M., Hobel, C. J., Glynn, L. M., & Sandman, C. A. (2008). Familialism, social support, and stress: Positive implications for pregnant Latinas. *Cultural Diversity & Ethnic Minority Psychology*, *14*(2), 155–162. https://doi.org/10.1037/1099-9809.14.2.155

Chen, C. H., Chen, H. M., & Huang, T. H. (1989). Stressors associated with pregnancy as perceived by pregnant women during three trimesters. *The Kaohsiung Journal of Medical Sciences*, *5*(9), 505–509.

Colón-Ramos, U., Racette, S., Ganiban, J., Nguyen, T., Kocak, M., Carroll, K., Völgyi, E., & Tylavsky, F. (2015). Association between dietary patterns during pregnancy and birth size measures in a diverse population in Southern US. *Nutrients*, *7*(2), 1318–1332. https://doi.org/10.3390/nu7021318

Coussons-Read, M. E., Lobel, M., Carey, J. C., Kreither, M. O., D'Anna, K., Argys, L., Ross, R. G., Brandt, C., & Cole, S. (2012). The occurrence of preterm delivery is linked to pregnancy-specific distress and elevated inflammatory markers across gestation. *Brain, Behavior, and Immunity*, *26*(4), 650–659. https://doi.org/10.1016/j.bbi.2012.02.009

Davis, D.-A. (2019). Obstetric racism: The racial politics of pregnancy, labor, and birthing. *Medical Anthropology*, *38*(7), 560–573. https://doi.org/10.1080/01459740.2018.1549389

Davis, E. P., & Sandman, C. A. (2012). Prenatal psychobiological predictors of anxiety risk in preadolescent children. *Psychoneuroendocrinology*, *37*(8), 1224–1233 https://doi.org/10.1016/j.psyneuen.2011.12.016

Ding, X. X., Wu, Y. Le, Xu, S. J., Zhu, R. P., Jia, X. M., Zhang, S. F., Huang, K., Zhu, P., Hao, J-H., & Tao, F. B. (2014). Maternal anxiety during pregnancy and adverse birth outcomes: A systematic review and meta-analysis of prospective cohort studies. *Journal of Affective Disorders*, *159*, 103–110. https://doi.org/10.1016/j.jad.2014.02.027

Dominguez, T. P., Dunkel-Schetter, C., Glynn, L. M., Hobel, C., & Sandman, C. A. (2008). Racial differences in birth outcomes: The role of general, pregnancy, and racism stress. *Health Psychology*, *27*(2), 194–203. https://doi.org/10.1037/0278-6133.27.2.194

Dunkel Schetter, C. (1998). Maternal stress and preterm delivery. *Prenatal Neonatal Medicine*, *3*, 39–42.

Dunkel Schetter, C. (2011). Psychological science on pregnancy: Stress processes, biopsychosocial models, and emerging research issues. *Annual Review of Psychology*, *62*(1), 531–558. https://doi.org/10.1146/annurev.psych.031809.130727

Dunkel Schetter, C., & Lobel, M. (2012). Pregnancy and birth outcomes: A multilevel analysis of prenatal maternal stress and birth weight. In A. Baum, T. A. Revenson, & J. Singer (Eds.), *Handbook of health psychology* (pp. 431–463). Psychology Press.

Dunkel Schetter, C., Niles, A. N., Guardino, C. M., Khaled, M., & Kramer, M. S. (2016). Demographic, medical, and psychosocial predictors of pregnancy anxiety. *Paediatric and Perinatal Epidemiology*, *30*(5), 421–429. https://doi.org/10.1111/ppe.12300

Dunkel Schetter, C., Schafer, P., Lanzi, R. G., Clark-Kauffman, E., Raju, T. N. K., & Hillemeier, M. M. (2013). Shedding light on the mechanisms underlying health disparities through community participatory methods: The stress pathway. *Perspectives on Psychological Science*, *8*(6), 613–633. https://doi.org/10.1177/1745691613506016

Dunkel Schetter, C., & Tanner, L. (2012). Anxiety, depression and stress in pregnancy: Implications for mothers, children, research, and practice. *Current Opinion in Psychiatry*, 25(2), 141–148. https://doi.org/10.1097/yco.0b013e3283503680

El-Den, S., O'Reilly, C. L., & Chen, T. F. (2015). A systematic review on the acceptability of perinatal depression screening. *Journal of Affective Disorders*, 188, 284–303. https://doi.org/10.1016/j.jad.2015.06.015

Engle, P. L., Scrimshaw, S. C., Zambrana, R. E., & Dunkel-Schetter, C. (1990). Prenatal and postnatal anxiety in Mexican women giving birth in Los Angeles. *Health Psychology*, 9(3), 285–299.

Evans, K., Spiby, H., & Morrell, C. J. (2015). A psychometric systematic review of self-report instruments to identify anxiety in pregnancy. *Journal of Advanced Nursing*, 71(9), 1986–2001. https://doi.org/10.1111/jan.12649

Field, T. (2017). Prenatal anxiety effects: A review. *Infant Behavior and Development*, 49, 120–128. https://doi.org/10.1016/j.infbeh.2017.08.008

Glazer, G. (1980). Anxiety levels and concerns among pregnant women. *Research in Nursing & Health*, 3(3), 107–113. https://doi.org/10.1002/nur.4770030305

Glover, V. (2014). Maternal depression, anxiety and stress during pregnancy and child outcome; what needs to be done. *Best Practice & Research Clinical Obstetrics & Gynaecology*, 28(1), 25–35. https://doi.org/10.1016/j.bpobgyn.2013.08.017

Grote, N. K., Bridge, J. A., Gavin, A. R., Melville, J. L., Iyengar, S., & Katon, W. J. (2010). A meta-analysis of depression during pregnancy and the risk of preterm birth, low birth weight, and intrauterine growth restriction. *Archives of General Psychiatry*, 67(10), 1012. https://doi.org/10.1001/archgenpsychiatry.2010.111

Grussu, P., Quatraro, R. M., & Nasta, M. T. (2005). Profile of mood states and parental attitudes in motherhood: Comparing women with planned and unplanned pregnancies. *Birth*, 32(2), 107–114. https://doi.org/10.1111/j.0730-7659.2005.00353.x

Guardino, C. M., & Dunkel Schetter, C. (2014). Understanding pregnancy anxiety: Concepts, correlates, and consequences. *Zero to Three*, 34(4), 12–21.

Guardino, C. M., Dunkel Schetter, C., Bower, J. E., Lu, M. C., & Smalley, S. L. (2014). Randomised controlled pilot trial of mindfulness training for stress reduction during pregnancy. *Psychology & Health*, 29(3), 334–349. https://doi.org/10.1080/08870446.2013.852670

Hillhouse, E. W., & Grammatopoulos, D. K. (2002). Role of stress peptides during human pregnancy and labour. *Reproduction*, 124(3), 323–329. https://doi.org/10.1530/rep.0.1240323

Hobel, C. J. (2004). Stress and preterm birth. *Clinical Obstetrics and Gynecology*, 47(4), 856–880. https://doi.org/10.1097/01.grf.0000142512.38733.8c

Huizink, A. C., Delforterie, M. J., Scheinin, N. M., Tolvanen, M., Karlsson, L., & Karlsson, H. (2016). Adaption of pregnancy anxiety questionnaire – revised for all pregnant women regardless of parity: PRAQ-R2. *Archives of Women's Mental Health*, (19), 125–132. https://doi.org/10.1007/s00737-015-0531-2

Huizink, A. C., Mulder, E. J. H., Robles de Medina, P. G., Visser, G. H. A., & Buitelaar, J. K. (2004). Is pregnancy anxiety a distinctive syndrome? *Early Human Development*, 79(2), 81–91. https://doi.org/10.1016/j.earlhumdev.2004.04.014

Huizink, A. C., Robles De Medina, P. G., Mulder, E. J. H., Visser, G. H. A., & Buitelaar, J. K. (2003). Stress during pregnancy is associated with developmental outcome in infancy. *Journal of Child Psychology and Psychiatry*, 44(6), 810–818. https://doi.org/10.1111/1469-7610.00166

Kaboli, S. K., Mahmoodi, Z., Mehdizadeh Tourzani, Z., Tehranizadeh, M., Kabir, K., & Dolatian, M. (2017). The effect of group counseling based on cognitive-behavioral approach on pregnancy-specific stress and anxiety. *Shiraz E-Medical Journal*, *18*(5), e13183. https://doi.org/10.5812/semj.45231

Kane, H. S., Dunkel Schetter, C., Glynn, L. M., Hobel, C. J., & Sandman, C. A. (2014). Pregnancy anxiety and prenatal cortisol trajectories. *Biological Psychology*, *100*, 13–19. https://doi.org/10.1016/j.biopsycho.2014.04.003

Kieffer, E. C., Willis, S. K., Arellano, N., & Guzman, R. (2002). Perspectives of pregnant and postpartum Latino women on diabetes, physical activity, and health. *Health Education & Behavior*, *29*(5), 542–556. https://doi.org/10.1177/109019802237023

Lederman, R. P. (1984). *Psychosocial adaptation in pregnancy: Assessment of seven dimensions of maternal development*. Prentice Hall.

Light, H. K., & Fenster, C. (1974). Maternal concerns during pregnancy. *American Journal of Obstetrics and Gynecology*, *118*(1), 46–50. https://doi.org/10.1016/S0002-9378(16)33644-4

Lindsay, J. R., & Nieman, L. K. (2005). The hypothalamic-pituitary-adrenal axis in pregnancy: Challenges in disease detection and treatment. *Endocrine Reviews*, *26*(6), 775–799. https://doi.org/10.1210/er.2004-0025

Lobel, M. (1994). Conceptualizations, measurement, and effects of prenatal maternal stress on birth outcomes. *Journal of Behavioral Medicine*, *17*, 225–272. https://doi.org/10.1007/bf01857952

Lobel, M., Cannella, D. L., Graham, J. E., DeVincent, C., Schneider, J., & Meyer, B. A. (2008). Pregnancy-specific stress, prenatal health behaviors, and birth outcomes. *Health Psychology*, *27*(5), 604–615. https://doi.org/10.1037/a0013242

Madhavanprabhakaran, G. K., D'Souza, M. S., & Nairy, K. S. (2015). Prevalence of pregnancy anxiety and associated factors. *International Journal of Africa Nursing Sciences*, *3*, 1–7. https://doi.org/10.1016/j.ijans.2015.06.002

Mahrer, N. E., Ramos, I. F., Guardino, C., Davis, E. P., Ramey, S. L., Shalowitz, M., & Dunkel Schetter, C. (2020). Pregnancy anxiety in expectant mothers predicts offspring negative affect: The moderating role of acculturation. *Early Human Development*, *141*, 104932. https://doi.org/10.1016/j.earlhumdev.2019.104932

Mancuso, R. A., Schetter, C. D., Rini, C. M., Roesch, S. C., & Hobel, C. J. (2004). Maternal prenatal anxiety and corticotropin-releasing hormone associated with timing of delivery. *Psychosomatic Medicine*, *66*(5), 762–769. https://doi.org/10.1097/01.psy.0000138284.70670.d5

McCoyd, J. L. M., Curran, L., & Munch, S. (2020). They say, "if you don't relax . . . you're going to make something bad happen": Women's emotion management during medically high-risk pregnancy. *Psychology of Women Quarterly*, *44*(1), 117–129. https://doi.org/10.1177/0361684319883199

McLean, M., Bisits, A., Davies, J., Woods, R., Lowry, P., & Smith, R. (1995). A placental clock controlling the length of human pregnancy. *Nature Medicine*, *1*(5), 460–463.

Meades, R., & Ayers, S. (2011). Anxiety measures validated in perinatal populations: A systematic review. *Journal of Affective Disorders*, *133*(1–2), 1–15. https://doi.org/10.1016/j.jad.2010.10.009

Meijer, J. L., Bockting, C. L. H., Stolk, R. P., Kotov, R., Ormel, J., & Burger, H. (2014). Associations of life events during pregnancy with longitudinal change in symptoms of antenatal anxiety and depression. *Midwifery*, *30*(5), 526–531. https://doi.org/10.1016/j.midw.2013.06.008

Mirabzadeh, A., Dolatian, M., Forouzan, A. S., Sajjadi, H., Majd, H. A., & Mahmoodi, Z. (2013). Path analysis associations between perceived social support, stressful life events and other psychosocial risk factors during pregnancy and preterm delivery. *Iranian Red Crescent Medical Journal*, *15*(6), 507–514. https://doi.org/10.5812/ircmj.11271

Mudra, S., Göbel, A., Barkmann, C., Goletzke, J., Hecher, K., Schulte-Markwort, M., Diemert, A., & Arck, P. (2020). The longitudinal course of pregnancy-related anxiety in parous and nulliparous women and its association with symptoms of social and generalized anxiety. *Journal of Affective Disorders*, *260*, 111–118. https://doi.org/10.1016/j.jad.2019.08.033

Mwape, L., McGuinness, T. M., Dixey, R., & Johnson, S. E. (2012). Socio-cultural factors surrounding mental distress during the perinatal period in Zambia: A qualitative investigation. *International Journal of Mental Health Systems*, *6*(1), 1–10. https://doi.org/10.1186/1752-4458-6-12

Nast, I., Bolten, M., Meinlschmidt, G., & Hellhammer, D. H. (2013). How to measure prenatal stress? A systematic review of psychometric instruments to assess psychosocial stress during pregnancy. *Paediatric and Perinatal Epidemiology*, *27*(4), 313–322. https://doi.org/10.1111/ppe.12051

Newham, J. J., Wittkowski, A., Hurley, J., Aplin, J. D., & Westwood, M. (2014). Effects of antenatal yoga on maternal anxiety and depression: A randomized controlled trial. *Depression and Anxiety*, *31*(8), 631–640. https://doi.org/10.1002/da.22268

Pierce, G. R. (1994). The quality of relationships inventory: Assessing the interpersonal context of social support. In B. R. Burleson, T. L. Albrecht, & I. G. Sarason (Eds.), *Communication of social support: Messages, interactions, relationships, and community* (pp. 247–264). Sage Publications, Inc.

Pleshette, N., Asch, S. S., & Chase, J. (1956). A study of anxieties during pregnancy, labor, the early and late puerperium. *Bulletin of the New York Academy of Medicine*, *32*(6), 436–455. www.ncbi.nlm.nih.gov/pubmed/13316338

Ponting, C., Mahrer, N. E., Zelcer, H., Dunkel Schetter, C., & Chavira, D. A. (2020). Psychological interventions for depression and anxiety in pregnant Latina and Black women in the United States: A systematic review. *Clinical Psychology and Psychotherapy*. https://doi.org/10.1002/cpp.2424

Ramos, I. F. (2020). *Cultural and psychobiological processes in pregnant Latina women* [Unpublished doctoral dissertation, UCLA]. ProQuest ID: Ramos_ucla_0031D_18585. Merritt ID: ark:/13030/m5d274zn. https://escholarship.org/uc/item/5n88j0vh

Ramos, I. F., Guardino, C. M., Mansolf, M., Glynn, L. M., Sandman, C. A., Hobel, C. J., & Dunkel Schetter, C. (2019). Pregnancy anxiety predicts shorter gestation in Latina and non-Latina white women: The role of placental corticotrophin-releasing hormone. *Psychoneuroendocrinology*, *99*, 166–173. https://doi.org/10.1016/j.psyneuen.2018.09.008

Reck, C., Zimmer, K., Dubber, S., Zipser, B., Schlehe, B., & Gawlik, S. (2013). The influence of general anxiety and childbirth-specific anxiety on birth outcome. *Archives of Women's Mental Health*, *16*(5), 363–369. https://doi.org/10.1007/s00737-013-0344-0

Rini, C. K., Dunkel-Schetter, C., Wadhwa, P. D., & Sandman, C. A. (1999). Psychological adaptation and birth outcomes: The role of personal resources, stress, and sociocultural context in pregnancy. *Health Psychology*, *18*(4), 333–345. https://doi.org/10.1037/0278-6133.18.4.333

Roesch, S. C., Schetter, C. D., Woo, G., & Hobel, C. J. (2004). Modeling the types and timing of stress in pregnancy. *Anxiety, Stress & Coping*, *17*(1), 87–102. https://doi.org/10.1080/1061580031000123667

Ross, K. M., Rook, K., Winczewski, L., Collins, N., & Dunkel Schetter, C. (2019). Close relationships and health: The interactive effect of positive and negative aspects. *Social and Personality Psychology Compass*, *13*(6). https://doi.org/10.1111/spc3.12468

Rubertsson, C., Hellström, J., Cross, M., & Sydsjö, G. (2014). Anxiety in early pregnancy: prevalence and contributing factors. *Archives of women's mental health*, *17*(3), 221–228. https://dx.doi.org/10.1007/s00737-013-0409-0

Rwakarema, M., Premji, S. S., Nyanza, E. C., Riziki, P., & Palacios-Derflingher, L. (2015). Antenatal depression is associated with pregnancy-related anxiety, partner relations, and wealth in women in Northern Tanzania: A cross-sectional study. *BMC Women's Health*, *15*(1), 1–10. https://doi.org/10.1186/s12905-015-0225-y

Sandman, C. A. (2015). Fetal exposure to placental corticotropin-releasing hormone (pCRH) programs developmental trajectories. *Peptides*, *72*, 145–153. http://dx.doi.org/10.1016/j.peptides.2015.03.020

Shin, D., Lee, K., & Song, W. (2015). Dietary patterns during pregnancy are associated with risk of gestational diabetes mellitus. *Nutrients*, *7*(11), 9369–9382. https://doi.org/10.3390/nu7115472

Sikkema, J. M., Robles de Medina, P. G., Schaad, R. R., Mulder, E. J., Bruinse, H. W., Buitelaar, J. K., Visser, G. H. A., & Franx, A. (2001). Salivary cortisol levels and anxiety are not increased in women destined to develop preeclampsia. *Journal of Psychosomatic Research*, *50*(1), 45–49. https://doi.org/10.1016/S0022-3999(00)00208-7

Sinesi, A., Maxwell, M., O'Carroll, R., & Cheyne, H. (2019). Anxiety scales used in pregnancy: Systematic review. *BJPsych Open*, *5*(1), e5. https://doi.org/10.1192/bjo.2018.75

Standley, K., Soule, B., & Copans, S. A. (1979). Dimensions of prenatal anxiety and their influence on pregnancy outcome. *American Journal of Obstetrics and Gynecology*, *135*(1), 22–26. www.ncbi.nlm.nih.gov/pubmed/474657

Stewart, R. C., Umar, E., Gleadow-Ware, S., Creed, F., & Bristow, K. (2015). Perinatal distress and depression in Malawi: An exploratory qualitative study of stressors, supports and symptoms. *Archives of Women's Mental Health*, *18*(2), 177–185. https://doi.org/10.1007/s00737-014-0431-x

Stoll, K., Swift, E. M., Fairbrother, N., Nethery, E., & Janssen, P. (2018). A systematic review of nonpharmacological prenatal interventions for pregnancy-specific anxiety and fear of childbirth. *Birth*, *45*(1), 7–18. https://doi.org/10.1111/birt.12316

Szekely, E., Neumann, A., Sallis, H., Jolicoeur-Martineau, A., Verhulst, F. C., Meaney, M. J., Pearson, R. M., Levitan, R. D., Kennedy, J. L., Lydon, J. E., Steiner, M., Greenwood, C. M. T., Tiemeier, H., Evans, J., & Wazana, A. (2021). Maternal prenatal mood pregnancy-specific worries, and early child psychopathology: Findings from the DREAM BIG consortium. *Journal of the American Academy of Child and Adolescent Psychiatry*, *60*(1), 186–197. https://doi.org/10.1016/j.jaac.2020.02.017

Tallis, F., Davey, G. C. L., & Bond, A. (1994). *The worry domains questionnaire.* John Wiley & Sons.

Tsartsara, E., & Johnson, M. P. (2006). The impact of miscarriage on women's pregnancy-specific anxiety and feelings of prenatal maternal – fetal attachment during the course of a subsequent pregnancy: An exploratory follow-up study. *Journal of Psychosomatic Obstetrics & Gynecology*, *27*(3), 173–182. https://doi.org/10.1080/01674820600646198

Urizar, G. G., Caliboso, M., Gearhart, C., Yim, I. S., & Dunkel Schetter, C. (2019). Process evaluation of a stress management program for low-income pregnant women: The SMART Moms/Mamás LÍSTAS Project. *Health Education & Behavior*, 109019811986055. https://doi.org/10.1177/1090198119860559

Van den Bergh, B. R. (1990). The influence of maternal emotions during pregnancy on fetal and neonatal behavior. *Journal of Prenatal & Perinatal Psychology & Health*, *5*(2), 119–130.

Van den Bergh, B. R. H. (1992). Maternal emotions during pregnancy and fetal and neonatal behaviour. *Fetal Behaviour: Developmental and Perinatal Aspects.* http://arno.uvt.nl/show.cgi?fid=94097

Van Den Bergh, B. R. H., Mulder, E. J. H., Mennes, M., & Glover, V. (2005). Antenatal maternal anxiety and stress and the neurobehavioural development of the fetus and child: Links and possible mechanisms. A review. *Neuroscience and Biobehavioral Reviews*, *29*(2), 237–258. https://doi.org/10.1016/j.neubiorev.2004.10.007

Wadhwa, P. D., Dunkel Schetter, C., Chicz-DeMet, A., Porto, M., & Sandman, C. A. (1996). Prenatal psychosocial factors and the neuroendocrine axis in human pregnancy. *Psychosomatic Medicine*, *58*(5), 432–446. https://doi.org/10.1097/00006842-199609000-00006

Wadhwa, P. D., Garite, T. J., Porto, M., Glynn, L., Chicz-DeMet, A., Dunkel Schetter, C., & Sandman, C. A. (2004). Placental corticotropin-releasing hormone (CRH), spontaneous preterm birth, and fetal growth restriction: A prospective investigation. *American Journal of Obstetrics & Gynecology*, *191*(4), 1063–1069. https://doi.org/10.1016/j.ajog.2004.06.070

Wadhwa, P. D., Sandman, C. A., Porto, M., Dunkel-Schetter, C., & Garite, T. J. (1993). The association between prenatal stress and infant birth weight and gestational age at birth: A prospective investigation. *American Journal of Obstetrics and Gynecology*, *169*(4), 858–865. https://doi.org/10.1016/0002-9378(93)90016-C

Westerneng, M., Witteveen, A. B., Warmelink, J. C., Spelten, E., Honig, A., & de Cock, P. (2017). Pregnancy-specific anxiety and its association with background characteristics and health-related behaviors in a low-risk population. *Comprehensive Psychiatry*, *75*, 6–13. https://doi.org/10.1016/j.comppsych.2017.02.002

Yim, I. S., Tanner Stapleton, L. R., Guardino, C. M., Hahn-Holbrook, J., & Dunkel Schetter, C. (2015). Biological and psychosocial predictors of postpartum depression: Systematic review and call for integration. *Annual Review of Clinical Psychology*. *11*, 99–137. https://doi.org/10.1146/annurev-clinpsy-101414-020426

Zhou, C., Weng, J., Tan, F., Wu, S., Ma, J., Zhang, B., & Yuan, Q. (2020). Pregnancy-related anxiety among Chinese pregnant women in mid-late pregnancy under the two-child policy and its significant correlates. *Journal of Affective Disorders*, *276*, 272–278. https://doi.org/10.1016/j.jad.2020.07.099

2 Pregnancy-related anxiety as distinct from state/trait anxiety and depression

Anja C. Huizink

Pregnancy-related anxiety as distinct from state/trait anxiety and depression

Pregnancy is an important transitional period in life, which can be accompanied with many pleasurable feelings and thoughts. At the same time, women can experience or develop feelings of anxiety that are specially related to pregnancy and birth. This chapter focuses on this type of anxiety, pregnancy-related anxiety, and how it is distinct from general anxiety and depression.

Normal patterns of change in mental health during pregnancy

For women who are pregnant for the first time, it is rather common to experience some changes in psychological well-being. Part of these changes in psychological well-being may be due to the fact that a major life transition is involved during (first-time) pregnancy: the transition to parenthood (Fox, 2009). This transition is regarded as a complex life event that may create many psychosocial challenges, which one needs to adapt to. This process of adaptation can involve a risk, such that mental health may be affected, at least to some extent. For instance, pregnant women can start to worry about new responsibilities associated with motherhood (Lederman, 1990) and they may anticipate negative changes in the partner relationship (Kroelinger & Oths, 2000). The demands of new parenthood are often accompanied with an increase in family stress, lack of intimacy, and insufficient communication between partners (Hansson & Ahlborg, 2016), as the former love partners have to make a shift to becoming parents with shared new responsibilities as well (Ngai & Ngu, 2016). Also, when couples already have a child, the next pregnancy can come with new transitions that may cause stress, and previous negative experiences with pregnancy and childbirth may be an additional source of stress (Westerneng et al., 2015). However, on average, nulliparous women report higher levels of pregnancy anxiety than multiparous women do (Bernazzani et al., 1997; Melender, 2002; Westerneng et al., 2015). Thus, pregnancy and becoming a parent are, in fact, two entwined life transitions. In general, such major life transitions can cause anxiety, depression, and stress. Indeed, mental

DOI: 10.4324/9781003014003-4

health problems during pregnancy are relatively common (Dunkel Schetter & Tanner, 2012).

Pregnancy can also be viewed from a developmental psychopathology perspective, as it represents a period of heightened vulnerability for mental health problems (Glynn et al., 2018; Huizink & de Rooij, 2018). Particularly anxiety and depression, but also stress, have been reported. In general, first-time pregnancy and new parenthood are acknowledged as a period of increased emotional vulnerability (Austin et al., 2010; Morse et al., 2000). For women experiencing a first pregnancy, feelings of anxiety and depression are quite common (Barnett & Parker, 1986; Dayan et al., 2006), although it should be noted that for most women, these feelings are transient and diminish over time across pregnancy (Don et al., 2014; Huizink et al., 2014). A recent systematic review and meta-analysis among pregnant women found prevalence rates for self-reported (general) anxiety ranging from 18.2% in the first trimester to 19.1% in the second, and 24.6% in the third trimester (Dennis et al., 2017). No differentiation was made between nulliparous and multiparous women, and both were included in the analysis. In the same study, a clinical diagnosis of any anxiety disorder during pregnancy was found in 15.2% of pregnant women, which indicates that for a significant proportion of women, there is a reason for concern about their mental health in pregnancy.

Studies are, however, somewhat inconsistent with regard to the normative patterns of change of (general) anxiety across pregnancy. While some studies suggest that self-reported symptoms of anxiety are relatively stable over the course of pregnancy (Grant et al., 2008), other studies report an increase in anxiety into the early postpartum period (Behringer et al., 2011; Whisman et al., 2011). Don et al. (2014) tested whether these different trajectories of anxiety across pregnancy and the transition to parenthood form distinct subgroups of parents, based on their general ability to adjust to, or adequately cope with, demanding situations. Their findings indeed suggest that distinct trajectories of anxiety can be identified in this important transitional phase. The majority of new parents (89.4%) was shown to start with low levels of anxiety in the beginning of pregnancy, which then declined following the birth of their first child. A smaller group, representing 10.6% of new parents, reported moderate anxiety levels during pregnancy that remained on the same level after the birth of their child. Membership to this latter, moderately anxious group, was predicted by higher levels of prenatal depression, lower expected parenting efficacy, and lower relationship satisfaction. In a large pregnancy cohort, including over 3,202 pregnant women and 2,076 expecting fathers, Korja et al. (2018) used latent growth mixture modeling to describe the trajectory of general anxiety across pregnancy and identified four different trajectories of anxiety symptoms among both expecting mothers and fathers. These trajectories could be described as consistently low levels of symptoms, consistently high levels of symptoms, high and decreasing levels of symptoms, and moderate and increasing levels of symptoms. The large majority (85.0%) of (expecting) parents showed consistently low levels of anxiety, with only 1.0% reporting consistently high levels of anxiety throughout pregnancy. The two other trajectories fitted best with each 7.0% of the participants.

Depression may also occur during pregnancy. Whereas numerous studies have focused on the development of postpartum depression in particular (see Shorey et al., 2018 for a meta-analysis), other studies have also examined the occurrence and trajectory of antenatal depression (e.g., Leight et al., 2010). The estimates of depression during pregnancy vary, ranging from 4.9% with a clinical diagnosis of a major depressive disorder to 16.0% for self-reported depressive symptoms (Leight et al., 2010). Based on a meta-analysis of 21 studies, a pooled prevalence for depression of 7.4%, 12.8%, and 12.0%, for the first, second, and third trimesters of pregnancy, respectively, was found (Bennett et al., 2004). A relatively similar prevalence rate was reported in a more recent meta-analysis, yielding a pooled prevalence estimate of perinatal depression (major depressive disorder) of 11.9%, with perinatal depression reflecting symptom onset during pregnancy or in the 4 weeks following delivery (Woody et al., 2017).

Not many studies can be found that examined the normative trajectory of depression across pregnancy. In the study of Korja et al. (2018), trajectories of depression were also examined in the same group of participants as described earlier. For depression, five different trajectories could be modeled, again with the majority of participants (67.0%) fitting best with a trajectory of consistently low scores on depression throughout pregnancy, and only 2.0% showing consistently high scores. For depression, however, almost a quarter (24.0%) reported stable moderate levels of depression throughout pregnancy. Another smaller study among 374 women, who were retrospectively interviewed shortly after birth, found that depressed mood showed elevations at the beginning and end of pregnancy, which the authors regarded as a normative pattern of change in symptom expression (Amiel Castro et al., 2017). An interesting Australian prospective cohort study used three waves of data from a large community sample in which data were collected from women before pregnancy and follow-up data during pregnancy were available from the same women (Leach et al., 2014). The authors examined whether pregnancy was associated with increases in levels of anxiety and depression, while being able to control for symptom levels before pregnancy. Their findings show that no increase in depression or anxiety was found due to pregnancy, although the level of depression and anxiety during pregnancy could not be differentiated into different trimesters. For anxiety, there was even a greater decline in anxiety from pre-pregnancy levels to pregnancy levels than for women who remained non-pregnant during the course of the study.

A number of studies have also consistently demonstrated a high rate of comorbidity between anxiety and depression in general (Lamers et al., 2011), and therefore, one can expect this comorbidity in pregnancy as well. Several general risk factors for this comorbidity, such as female gender, low socioeconomic status, and low education level, are also related to increased levels of either anxiety or depression in pregnancy (Austin & Lumley, 2003; Martini et al., 2015). In a meta-analysis based on in total 66 studies and 162,120 women, Falah-Hassani et al. (2017) reported a prevalence ranging from 6.3% to 9.5% for self-reported comorbid depressive symptoms and anxiety symptoms during pregnancy. Even for clinical diagnoses of any anxiety disorder and depression, the comorbidity rate was 9.3%.

Finally, stress during pregnancy, or prenatal stress, may also occur and several studies have reported prevalence rates ranging from 6.0% of pregnant women experiencing high levels of stress to as much as 78.0% reporting low-to-moderate psychosocial stress (Woods et al., 2010). It is important to mention that in most of these studies, prenatal stress is regarded and measured as psychosocial stress. Psychosocial stress can be described as a result of being exposed to a stressful situation that is considered to be too difficult to deal with, exceeding one's capacity to cope, which in turn causes feelings of tension or stress. Thus, the actual physiological stress response of one's body is often not considered or assessed, but rather, questionnaires are used to assess the level of psychosocial stress such as the Perceived Stress Scale (PSS; Cohen et al., 1983) or similar instruments. In fact, studies have shown that measures of psychosocial stress and physiological stress, most often indexed by saliva or hair cortisol, are not consistently associated (Baibazarova et al., 2013; Kramer et al., 2009; Mustonen et al., 2019). No systematic research has been done to determine accurate prevalence rates and normative patterns of change in psychosocial stress levels. This type of descriptive and epidemiological research is also hampered by the fact that other aspects of maternal emotions or maternal adversities are often used under the umbrella term "prenatal distress," collectively referring to a negative psychological state of well-being. This may include perceived stress, perhaps the best index of psychosocial stress, but it may also include maternal trait and state anxiety, pregnancy-specific anxiety, and even symptoms of depression. Hence, the rates of reported maternal distress may reflect anxiety or depression as well.

In sum, pregnancy is associated with some normative patterns of change in mental health, particularly observed in an increase in (general) anxiety, and perhaps depression and stress as well. These changes may be due to major life transition that is involved in pregnancy: the transition to parenthood, with associated new roles and responsibilities. Adaptation to these changes can create a challenge to some women that in turn may lead to increased feelings of anxiety, depression, or stress.

Occurrence of pregnancy-related anxiety

Although general measures of mental health problems, including anxiety, depression, and stress, show that such mental health problems appear to emerge during pregnancy relatively often, these general measures may not sufficiently detect feelings of anxiety and stress that are unique during pregnancy (Bayrampour et al., 2016). Other concerns and worries may arise across the period of pregnancy that are specifically related to this unique transitional phase in life, which are often referred to as pregnancy-related anxiety or pregnancy-specific anxiety. Indeed, several studies have shown that pregnancy-related anxiety may be regarded as a distinct concept from general anxiety (see for a review, Bayrampour et al., 2016). Examples of pregnancy-related anxiety include worries about the health (and sometimes development) of one's (unborn) baby, which can include worries about fetal loss, concerns and fears about the upcoming delivery and the pain and loss of control it may cause, and worries about the body changes women experience in pregnancy, but also concerns about parenting and newborn care, although the latter concepts fit better with parental self-efficacy or parenting stress (Bayrampour et al., 2016; Huizink et al., 2004; Sjögren, 1997). Most of these worries are specifically related to pregnancy and reflect an emotional state that is clearly contextually based. Per definition this type of anxiety is transient as these worries naturally subside after birth. It has been suggested that measures of pregnancy-related anxiety could be more sensitive to capture variability in mood and emotion than more general and less context-dependent questions that are included in general anxiety or depression assessments (Robertson-Blackmore et al., 2016).

These pregnancy-related anxieties have often been reported, ranging from 7.5%–13.1% for fear of childbirth to 14.8% for a more comprehensive measure of pregnancy-related anxiety (Poikkeus et al., 2006). Several measures of pregnancy-related anxiety are available (for an overview and critical evaluation, see Brunton et al., 2015), of which the 10-item Pregnancy-Related Anxiety Questionnaire-Revised (PRAQ-R) is often used. The PRAQ-R is a shortened version of the PRAQ and has shown good psychometric values (Huizink et al., 2004). The PRAQ-R is brief and therefore a feasible instrument to use in both scientific (larger scale) studies, but also in clinical practice (Witteveen et al., 2016). The disadvantage of this measure, however, is that it is developed for first-time mothers only. Therefore, Huizink et al. (2016) tested whether rephrasing of one item would yield factorial invariance across nulliparous and multiparous Finnish pregnant women. The results showed that, indeed, changing one item and, therefore, revising the questionnaire into the adapted version PRAQ-R2 made the instrument valid for all pregnant women regardless of parity. This finding was replicated by Dellagiulia et al. (2019) using a large Italian sample of both nulliparous and multiparous pregnant women and cross-validating the factorial structure of the PRAQ-R2 with the original Finnish sample of the study of Huizink et al. (2016). Dellagiulia et al. (2019) concluded that the Italian version had satisfying psychometric properties, and invariance across two countries was confirmed. Additionally, Mudra et al. (2019) tested the psychometric properties of the German version of the PRAQ-R2 in the third trimester pregnancy and concluded that its validity and reliability were satisfactory.

Only a few studies have actually examined the (normative) course of pregnancy-related anxiety across pregnancy. Mudra et al. (2020) used the PRAQ-R2 in each trimester of pregnancy to measure pregnancy-related anxiety in a sample of 180 pregnant women (54.2% nulliparous), who were on average well educated with an average to high income. The total score of this instrument showed a stable and relatively low level of anxiety across pregnancy. However, fear of giving birth, one of the subscales of the PRAQ-R2, was found to increase over time, when delivery was approaching. In contrast, worries about the health of the child, another subscale of the PRAQ-R2, showed a declining trajectory. These findings are mostly in line with other studies, reporting a stable level of total pregnancy-related anxiety across pregnancy (Huizink et al., 2014), and a decrease in fear of giving birth and worries about the health of the child across pregnancy (Huizink et al., 2014; Robertson-Blackmore et al., 2016). According to Mudra et al. (2020), this decrease across pregnancy may be explained by growing confidence of the mother regarding the health of the fetus she is carrying after several medical check-ups, ultrasounds, and feeling the baby move in her womb.

Pregnancy-related anxiety as a distinct concept

It can be assumed that women who tend to worry in general may also report high levels of pregnancy-related anxiety. Such a tendency to worry may be reflected in high scores on general (trait) anxiety or in high levels of depressive symptoms. In particular, during an important new life phase such as becoming a parent, with its new challenges and responsibilities, women with a predisposition toward anxiety and depression, or women who are already anxious or depressed, may develop new worries and fears related to pregnancy as well (Huizink et al., 2014). In a first study to examine the interrelations between general anxiety and pregnancy-related anxiety, Huizink et al. (2004) concluded that pregnancy-related anxieties could be regarded as a relative distinct phenomenon that develops in some women across pregnancy. This conclusion was based on a study among 230 nulliparous pregnant women, in which it was found that only a small to moderate (8.0%–27.0%) portion of the variance of pregnancy-related anxiety, measured with the ten-item PRAQ-R, was explained by general anxiety and depression in early and mid-pregnancy. In the last trimester of pregnancy, no linear association was found between general anxiety or depression and pregnancy anxiety.

More recently, Huizink et al. (2014) studied the interrelationship between pregnancy-related anxiety and general trait and state anxiety across pregnancy in another, larger sample ($N = 1,309$) of pregnant women. In this study, it was hypothesized that an increase or decrease in pregnancy-related anxiety during the course of pregnancy also affected general anxiety levels, both state and trait anxiety. Alternatively, it was hypothesized that changes in state and trait anxiety could also affect the level of pregnancy-related anxiety across pregnancy. The cross-sectional correlation coefficients between pregnancy-related anxiety (PRAQ-R) and trait and state anxiety in each trimester ranged between 0.54 and 0.62, suggesting that there is some overlap but also some specificity in these different measures of anxiety.

Furthermore, in this study, cross-lagged, cross-time pathways were analyzed between scores on pregnancy-related anxiety and trait and state anxiety, assessed at 12, 22, and 32 weeks of gestation. The results show that pregnancy-related anxiety predicted both state and trait anxiety longitudinally, whereas only trait anxiety, but not state anxiety, predicted pregnancy-related anxiety over time. Thus, these findings imply that specific anxieties associated with pregnancy may have an impact on general feelings of anxiety as well, and that high levels of trait anxiety may lead to more pregnancy-related anxiety. It is important to note that the overall level of pregnancy-related anxiety in the study sample was stable, whereas trait anxiety decreased during pregnancy for most women. Thus, the findings most likely reflected an interrelationship between higher levels of pregnancy-related anxiety and trait anxiety for a group of women who were at risk to develop anxiety symptoms across pregnancy. The conclusion from this study was that it can be useful to measure both pregnancy-related anxiety and trait anxiety across pregnancy, to get a more comprehensive picture of pregnant women's emotional well-being.

Dellagiulia et al. (2019) tested for the convergent validity of the Italian version of the PRAQ-R2 and found moderate associations between the PRAQ-R2 scores and general trait anxiety and depression scores. These findings are in line with previous studies (e.g., Huizink et al., 2014), providing further evidence for the proposition idea that the PRAQ-R2 captures unique anxieties during the period of pregnancy.

Finally, Robertson-Blackmore et al. (2016) set out to study whether pregnancy-related anxiety is distinct from general anxiety and, more particularly, from clinically significant anxiety as assessed with a structured clinical interview twice during pregnancy (at 20 and 32 weeks of gestation) and twice in the postpartum period (8 weeks and 6 months postnatally). First, they examined the overlap between pregnancy-related anxiety and self-reported questionnaires on anxiety (Penn State Worry Questionnaire) and depression (Edinburgh Postnatal Depression Scale). Pregnancy-related anxiety was assessed with a self-designed 7-item questionnaire that tapped into worries about birth, and about the baby's health and development. Correlation coefficients between pregnancy-related anxiety and self-reported general anxiety varied between 0.22 to 0.42 at gestational weeks 20 and 32, while somewhat lower correlations were found between pregnancy-related anxiety and clinical reports based on the structured interview (0.09–0.24). For the self-reported depression, modest associations (r's ranging between 0.21 and 0.36) were found with pregnancy-related anxiety.

Second, they tested whether pregnancy-related anxiety showed a distinct course in pregnancy. Longitudinal analyses showed a reduction in pregnancy-related anxiety from gestational week 20 to week 32 for the worries about baby's health and development, but no reduction in worries about birth, or in general anxiety or depression. Finally, it was examined whether pregnancy-related anxiety had different associations with external factors, such as parity and preterm birth, as compared to general anxiety and depression. The findings of this part of their study are described in the next section.

Based on these studies, one can conclude that pregnancy-related anxiety reflects a distinct pattern of anxiety that can develop during pregnancy. Pregnancy-related anxiety and general anxiety, but also depression, are not the same, although they are moderately related to each other. Moreover, pregnancy-related anxiety and in particular trait anxiety seem to influence each other over time.

Predictive validity of pregnancy-related anxiety as compared to prenatal general anxiety and depression

There is ample evidence for the association between maternal anxiety, depression, or stress during pregnancy, and affected birth outcome (e.g., lower birth weight, shorter gestational age at birth), developmental delays, and behavioral problems of the child (e.g., Dunkel Schetter & Tanner, 2012; Huizink et al., 2002; Reck et al., 2013). One can question whether pregnancy-related anxiety would have a stronger predictive value for these birth and child outcomes than prenatal general anxiety and depression?

Before answering that empirical question, it is important to mention that most of this type of research is embedded in the framework of fetal programming, which is also referred to as the developmental origins of (mental) health and disease (DoHaD) hypothesis (O'Donnell & Meaney, 2017). The basic assumption of this hypothesis is that the fetal environmental programs the individual vulnerability to a range of adverse health outcomes. From the numerous studies that were conducted, two general conclusions can be drawn. First, the principle of multifinality, in which one specific factor may have differential effects on developmental psychopathology (Cicchetti & Rogosch, 1996; Nolen-Hoeksema & Watkins, 2011), complicates the search for underlying mechanisms that explain the potential effect of pregnancy-related anxiety on the offspring. In other words, if the outcomes related to high levels of pregnancy-related anxiety vary to a large extent, there is little reason to assume that a specific mechanism can be responsible for the harmful effects of pregnancy-related anxiety on the offspring. Rather, pregnancy-related anxiety may be a proxy of general vulnerability of both the mother and her (un)born child. Second, evidence also supports the concept of equifinality (Cicchetti & Rogosch, 1996), in which different risk factors such as prenatal maternal depression versus pregnancy-related anxiety, or even prenatal maternal smoking, lead to the same adverse outcomes. Equifinality is also referred to as divergent trajectories (Nolen-Hoeksema & Watkins, 2011), which is particularly relevant to get a better understanding of whether pregnancy-related anxiety can actually be regarded as a stronger or more robust predictor of adverse offspring outcomes, as compared to relatively similar prenatal influences, such as maternal anxiety or depression. Both multifinality and equifinality can be assumed to best describe the consequences of prenatal influences for the offspring (Huizink & De Rooij, 2018), which implies that the predictive value of pregnancy-related anxiety with regard to birth and child outcomes is probably rather similar to the predictive value of other maternal factors that may share part of the underlying mechanisms. These mechanisms may relate to increased exposure to high levels of maternal cortisol during pregnancy (Davis et al., 2007; Gitau et al., 2001), epigenetic pathways (Cao-Lei et al., 2017; Oberlander et al., 2008), changes in 11β-HSD2 methylation (Chapman et al., 2013; Monk et al., 2016), or altered brain development (Buss et al., 2012). Furthermore, pregnancy-related anxiety, similar to general anxiety or depression, may transfer to high levels of postnatal parenting stress or altered maternal behavior, both of which may sub-sequently negatively impact mother-child interaction and infant and child out-comes (Huizink et al., 2017; Kataja et al., 2017).

With this theoretical reasoning in mind, it is surprising to observe that preg-nancy-related anxiety seems to be a robust predictor of birth (DiPietro et al., 2004; Dunkel Schetter & Tanner, 2012) and infant and child outcomes (Davis & Sandman, 2010; Huizink et al., 2003; Nolvi et al., 2016), when compared with more general anxiety measures during pregnancy. Robertson-Blackmore et al. (2016) also reported a stronger association with parity, maternal age at first preg-nancy, and maternal race for pregnancy-related anxiety as compared to the other mental health measures, including clinical data on anxiety. Finally, in their study, pregnancy-related anxiety, particularly about the health and development of the baby, was an independent predictor of birth weight and gestational age at birth, and notably also predicted postpartum general anxiety disorder.

Hence, as stated before, it seems that measures of pregnancy-related anxiety are more sensitive to capture subtle but relevant changes in feelings of anxiety and stress during the course of pregnancy, which in turn could lead to their stronger predictive value. As pregnancy-related anxiety cannot easily be modeled in animal studies, we lack a clear understanding of potential physiological mechanisms that could be responsible for these associations. Nevertheless, it is likely that these mechanisms are similar to those underlying general anxiety or depression effects on the offspring, although evidence can be derived from human studies only.

Two human studies examined the association between pregnancy-related anxi-ety and maternal saliva cortisol levels. Davis and Sandman (2010) reported no significant cross-sectional associations between pregnancy-related anxiety and maternal cortisol levels at five different time points. The study of Kane et al. (2014) applied a longitudinal analysis of pregnancy-related anxiety and cortisol across pregnancy and found that women with higher mean levels of pregnancy-related anxiety across the prenatal period more often had steeper increases in cortisol, as compared to women with low levels of pregnancy-related anxiety. This study provides some first evidence explaining how pregnancy-related anxiety can impact the developing fetus and, subsequently, birth and child outcomes. In addition, one study examined the association of pregnancy-related anxiety with hair cortisol levels, and after adjustment for covariates, found no significant rela-tion (Mustonen et al., 2019). It is of interest that thus far for more general anxiety or stress measures during pregnancy, and now also for hair cortisol in relation to pregnancy-related anxiety, there is no consistent evidence to support the hypothesis that maternal cortisol could mediate their association with adverse birth and offspring outcomes (Zijlmans et al., 2015).

When looking at the research support for the impact of pregnancy-related anxiety on birth outcome and infant and child development, the following find-ings have been reported. With regard to delivery aspects and birth outcomes, pregnancy-related anxiety has been associated with preliminary requests for pain relief and elective cesarean section (Andersson et al., 2004; Atiba et al., 1993), increased risk of emergency cesarean section (Ryding et al., 1998), preterm birth, and low birth weight (Dunkel Schetter & Tanner, 2012). In particular, third tri-mester pregnancy-related anxiety may be related to preterm birth, as was shown in a prospective study of 208 pregnant women (Khalesi & Bokai, 2018). With regard to infant outcomes, more difficult temperament (Gutteling et al., 2005; Nolvi et al., 2016) as well as motor and mental developmental delays in infancy (Huizink et al., 2003) have been reported. Moreover, behavioral and emotional problems in childhood (Huizink et al., 2002; Van den Bergh et al., 2005) have been associated with pregnancy-related anxiety, as well as with changes in brain gray matter volume (Buss et al., 2010). The latter changes in the brain may mediate the higher levels of impulsivity (or lack of self-regulation) and emotional problems in children after being exposed to prenatal maternal anxiety.

Besides predicting birth and child outcomes, pregnancy-related anxiety was also recently related to parenting stress. In a pregnancy cohort study, it was found that both trait anxiety and pregnancy-related anxiety, but not depression, were independent predictors of parenting stress at 3 months postpartum (Huizink et al., 2017). Parenting stress was assessed with the self-reported questionnaire (Nijmeegse Ouderlijke Stress Index [NOSI], de Brock et al., 1992), which included sense of competence, role restriction, depression, experience of health, and relationship with spouse. Thus, feelings of anxiety and concern were trans-ferred to the postpartum, in first-time parenthood. It can be assumed that women who tend to worry a lot during pregnancy will continue to worry as a parent of their newborn child, and hence may report higher levels of parenting stress. This could reflect an inability to adequately cope with the entwined life transitions of both pregnancy and new parenthood. This in turn could lead to a perceived discrepancy between the demands of new parenthood and the individual available resources to meet with those demands.

Conclusion

It can be concluded, based on the findings from a number of studies, that preg-nancy-related anxiety is a relatively distinct phenomenon that develops during pregnancy in some women. Although some small to moderate associations have been found with general anxiety measures and depression, evidence also shows that pregnancy-related anxiety is largely independent of these general indices of mental health and also differs from clinical assessments of general anxiety. It may be that pregnancy-related anxiety reflects a more sensitive measure of variabil-ity in mood across pregnancy, as by nature, pregnancy-related anxiety is very context-specific. Pregnancy-related anxiety also shows a distinct pattern across pregnancy, with a relatively low and stable pattern of overall pregnancy-related anxiety scores, a decrease in the level of concern about the health of the baby, and either an increase or a decrease in fear for childbirth when pregnancy is progress-ing. Finally, pregnancy-related anxiety's predictive validity has been shown in a number of studies, by robust relationships with birth, infant and child outcomes, and also with maternal mood and parenting stress. An increase in maternal cor-tisol levels associated with pregnancy-related anxiety may be involved in the underlying psychobiological pathway that could explain this range of outcomes, although consistent evidence for this association is lacking. It is therefore recommended to assess levels of pregnancy-related anxiety along with other measures of maternal mental mood during pregnancy to get the most comprehensive picture of women's mental health. Furthermore, for women suffering from high levels of these types of pregnancy-related anxieties, there is a need to develop and test the effectiveness of interventions to reduce particularly high levels of pregnancy-related anxiety, as this may not only be beneficial for the pregnant women themselves but also for their child's development.

References

Amiel Castro, R. T., Pinard Anderman, C., Glover, V., O'Connor, T. G., Ehlert, U., & Kammerer, M. (2017). Associated symptoms of depression: Patterns of change during pregnancy. *Archives of Women's Mental Health*, *20*(4), 123–128. https://doi.org/ 10.1007/s00737-016-0685-6

Andersson, L., Sundstrom-Poromaa, I., Wulff, M., Aström, M., & Bixo, M. (2004). Neonatal outcome following maternal antenatal depression and anxiety: A population-based study. *American Journal of Epidemiology*, *159*, 872–881. https://doi. org/10.1093/aje/kwh122

Atiba, E. O., Adeghe, A. J., Murphy, P. J., Felmingham, J. E., & Scott, G. I. (1993). Patients' expectation and caesarean section rate. *Lancet*, *341*, 246. https://doi. org/10.1016/0140-6736(93)90111-s

Austin, M. P., Hadzi-Pavlovic, D., Priest, S. R., Reilly, N., Wilhelm, K., Saint, K., & Parker, G. (2010). Depressive and anxiety disorders in the postpartum period: How prevalent are they and can we improve their detection? *Archives of Women's Mental Health*, *13*(5), 395–401. https://doi.org/10.1007/s00737-010-0153-7

Austin, M. P., & Lumley, J. (2003). Antenatal screening for postnatal depression: A systematic review. *Acta Psychiatrica Scandinavia*, *107*, 10–17. https://doi.org/ 10.1034/j.1600-0447.2003.02024.x

Baibazarova, E., van de Beek, C., Cohen-Kettenis, P. T., Buitelaar, J., Shelton, K. H., & van Goozen, S. H. (2013). Influence of prenatal maternal stress, maternal plasma cortisol and cortisol in the amniotic fluid on birth outcomes and child temperament at 3 months. *Psychoneuroendocrinology*, *38*, 907–915. https://doi.org/10.1016/j.psyneuen. 2012.09.015

Barnett, B., & Parker, G. (1986). Possible determinants, correlates and consequences of high levels of anxiety in primiparous mothers. *Psychological Medicine*, *16*, 177–185. https://doi.org/ 10.1017/s0033291700002610

Bayrampour, H., Ali, E., McNeil, D. A., Benzies, K., MacQueen, G., & Tough, S. (2016). Pregnancy-related anxiety: A concept analysis. *International Journal of Nursing Studies*, *55*, 115–130. https://doi.org/10.1016/j.ijnurstu.2015.10.023

Behringer, J., Reiner, I., & Spangler, G. (2011). Maternal representations of past and current attachment relationships, and emotional experience across the transition to motherhood: A longitudinal study. *Journal of Family Psychology*, *25*, 210–219. https://doi.org/10.1037/a0023083

Bennett, H. A., Einarson, A., Taddio, A., Koren, G., & Einarson, T. R. (2004). Prevalence of depression during pregnancy: Systematic review. *Obstetrics and Gynecology*,

103(4), 698–709. Erratum in: *Obstetrics and Gynecology, 103*(6), 1344. https://doi.org/10.1097/01.AOG.0000116689.75396.5f

Bernazzani, O., Saucier, J. F., David, H., & Borgeat, F. (1997). Psychosocial factors related to emotional disturbances during pregnancy. *Journal of Psychosomatic Research, 42,* 391–402. https://doi.org/10.1016/s0022-3999(96)00371-6

Brunton, R. J., Dryer, R., Saliba, A., & Kohlhoff, J. (2015). Pregnancy anxiety: A systematic review of current scales. *Journal of Affective Disorders, 176,* 24–34. https://doi.org/10.1016/j.jad.2015.01.039

Buss, C., Davis, E. P., Muftuler, L. T., Head, K., & Sandman, C. A. (2010). High pregnancy anxiety during mid-gestation is associated with decreased gray matter density in 6-9-year-old children. *Psychoneuroendocrinology, 35,* 41–53. https//doi.org:10.1016/j.psyneuen.2009.07.010.

Buss, C., Davis, E. P., Shahbaba, B., Pruessner, J. C., Head, K., & Sandman, C. A. (2012). Maternal cortisol over the course of pregnancy and subsequent child amygdala and hippocampus volumes and affective problems. *Proceedings of the National Academy of Sciences of the United States of America, 109,* E1312–E1319. https://doi.org/10.1073/pnas.1201295109

Cao-Lei, L., de Rooij, S. R., King, S., Matthews, S. G., Metz, G. A. S., Roseboom, T. J., & Szyf, M. (2017). Prenatal stress and epigenetics. *Neuroscience & Biobehavioral Reviews, S0149–S7634*(16), 30726. https://doi.org/10.1016/j.neubiorev.2017.05.016

Chapman, K., Holmes, M., & Seckl, J. (2013). 11b-hydroxysteroid dehydrogenases: Intracellular gate-keepers of tissue glucocorticoid action. *Physiological Reviews, 93,* 1139–1206. https://doi.org/10.1152/physrev.00020.2012

Cicchetti, D., & Rogosch, F. A. (1996). Equifinality and multifinality in developmental psychopathology. *Development and Psychopathology, 8,* 597–600. https://doi.org/10.1017/S0954579400007318

Cohen, S., Kamarck, T., & Mermelstein, R. (1983). A global measure of perceived stress. *Journal of Health and Social Behavior, 24,* 385–396. https://doi.org/10.2307/2136404

Davis, E. P., Glynn, L. M., Schetter, C. D., Hobel, C., Chicz-Demet, A., & Sandman, C. A. (2007). Prenatal exposure to maternal depression and cortisol influences infant temperament. *Journal of the American Academy of Child & Adolescent Psychiatry, 46,* 737–746. https://doi.org/10.1097/chi.0- b013e318047b775

Davis, E. P., & Sandman, C. A. (2010). The timing of prenatal exposure to maternal cortisol and psychosocial stress is associated with human infant cognitive development. *Child Development, 81,* 131–148. https://doi.org/10.1111/j.1467-8624.2009.01385.x

Dayan, J., Creveuil, C., Marks, M. N., Conroy, S., Herlicoviez, M., Dreyfus, M., & Tordjman, S. (2006). Prenatal depression, prenatal anxiety, and spontaneous preterm birth: A prospective cohort study among women with early and regular care. *Psychosomatic Medicine, 68*(6), 938–946. https://doi.org/10.1097/01.psy.0000244025.20549.bd

de Brock, A. J. L. L., Vermulst, A. A., Gerris, J. R. M., & Abidin, R. R. (1992). *NOSI, manual experimental version [Nijmeegse Ouderlijke Stress Index (NOSI), handleiding experimentele versie].* Pearson.

Dellagiulia, A., Lionetti, F., Pastore, M., Karlsson, L., Karlsson, H., & Huizink, A. C. (2019). The pregnancy anxiety questionnaire revised – 2: A contribution to its validation *European Journal of Psychological Assessment, 36*(5), 787–795. https://doi.org.au/10.1027/1015-5759/a000559

Dennis, C. L., Falah-Hassani, K., & Shiri, R. (2017). Prevalence of antenatal and postnatal anxiety: Systematic review and meta-analysis. *The British Journal of Psychiatry, 210,* 315–323. https://doi.org/10.1192/bjp.bp.116.187179

DiPietro, J. A., Ghera, M. M., Costigan, K., & Hawkins, M. (2004). Measuring the ups and downs of pregnancy stress. *Journal of Psychosomatic Obstetrics and Gynaecology, 25*(3–4), 189–201. https://doi.org/10.1080/01674820400017830

Don, B. P., Chong, A., Biehle, S. N., Gordon, A., & Mickelson, K. D. (2014). Anxiety across the transition to parenthood: Change trajectories among low-risk parents. *Anxiety Stress Coping, 27*(6), 633–649. https://doi.org/10.1080/10615806.2014.903473

Dunkel Schetter, C., & Tanner, L. (2012). Anxiety, depression and stress in pregnancy: Implications for mothers, children, research, and practice. *Current Opinion in Psychiatry, 25,* 141–148. https://doi.org/10.1097/YCO.0b013e3283503680

Falah-Hassani, K., Shiri, R., & Dennis, C.-L. (2017). The prevalence of antenatal and postnatal co-morbid anxiety and depression: A meta-analysis. *Psychological Medicine, 47,* 2041–2053. https://doi.org/10.1017/S0033291717000617

Fox, B. (2009). *When couples become parents. The creation of gender in the transition to parenthood.* University of Toronto Press.

Gitau, R., Fisk, N. M., & Glover, V. (2001). Maternal stress in pregnancy and its effect on the human foetus: An overview of research findings. *Stress, 4,* 195–203. https://doi.org/ 10.3109/10253890109035018

Glynn, L. M., Howland, M. A., & Fox, M. (2018). Maternal programming: Application of a developmental psychopathology perspective. *Development and Psychopathology, 30*(3), 905–919. https://doi.org/10.1017/s0954579418000524

Grant, K. A., McMahon, C., & Austin, M. P. (2008). Maternal anxiety during the transition to parenthood: A prospective study. *Journal of Affective Disorders, 108,* 101–111. https://doi.org/10.1016/j.jad.2007.10.002

Gutteling, B. M., de Weerth, C., Willemsen-Swinkels, S. H., Huizink, A. C., Mulder, E. J., Visser, G. H., & Buitelaar, J. K. (2005). The effects of prenatal stress on temperament and problem behavior of 27-month-old toddlers. *European Child & Adolescent Psychiatry, 14,* 41–51. https://doi.org/10.1007/s00787-005-0435-1

Hansson, M., & Ahlborg, T. (2016). Factors contributing to separation/divorce in parents of small children in Sweden. *Nordic Psychology, 68,* 40–57. https://doi.org/10.1080/19012276.2015.1071201

Huizink, A., Mulder, E., de Medina, P., Visser, G., & Buitelaar, J. (2004). Is pregnancy anxiety a distinctive syndrome? *Early Human Development, 79,* 81–91. https://doi.org/10.1016/j.earlhumdev.2004.04.014

Huizink, A. C., Delforterie, M. J., Scheinin, N. M., Tolvanen, M., Karlsson, L., & Karlsson, H. (2016). Adaption of pregnancy anxiety questionnaire-revised for all pregnant women regardless of parity: PRAQ-R2. *Archives of Women's Mental Health, 19*(1), 125–132. https://doi.org/ 10.1007/s00737-015-0531-2

Huizink, A. C., de Medina, P. G., Mulder, E. J., Visser, G. H., & Buitelaar, J. K. (2002). Psychological measures of prenatal stress as predictors of infant temperament. *Journal of the American Academy of Child & Adolescent Psychiatry, 41*(9), 1078–1085. https://doi.org/10.1097/00004583-200209000-00008

Huizink, A. C., de Medina, P. G., Mulder, E. J., Visser, G. H., & Buitelaar, J. K. (2003). Stress during pregnancy is associated with developmental outcome in infancy. *Journal of Child Psychology and Psychiatry*, *44*, 810–818. https://doi.org/10.1111/1469-7610.00166

Huizink, A. C., & de Rooij, S. R. (2018). Prenatal stress and models explaining risk for psychopathology revisited: Generic vulnerability and divergent pathways. *Development and Psychopathology*, *30*(3), 1041–1062. https://doi.org/10.1017/S0954579418000354

Huizink, A. C., Menting, B., De Moor, M. H. M., Verhage, M. L., Kunseler, F. C., Schuengel, C., & Oosterman, M. (2017). From prenatal anxiety to parenting stress: A longitudinal study. *Archives of Women's Mental Health*, *20*(5), 663–672. https://doi.org/10.1007/s00737-017-0746-5

Huizink, A. C., Menting, B., Oosterman, M., Verhage, M. L., Kunseler, F. C., & Schuengel, C. (2014). The interrelationship between pregnancy-specific anxiety and general anxiety across pregnancy: A longitudinal study. *Journal of Psychosomatic Obstetrics and Gynaecology*, *35*(3), 92–100. https://doi.org/10.3109/0167482X.2014.944498

Kane, H., Schetter, C., Glynn, L., Hobel, C., & Sandman, C. (2014). Pregnancy anxiety and prenatal cortisol trajectories. *Biological Psychology*, *100*, 13–19. https://doi.org/10.1016/j.biopsycho.2014.04.003

Kataja, E. L., Karlsson, L., Huizink, A. C., Tolvanen, M., Parsons, C., Nolvi, S., & Karlsson, H. (2017). Pregnancy-related anxiety and depressive symptoms are associated with visuospatial working memory errors during pregnancy. *Journal of Affective Disorders*, *218*, 66–74. https://doi.org/10.1016/j.jad.2017.04.033

Khalesi, Z. B., & Bokai, M. (2018). The association between pregnancy-specific anxiety and preterm birth: A cohort study. *African Health Sciences*, *18*(3), 569–575. https://doi.org/10.4314/ahs.v18i3.14

Korja, R., Nolvi, S., Kataja, E. L., Scheinin, N., Junttila, N., Lahtinen, H., Saarni, S., Karlsson, L., & Karlsson, H. (2018). The courses of maternal and paternal depressive and anxiety symptoms during the prenatal period in the finnbrain birth cohort study. *PLoS One*, *13*(12), 1–19. https://doi.org/10.1371/journal.pone.0207856

Kramer, M., Lydon, J., Seguin, L., Goulet, L., Kahn, S., McNamara, H., Genest, J., Dassa, C., Chen, M. F., Sharma, S., Meaney, M. J., Thomson, S., Van Uum, S., Koren, G., Dahhou, M., Lamoureux, J., & Platt, R. (2009). Stress pathways to spontaneous preterm birth: The role of stressors, psychological distress, and stress hormones. *American Journal of Epidemiology*, *169*, 1319–1326. https://doi.org/10.1093/aje/kwp061

Kroelinger, C. D., & Oths, K. S. (2000). Partner support and pregnancy wantedness. *Birth*, *27*, 112–119. https://doi.org/10.1046/j.1523-536x.2000.00112.x

Lamers, F., van Oppen, P., Comijs, H. C., Smit, J. H., Spinhoven, P., van Balkom, A. J., Nolen, W. A., Zitman, F. G., Beekman, A. T., & Penninx, B. W. (2011). Comorbidity patterns of anxiety and depressive disorders in a large cohort study: The Netherlands study of depression and anxiety (NESDA). *Journal of Clinical Psychiatry*, *72*, 341–348. https://doi.org/10.4088/JCP.10m06176blu

Leach, L. S., Christensen, H., & Mackinnon, A. (2014). Pregnancy and levels of depression and anxiety: A prospective cohort study of Australian women. *Australian & New Zealand Journal of Psychiatry*, *48*(10), 944–951. https://doi.org/10.1177/0004867414533013

Lederman, R. P. (1990). Anxiety and stress in pregnancy: Significance and nursing assessment. *NAACOG's Clinical Issues in Perinatal Women's Health Nursing*, *1*, 279–288.

Leight, K. L., Fitelson, E. M., Weston, C. A., & Wisner, K. L. (2010). Childbirth and mental disorders. *International Review of Psychiatry*, 22, 453–471. https://doi.org/10.3109/09540261.2010.514600

Martini, J., Petzoldt, J., Einsle, F., Beesdo-Baum, K., Höfler, M., & Wittchen, H.-U. (2015). Risk factors and course patterns of anxiety and depression disorders during pregnancy and after delivery: A prospective-longitudinal study. *Journal of Affective Disorders*, 175, 385–395. https://doi.org/10.1016/j.jad.2015.01.012

Melender, H. L. (2002). Experiences of fears associated with pregnancy and childbirth: A study of 329 pregnant women. *Birth*, 29(2), 101–111. https://doi.org/10.1046/j.1523-536x.2002.00170.x

Monk, C., Feng, T., Lee, S., Krupska, I., Champagne, F. A., & Tycko, B. (2016). Distress during pregnancy: Epigenetic regulation of placenta glucocorticoid-related genes and fetal neurobehavior. *American Journal of Psychiatry*, 173, 705–713. https://doi.org/10.1176/appi.ajp.2015.15091171

Morse, C. A., Buist, A., & Durkin, S. (2000). First-time parenthood: Influences on pre- and postnatal adjustment in fathers and mothers. *Journal of Psychosomatic Obstetrics and Gynaecology*, 21(2), 109–120. https://doi.org/10.3109/01674820009075616

Mudra, S., Göbel, A., Barkmann, C., Goletzke, J., Hecher, K., Schulte-Markwort, M., Diemert, A., & Arck, P. (2020). The longitudinal course of pregnancy-related anxiety in parous and nulliparous women and its association with symptoms of social and generalized anxiety. *Journal of Affective Disorders*, 260, 111–118. https://doi.org/10.1016/j.jad.2019.08.033

Mudra, S., Göbel, A., Barthel, D., Hecher, K., Schulte-Markwort, M., Goletzke, J., Arck, P., & Diemert, A. (2019). Psychometric properties of the German version of the pregnancy-related anxiety questionnaire-revised 2 (PRAQ-R2) in the third trimester of pregnancy. *BMC Pregnancy & Childbirth*, 19(1), 242. https://doi.org/10.1186/s12884-019-2368-6

Mustonen, P., Karlsson, L., Kataja, E-L., Scheinin, N. M., Korteslouma, S., Coimbra, B., Rodrigues, A. J., Sousa, N., & Karlsson, H. (2019). Maternal prenatal hair cortisol is associated with prenatal depressive symptom trajectories. *Psychoneuroendocrinology*, 109, 104383. https://doi.org/10.1016/j.psyneuen.2019.104383

Ngai, F. W., & Ngu, S. F. (2016). Family sense of coherence and family and marital functioning across the perinatal period. *Sexual & Reproductive HealthCare*, 7, 33–37. https://doi.org/10.1016/j.srhc.2015.11.001

Nolen-Hoeksema, S., & Watkins, E. R. (2011). A heuristic for developing transdiagnostic models of psychopathology: Explaining multifinality and divergent trajectories. *Perspectives on Psychological Science*, 6, 589–609. https://doi.org/10.1177/1745691611419672

Nolvi, S., Karlsson, L., Bridgett, D. J., Korja, R., Huizink, A. C., Kataja, E. L., & Karlsson, H. (2016). Maternal prenatal stress and infant emotional reactivity six months postpartum. *Journal of Affective Disorders*, 199, 163–170. https://doi.org/10.1016/j.jad.2016.04.020

Oberlander, T. F., Weinberg, J., Papsdorf, M., Grunau, R., Misri, S., & Devlin, A. M. (2008). Prenatal exposure to maternal depression, neonatal methylation of human glucocorticoid receptor gene (NR3C1) and infant cortisol stress responses. *Epigenetics*, 3, 97–106. https://doi.org/10.4161/epi.3.2.6034

O'Donnell, K. J., & Meaney, M. J. (2017). Fetal origins of mental health: The developmental origins of health and disease hypothesis. *American Journal of Psychiatry*, 174, 319–328. https://doi.org/10.1176/appi.ajp.2016.16020138

Poikkeus, P., Saisto, T., Unkila-Kallio, L., Punamaki, R. L., Repokari, L., Vilska, S., Tiitinen, A., & Tulppala, M. (2006). Fear of childbirth and pregnancy-related anxiety in women conceiving with assisted reproduction. *Obstetrics and Gynecology*, *108*, 70–76. https://doi.org/10.1097/01.AOG.0000222902.37120.2f

Reck, C., Zimmer, K., Dubber, S., Zipser, B., Schlele, B., & Gawlik, S. (2013). The influence of general anxiety and childbirth-specific anxiety on birth outcome. *Archives of Women's Mental Health*, *16*, 363–369. https://doi.org/10.1007/s00737-013-0344-0

Robertson-Blackmore, E., Gustafsson, H., Gilchrist, M., Wyman, C., & O'Connor, T. G. (2016). Pregnancy-related anxiety: Evidence of distinct clinical significance from a prospective longitudinal study. *Journal of Affective Disorders*, *197*, 251–258. https://doi.org/10.1016/j.jad.2016.03.008

Ryding, E. L., Wijma, B., Wijma, K., & Rudhstrom, H. (1998). Fear of childbirth during pregnancy may increase the risk of emergency cesarean section. *Acta Obstetricia et Gynecologica Scandinavica*, *77*, 542–547.

Shorey, S., Chee, C. Y. I., Ng, E. D., Chan, Y. H., Tam, W. W. S., & Chong, Y. S. (2018). Prevalence and incidence of postpartum depression among healthy mothers: A systematic review and meta-analysis. *Journal of Psychiatric Research*, *104*, 235–248. https://doi.org/10.1016/j.jpsychires.2018.08.001

Sjögren, B. (1997). Reasons for anxiety about childbirth in 100 pregnant women. *Journal of Psychosomatic Obstetrics and Gynaecology*, *18*, 266–272. https://doi.org/10.3109/01674829709080698

Van den Bergh, B. R. H., Mennes, M., Oosterlaan, J., Stevens, V., Stiers, P., Marcoen, A., & Lagae, L. (2005). High antenatal maternal anxiety is related to impulsivity during performance on cognitive tasks in 14- and 15-year-olds. *Neuroscience & Biobehavioral Review*, *20*, 259–269. https://doi.org/10.1016/j.neubiorev.2004.10.010

Westerneng, M., de Cock, P., Spelten, E., Honig, A., & Hutton, E. (2015). Factorial invariance of pregnancy-specific anxiety dimensions across nulliparous and parous pregnant women. *Journal of Health Psychology*, *20*, 164–172. https://doi.org/10.1177%2F1359105313500684

Whisman, M. A., Davila, J., & Goodman, S. H. (2011). Relationship adjustment, depression, and anxiety during pregnancy and the postpartum period. *Journal of Family Psychology*, *25*, 375–383. https://doi.org/10.1037/a0023790

Witteveen, A. B., De Cock, P., Huizink, A. C., De Jonge, A., Klomp, T., Westerneng, M., & Geerts, C. C. (2016). Pregnancy related anxiety and general anxious or depressed mood and the choice for birth setting: A secondary data-analysis of the DELIVER study. *BMC Pregnancy and Childbirth*, *16*(1), 363. https://doi.org/10.1186/s12884-016-1158-7

Woods, S. M., Melville, J. L., Guo, Y., Fan M-Y., & Gavin, A. (2010). Psychosocial stress during pregnancy. *American Journal of Obstetrics and Gynecology*, *202*, 61e1–61e7. https://doi.org/10.1016/j.ajog.2009.07.041

Woody, C. A., Ferrari, A. J., Siskind, D. J., Whiteford, H. A., & Harris, M. G. (2017). A systematic review and meta-regression of the prevalence and incidence of perinatal depression. *Journal of Affective Disorders*, *219*, 86–92. https://doi.org/10.1016/j.jad.2017.05.003

Zijlmans, M. A., Korpela, K., Riksen-Walraven, J. M., de Vos, W. M., & de Weerth, C. (2015). Maternal prenatal stress is associated with the infant intestinal microbiota. *Psychoneuroendocrinology*, *53*, 233–245. https://doi.org/10.1016/j.psyneuen.2015.01.006

3 Pregnancy-related anxiety and affective disorders in pregnancy

Thomas G O'Connor, Ntemena Kapula, Allison Cunning, Hannah Murphy, Jessica Brunner, and Emma Robertson-Blackmore

Pregnancy-related anxiety and affective disorders in pregnancy

Introduction and context

There is a long history of clinical research suggesting that the dramatic social, psychological, and biological changes that accompany pregnancy and childbirth have a particular impact on maternal mental health throughout the perinatal period. Detailed clinical observations date back over a century. One of the most notable figures was the French Psychiatrist Louis Victor Marcé. His volume on mental health in relation to pregnancy and childbearing in 1858 arguably initiated this field; fittingly, the leading international society of perinatal mental health was named for him when it was founded in 1980. A great many papers on postpartum depression, psychosis, and other forms of mental illness have since generated an impressive and influential clinical and scientific literature. One of the clearest signs of success of this work is the number of professional and clinical societies dedicated to perinatal mental illness, the penetration of this information into routine clinical practices, and a well-known and widely distributed measure of symptoms that is used around the world (Cox et al., 1987).

One of the most fundamental questions that remains is the degree to which the expression and prevalence of mental illness in the perinatal period differs from other periods of the life cycle (and, if so, what accounts for this). There is little doubt that postpartum psychosis is distinct (e.g., Blackmore et al., 2013; Sit et al., 2006), and the evidence supporting a particular treatment mechanism for postpartum illnesses provides further evidence for their clinical distinction (Kanes et al., 2017). In contrast, evidence for clinical distinctiveness is nowhere near as certain for non-psychotic affective symptoms – although this remains an active area of investigation and hypothesizing (Di Florio & Meltzer-Brody, 2015; Guintivano et al., 2018; Schiller et al., 2015).

This is the context for our discussion of pregnancy-related anxiety. In this chapter, we examine pregnancy-related anxiety in relation to diagnostic assessments of affective disorders, focusing particularly on those clinical areas that have attracted

DOI: 10.4324/9781003014003-5

the most attention, namely, depression, anxiety, and trauma. Before reviewing those data, we first review the construct of pregnancy-related anxiety and in a variety of forms.

Pregnancy-related anxiety has emerged as a commonly assessed construct in the past decade or so. It does, however, have a rather longer history, at least in some forms. One specific expression of pregnancy-related anxiety, tokophobia or the excessive fear of childbirth, was formally introduced to the clinical literature somewhat recently (Hofberg & Brockington, 2000), but it was described a century ago by Knauer. The broader construct of pregnancy-related anxiety is, however, much broader than fear of childbirth and, insofar as we understand the term, there is a general consensus on its meaning. Pregnancy-related anxiety refers to worry or distress particular to pregnancy and childbirth, including the health of the developing child. This includes routine, inevitable, and seemingly normative changes, such as those in physical appearance; common worries that could be reality-based, excessive and/or distorted, such as fear about the child's health; and fears about pain of childbirth. Agreement about the construct is evident – perhaps despite the existence of a long list of proposed measures (Blackmore et al., 2016; Brunton et al., 2018; Cote-Arsenault, 2003; DiPietro et al., 2008; Huizink et al., 2004; Lobel et al., 2008; Rini et al., 1999; Somerville et al., 2014; Van den Bergh, 1990). Reviews of the literature appear often and confirm the place of pregnancy-related anxiety as a clinical construct that has attracted sizable interest (Alderdice et al., 2012; Bayrampour et al., 2016; Brunton et al., 2015; Dunkel Schetter & Tanner, 2012; Meades & Ayers, 2011; Sinesi et al., 2019).

Agreement on the construct and measurement of pregnancy-related anxiety is a precondition for assessing its prevalence, one kind of clinical significance. Rates of tokophobia, one particular form of pregnancy-related anxiety, will differ by standard of definition and methodology, but in this regard there is a high degree of consistency, with most studies assessing extreme fear of childbirth using the Wijma Delivery Expectancy/Experience Questionnaire (Rouhe et al., 2009). One study reported a rate of 7.5% (Adams et al., 2012), and rates twice as high have been reported in a study comparing rates across counties (Nilsson et al., 2018). Prevalence rates of the broader phenotype of pregnancy-related anxiety – particularly as distinct from conventional measures of anxiety – are not derivable from published studies. Accordingly, it is not yet clear if the rates would mimic what has been reported for more traditional affective disorders in the perinatal period (e.g., Buist et al., 2011). For example, a recent meta-analytic review (Fawcett et al., 2019) of 26 studies of prevalence found rates of any anxiety disorder to range from 17% to 25%, with specific disorders ranging from 1% (PTSD) to 5% (specific phobia). There is no widely accepted diagnostic threshold for pregnancy-related anxiety; prevalence rates cited earlier for tokophobia have been reported but based on an arbitrary cut-points and some variation in methodology. One of the leading factors in determining a disorder – for the purposes of estimating prevalence but also for the purposes of defining the need for treatment – is the presence of impairment. Perhaps a next step in this area for pregnancy-related anxiety may be to move from describing the symptoms to defining the way in which pregnancy-related anxiety symptoms are associated with impairments in work, relationships, and other conventional markers of adjustment and well-being, that is, apart from more general symptoms of anxiety. That kind of work will help affirm and confirm rates of prevalence that will be a major factor in establishing treatment approaches and priorities.

Another basic descriptive question concerns the course of pregnancy-related anxiety. Changes within pregnancy have been reported (and are considered later), but the more perplexing question is whether or not there is a modification to a particular form of worry in the *post*natal period; the construct of maternal-child bonding is one possible candidate (Gobel et al., 2018). In any event, we do not yet have a clear understanding of the developmental outcome of pregnancy-related anxiety post-pregnancy; it may resolve or find alternative expression. Limited evidence does not favor the former (Blackmore et al., 2011a, 2016) and evidence of the latter is largely absent. These are areas needing further interrogation, an issue to which we return in a later section of the chapter.

Associations with affective disorders and associated features

A key tenet of studies of pregnancy-related anxiety is that it does more than describe the *content* of pregnant women's worries. That is, if it is to have scientific and clinical impact, pregnancy-related anxiety must be shown to be a distinct clinical entity with construct and discriminant validity (e.g., Blackmore et al., 2016; Brunton et al., 2015; Huizink et al., 2004). This has been a focus for our research in this area.

Our work on perinatal anxiety and depression dates back to nearly two decades (Heron et al., 2004; O'Connor et al., 2002). We have included direct measures of pregnancy-related anxiety in cohort studies for many years, but our earlier work in the Avon Longitudinal Study of Parents and Children (ALSPAC) sample relied on a surrogate marker of pregnancy-related anxiety and depression: a history of miscarriage and still birth (Blackmore et al., 2011a). In that large community sample of over 13,000 pregnant women based in the west of England, we found that each pre-pregnancy loss was associated with a 0.25 standard deviation increase in mood symptoms in the current pregnancy – effects were comparable for prenatal anxiety and depression. This finding was notable but not especially novel (Hughes et al., 1999; Janssen et al., 1996; Theut et al., 1988). The more novel question that interested us was whether or not previous losses that predated the current pregnancy *continued* to be associated with an increase in anxiety and depression into the postnatal period, that is, even after the birth of a healthy child. It was: previous perinatal loss was associated with an increase in anxiety and depression in a subsequent pregnancy and this effect continued to that child's third birthday, the endpoint of our analysis. The study questioned the degree to which increased prenatal distress associated with prior loss "resolved," and suggested that the distress or trauma associated with prior perinatal loss may be a more intransigent distress. These and other results (Turton et al., 2001) support the notion that previous perinatal loss may constitute a traumatic event that requires special consideration in clinical research and theorizing on pregnancy-related anxiety.

In our prior paper that specifically targeted pregnancy-related anxiety in relation to diagnosed psychiatric syndromes, we (Blackmore et al., 2016) combined two separate cohorts based in Rochester that used parallel clinical protocols. The combined sample was composed of pregnant women receiving obstetrical care from a hospital-based practice serving a predominantly low-income, inner-city population. The aim was to enroll women at high psychosocial risk but not greater than normal obstetric risk. Key inclusion criteria were a confirmed singleton pregnancy <18 weeks gestation; 19–34 years of age; and low to medium obstetric risk. In those analyses, we subsequently excluded women who did not experience a live birth or delivered a baby of very low birth weight (<2,500 g) because of our interest in studying normal-risk pregnancies (that also avoided the confound of prenatal distress reflecting suspected or confirmed health concerns about the child, e.g., from health care providers).

A major novelty of that study was the inclusion of diagnostic assessments alongside continuous measures of symptoms, plus a measure of pregnancy-related anxiety. We administered the Structured Clinical Interview for DSM-IV (SCID) (First et al., 1995) at 18 and 32 weeks gestation (on average), as well as at multiple time points in the postnatal period. Diagnostic assessments were administered by trained clinical interviews, and we employed the usual set of quality control checks to ensure reliability of the diagnoses.

Pregnancy-related anxiety was collected using a modified version of items previously used (e.g., Huizink et al., 2004, 2015; Van den Bergh, 1990). Modifications of the pregnancy-related anxiety items were implemented to preempt any item from including reference to a first pregnancy – so as not to confound the measure with parity. We also modified wording of the items from other measures so that each question assessed a single dimension (e.g., "or" statements were eliminated). Our final list of items were the following: I am worried about the pain of contractions; I am worried about the pain of delivery; I am worried about not being able to control myself during labor; I am afraid that something will be wrong with my baby physically; I am afraid that something will be wrong with my baby mentally; I am afraid that my baby will be stillborn; I worry that my child will be in poor health. Responses were given on a 5-point Likert scale ranging from not at all, a little, somewhat, quite a bit, and very much.

Several findings from the analyses stood out. The first is that a clear two-factor structure emerged that distinguished items pertaining to worries about the child's health and items concerning childbirth; each of these two subscales showed high internal consistency. The distinction between worries about the child and worries about childbirth replicates prior studies and is reminiscent of studies that specifically targeted fear of childbirth. Importantly, the distinction between dimensions was also found longitudinally: whereas there was a sizable decline in worry about the child's health from the second to the third trimester, amounting to ¼ of a standard deviation, there was a slight increase in worry about childbirth over the same period. We have since replicated this factor structure and longitudinal pattern in pregnancy in an ongoing study of a new cohort of over 300 women, selected to ensure variation in stress exposure, socioeconomic status, and race and ethnicity (O'Connor et al., 2021).

The second, more novel finding from our previous study was a pattern of findings that distinguished pregnancy-related anxiety (as regards the child and childbirth) from conventional measures of symptoms – a particular feat given that the extensive assessment of symptoms included diagnostic assessments from independent assessors and maternal self-reports. Significantly *differential* patterns of association between pregnancy-related anxiety and other symptom measures were found for parity, age at first pregnancy, and number of miscarriages. These differential patterns of association complement and extend prior work showing mean differences in levels of pregnancy-related anxiety, for example, between experienced and nulliparous pregnant women (Huizink et al., 2015). Perhaps more impressive was that pregnancy-related anxiety (and items pertaining to the child in particular) predicted birth weight and postnatal anxiety disorder independent of prenatal anxiety disorder and the usual covariates. That was an important advance over prior studies showing that there is continuity of symptoms and disorders across the perinatal period (e.g., Freeman et al., 2018; Heron et al., 2004). The overall pattern of associations and predictions indicated that pregnancy-related anxiety could be distinguished from more conventional and general measures of anxiety (Blackmore et al., 2016).

For this chapter, we have analyzed the data in more detail to extend the research on pregnancy-related anxiety in relation to the main diagnostic categories in our work, namely, current and history of Major Depression, current Generalized Anxiety Disorder (GAD) and current post-traumatic stress disorder (PTSD), and the exposure to trauma as assessed from diagnostic interview. For the sake of simplicity, we here report findings assessing disorder at any stage in pregnancy (differences in diagnostic status between the two assessments was predictably trivial). We report analyses using a stem-leaf plot to show effect sizes, that is, the mean difference in pregnancy-related anxiety according to the diagnostic or trauma exposure groups. Figure 3.1 reports on pregnancy-related anxiety concerning the child and Figure 3.2 reports for pregnancy-related anxiety concerning childbirth.

Three novel patterns emerged. The first was that pregnancy-related anxiety was similarly related to GAD and Major Depression, and somewhat less related to diagnosed PTSD and a history of a major traumatic event. The second, unanticipated pattern was that the effect sizes were consistently greater for pregnancy-related anxiety concerning the health of the child than concerning childbirth. The third was that distress, trauma, and significant symptoms of depression that preceded pregnancy predicted "onset" of pregnancy-related anxiety. That is, for example, women with a history of depression (regardless of their current Major Depression status in pregnancy) exhibited more pregnancy-related anxiety than those without a positive history, with the effect somewhat stronger with respect to fears about the child than fears about childbirth. Similarly, a history of trauma (which by design preceded the current pregnancy) increased the risk for subsequent pregnancy-related anxiety, with the effect more marked for fears about the child.

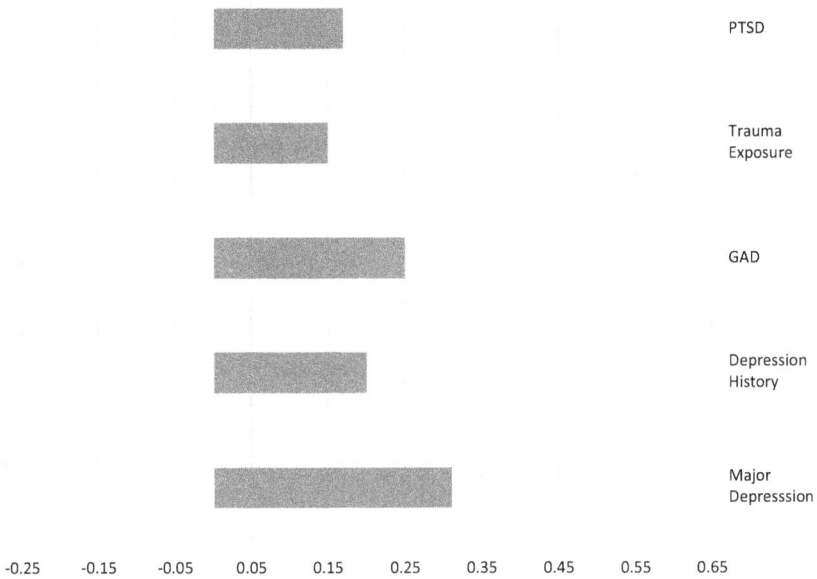

Figure 3.1 Effect sizes showing associations between select disorders and pregnancy-related anxiety (Worries about the Child, 32 weeks gestation)

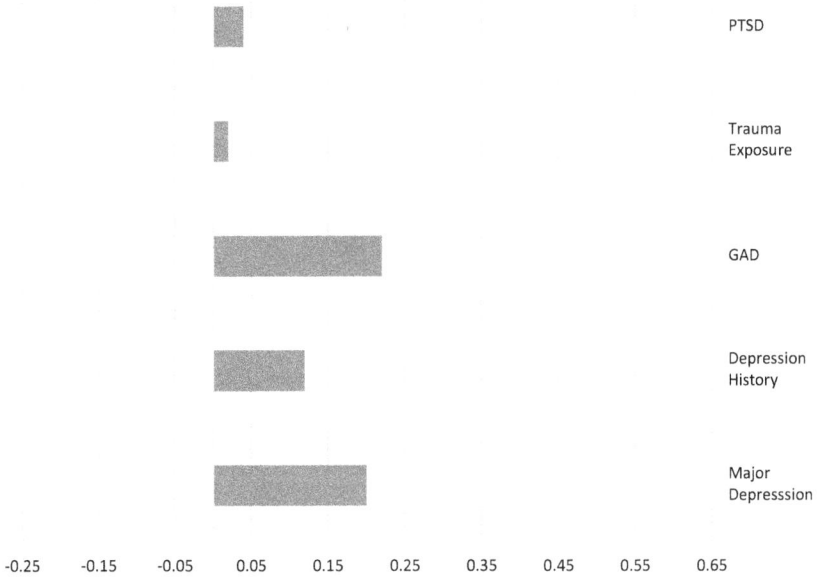

Figure 3.2 Effect sizes showing associations between select disorders and pregnancy-related anxiety (Worries about the Self, 32 weeks gestation)

These novel findings provide insight into the broad-based overlap between pregnancy-related anxiety and multiple diagnostic categories; these findings complement our previous analyses that showed that distinctions between pregnancy-related anxiety and other syndromes and disorders may be more apparent when predicting to outcomes, including both perinatal and postnatal health outcomes. And, in contrast to the concerted research on fear of childbirth/tokophobia, these results indicate that pregnancy-related anxiety concerning the health of the child may be more infused with general clinical distress and more likely to signal potential need for intervention. Quite how the symptom pattern concerning anxiety about the child is carried forward into the postnatal period to alter the formation of parental bonding and child-parent attachment requires additional research attention (McFarland et al., 2011). An important hypothesis is that pregnancy-related anxiety about the child may have a more persistent course into the postnatal period.

Several other kinds of studies are needed to push forward research on pregnancy-related anxiety and affective disorders. In particular, what has not yet been demonstrated is that pregnancy-specific anxiety and worries have a differential association with maternal biology than other disorders or symptom clusters. For example, there was not clear evidence in our study that pregnancy-related anxiety had a significantly different pattern of associations with maternal prenatal biology, based principally on cortisol. That line of work will require more attention and could help establish the distinctiveness of pregnancy-related anxiety. Stronger integration with maternal-fetal-placenta biology – that is, going beyond maternal biology to the interaction of maternal and child biology – is also a key next step for this work.

Another area of clinical interest, which was suggested in the results reported earlier, is the developmental origins of pregnancy-related anxiety. To question the origins of "pregnancy-related" anxiety is not intended as a paradox nor an irony but rather a hypothesis. That is, the term implies that the anxiety is pregnancy related, and the item content is exclusively about pregnancy and childbirth. However, it may be that the pregnancy-related anxiety derives from experiences and exposures that predate the (current) pregnancy. That, in fact, was a cornerstone idea in our earlier analyses on miscarriage in the ALSPAC study and in the earlier analyses on pre-pregnancy depression and trauma exposure. Importantly, other studies also suggest that pregnancy-related anxiety may have pre-pregnancy origins. For example, extreme fear of childbirth was reported to be greater in nulliparous women than women with a previous birth, and in women who experienced a prior cesarean section (Rouhe et al., 2009). The important point here is that studies of pregnancy-related anxiety may be too focused on prenatal anxiety and not fully appreciate that pre-pregnancy/pre-conception experiences may shape maternal risk for prenatal anxiety and stress biology – in a way that may hold substantial implications for perinatal and child health. Several groups are pursuing the hypothesis that trauma in early childhood may alter maternal psychology and biology (Blackmore et al., 2011b; Moog et al., 2016), and the effects may also carry forward to our conceptions and measurement of pregnancy-related anxiety.

Some applications for intervention

One measure of the significance and distinctiveness of the construct of preg-nancy-related anxiety may be its ability to attract specific treatment attention. That is the case for fear of childbirth, which has been targeted in several treat-ment modalities (Rondung et al., 2018; Rouhe et al., 2015) and is the sub-ject of several reviews (O'Connell et al., 2020; Smith et al., 2019; Stoll et al., 2018; Striebich et al., 2018). Less particular, and broader forms of a putative pregnancy-related anxiety phenotype have not attracted as much attention. How-ever, treatments for prenatal anxiety are increasing rapidly and already compose a diverse set of approaches and paradigms (O'Connor et al., 2014). It might be expected, therefore, that the range of treatment modalities and specificity of symptom expression may increase in the near term, along with efforts to assess biological and psychological mechanisms of treatment effects; to identify treat-ment modifiers; and to judge the impact of confounding comorbid conditions, from trauma to specific medical vulnerabilities.

One clinical application with special relevance to this chapter is the treatment decision concerning who might require intervention. That decision often hinges on evidence of impairment. However, the notion of impairment has not yet fea-tured in studies of pregnancy-related anxiety; in contrast, this is a central concern for affective disorder diagnoses. In fact, to date, pregnancy-related anxiety has been considered as a continuously distributed trait, without systematic attempt to define "elevated" symptomatology or assess evidence of impairment secondary to pregnancy-related anxiety. That may not necessarily be a limitation insofar as reduction in *experienced* pregnancy-related anxiety may, *ipso facto*, be sufficient reason to encourage treatment, that is, independent of any potential benefit for the health of the pregnancy or child. On the other hand, interventions for mood disturbance are rarely (successfully) applied to the entire continuum of distress. Moreover, even if there were an interest in applying an intervention to the entire continuum of symptoms, the limits of resources inevitably mean that non-uni-versal treatment decisions need to follow some practical guidance concerning prioritizing – and that usually implies severity/impairment.

The point here is not to argue that there needs to be a diagnostic end point for research on the construct of pregnancy-related anxiety. Indeed, attempts to insert the perinatal context into diagnostic decisions are rare and the process may not be fulfilling – witness the modest change for Major Depression from a "with postpartum onset" qualifier in DSM-IV to "with peripartum onset" in DSM-V. That modest change is notable insofar as there is now inclusion of the *pre*natal period, but the change was nowhere near as dramatic as many had suggested or hoped for. It is a tall order to require substantive changes in symptom expres-sion and timing in its expression within the perinatal period for any diagnostic system (notably, specific phobia can already capture tokophobia). Nevertheless, whether or not the consideration of pregnancy-related anxiety into a diagnostic manual is the aim, the blue print for this effort would offer a valuable framework for advancing research on pregnancy-related anxiety vis-à-vis affective disorders.

Conclusions and future directions

Some authors suggest that pregnancy and childbirth may be conceptualized as a major stressor that, like other stressors, may increase the risk for affective illness (Brockington, 1996). A complementary view is that pregnancy and childbirth provide a natural experiment that offers special and peculiar leverage for assessing how changes in social, psychological, immune, and neuroendocrine systems may correspond with changes in mental health and illness. Distress in pregnancy has, in any event, generated substantial clinical, scientific, and public health interest because mental illness during this period may have lasting consequences for the health of the mother and child. Further progress in this area will be strengthened by greater understanding of the distinct features of pregnancy-related anxiety as regards symptom expression, causes, and sequelae. That is the demanding task for research on pregnancy-related anxiety: it must reveal novel insights into perinatal mental health and its influence on the child. This volume indicates the momentum in this field and several specific marks of progress.

There are, however, matters that still need to be resolved. For example, many studies report associations between prenatal maternal affective disturbance and potential biological markers and mechanisms, with major candidates found in the autonomic, neuroendocrine, and immune systems. Although we do have data suggesting that pregnancy-related anxiety may be clinically distinguished from other forms of affective distress, we do not have evidence of any biological distinctiveness. Applications to maternal-fetal-*placenta* biology are especially missing. Integration of research on pregnancy-related anxiety with clinical service, health care utilization, and cost are also areas now needing concerted attention. This kind of work would place pregnancy-related anxiety in a practical and financial context – a precondition for its widespread acceptance. There also remains some uncertainty about how pregnancy-related anxiety interdigitates with common and likely related experiences and dispositions, such as planfulness of pregnancy, PTSD associated with sexual trauma prior to the pregnancy, and prior experience of miscarriage and stillbirth. Finally, there is the matter of clinical course. It seems unwise to presume that pregnancy-related anxiety will resolve with the birth of a healthy child, and that its burden on clinical services and health care costs are limited to obstetric care. Our report indicating that pregnancy-related anxiety predicted GAD in the postpartum period independent of prenatal GAD is one illustration of this (Blackmore et al., 2016). Some kind of spillover into the postnatal period is not inevitable, but neither is it implausible. These are the topics that will likely drive research on pregnancy-related anxiety for the next several years and illustrate the manner in which these studies will help promote maternal and child health.

Acknowledgments

Funding was provided in part by MH097293, MH073019, MH073842, UG3OD023349, UH3OD023349, and the Wynne Center for Family Research.

References

Adams, S. S., Eberhard-Gran, M., & Eskild, A. (2012). Fear of childbirth and duration of labour: A study of 2206 women with intended vaginal delivery. *BJOG, 119*(10), 1238–1246. https://doi.org/10.1111/j.1471-0528.2012.03433.x

Alderdice, F., Lynn, F., & Lobel, M. (2012). A review and psychometric evaluation of pregnancy-specific stress measures. *Journal of Psychosomatic Obstetrics and Gynaecology, 33*(2), 62–77. https://doi/10.3109/0167482X.2012.673040

Bayrampour, H., Ali, E., McNeil, D. A., Benzies, K., MacQueen, G., & Tough, S. (2016). Pregnancy-related anxiety: A concept analysis. *International Journal of Nursing Studies, 55*, 115–130. https://doi/10.1016/j.ijnurstu.2015.10.023

Blackmore, E. R., Cote-Arsenault, D., Tang, W., Glover, V., Evans, J., Golding, J., & O'Connor, T. G. (2011a). Previous prenatal loss as a predictor of perinatal depression and anxiety. *British Journal of Psychiatry, 198*(5), 373–378. https://doi/10.1192/bjp.bp.110.083105

Blackmore, E. R., Gustafsson, H., Gilchrist, M., Wyman, C., & O'Connor, T. G. (2016). Pregnancy-related anxiety: Evidence of distinct clinical significance from a prospective longitudinal study. *Journal of Affective Disorders, 197*, 251–258. https://doi.org/10.1016/j.jad.2016.03.008

Blackmore, E. R., Moynihan, J. A., Rubinow, D. R., Pressman, E. K., Gilchrist, M., & O'Connor, T. G. (2011b). Psychiatric symptoms and proinflammatory cytokines in pregnancy. *Psychosomatic Medicine, 73*(8), 656–663. https://doi.org/10.1097/PSY.0b013e31822fc277

Blackmore, E. R., Rubinow, D. R., O'Connor, T. G., Liu, X., Tang, W., Craddock, N., & Jones, I. (2013). Reproductive outcomes and risk of subsequent illness in women diagnosed with postpartum psychosis. *Bipolar Disorders, 15*(4), 394–404. https://doi.org/10.1111/bdi.12071

Brockington, I. F. (1996). *Motherhood and mental health.* Oxford University Press.

Brunton, R. J., Dryer, R., Krägeloh, C., Saliba, A., Kohlhoff, J., & Medvedev, O. (2018). The pregnancy-related anxiety scale: A validity examination using Rasch analysis. *Journal of Affective Disorders, 236*, 127–135. https://doi.org/10.1016/j.jad.2018.04.116

Brunton, R. J., Dryer, R., Saliba, A., & Kohlhoff, J. (2015). Pregnancy anxiety: A systematic review of current scales. *Journal of Affective Disorders, 176*, 24–34. https://doi.org/10.1016/j.jad.2015.01.039

Buist, A., Gotman, N., & Yonkers, K. A. (2011). Generalized anxiety disorder: Course and risk factors in pregnancy. *Journal of Affective Disorders, 131*(1–3), 277–283. https://doi.org/10.1016/j.jad.2011.01.003

Cote-Arsenault, D. (2003). The influence of perinatal loss on anxiety in multigravidas. *Journal of Obstetric, Gynecologic, and Neonatal Nursing, 32*(5), 623–629. https://doi.org/10.1177/0884217503257140

Cox, J. L., Holden, J. M., & Sagovsky, R. (1987). Detection of postnatal depression. Development of the 10-item Edinburgh Postnatal Depression Scale. *British Journal of Psychiatry, 150*, 782–786.

Di Florio, A., & Meltzer-Brody, S. (2015). Is postpartum depression a distinct disorder? *Current Psychiatry Reports, 17*(10), 76. https://doi.org/10.1007/s11920-015-0617-6

DiPietro, J. A., Christensen, A. L., & Costigan, K. A. (2008). The pregnancy experience scale-brief version. *Journal of Psychosomatic Obstetrics and Gynaecology, 29*(4), 262–267. https://doi.org/10.1080/01674820802546220

Dunkel Schetter, C., & Tanner, L. (2012). Anxiety, depression and stress in pregnancy: Implications for mothers, children, research, and practice. *Current Opinion in Psychiatry*, *25*(2), 141–148. https://doi.org/10.1097/YCO.0b013e3283503680

Fawcett, E. J., Fairbrother, N., Cox, M. L., White, I. R., & Fawcett, J. M. (2019). The prevalence of anxiety disorders during pregnancy and the postpartum period: A multivariate Bayesian meta-analysis. *Journal of Clinical Psychiatry*, *80*(4). https://doi.org/10.4088/JCP.18r12527

First, M. B., Spitzer, R. L., Gibbon, M., & Williams, J. B. W. (1995). *Structured clinical interview for DSM-IV*. American Psychiatric Press.

Freeman, M. P., Claypoole, L. D., Burt, V. K., Sosinsky, A. Z., Moustafa, D., Noe, O. B., Cheng, L. J., & Cohen, L. S. (2018). Course of major depressive disorder after pregnancy and the postpartum period. *Depression & Anxiety*, *35*(12), 1130–1136. https://doi.org/10.1002/da.22836

Gobel, A., Stuhrmann, L. Y., Harder, S., Schulte-Markwort, M., & Mudra, S. (2018). The association between maternal-fetal bonding and prenatal anxiety: An explanatory analysis and systematic review. *Journal of Affective Disorders*, *239*, 313–327. https://doi.org/10.1016/j.jad.2018.07.024

Guintivano, J., Sullivan, P. F., Stuebe, A. M., Penders, T., Thorp, J., Rubinow, D. R., & Meltzer-Brody, S. (2018). Adverse life events, psychiatric history, and biological predictors of postpartum depression in an ethnically diverse sample of postpartum women. *Psychological Medicine*, *48*(7), 1190–1200. https://doi.org/10.1017/S0033291717002641

Heron, J., O'Connor, T. G., Evans, J., Golding, J., & Glover, V. (2004). The course of anxiety and depression through pregnancy and the postpartum in a community sample. *Journal of Affective Disorders*, *80*(1), 65–73. https://doi.org/10.1016/j.jad.2003.08.004

Hofberg, K., & Brockington, I. (2000). Tokophobia: An unreasoning dread of childbirth. A series of 26 cases. *British Journal of Psychiatry*, *176*, 83–85. https://doi.org/10.1192/bjp.176.1.83

Hughes, P. M., Turton, P., & Evans, C. D. (1999). Stillbirth as risk factor for depression and anxiety in the subsequent pregnancy: Cohort study. *BMJ*, *318*(7200), 1721–1724. https://doi.org/10.1136/bmj.318.7200.1721

Huizink, A. C., Delforterie, M. J., Scheinin, N. M., Tolvanen, M., Karlsson, L., & Karlsson, H. (2015). Adaption of pregnancy anxiety questionnaire-revised for all pregnant women regardless of parity: PRAQ-R2. *Archives of Women's Mental Health*, *19*, 125–132. https://doi.org/10.1007/s00737-015-0531-2

Huizink, A. C., Mulder, E. J., Robles de Medina, P. G., Visser, G. H., & Buitelaar, J. K. (2004). Is pregnancy anxiety a distinctive syndrome? *Early Human Development*, *79*(2), 81–91. https://doi.org/10.1016/j.earlhumdev.2004.04.014

Janssen, H. J., Cuisinier, M. C., Hoogduin, K. A., & de Graauw, K. P. (1996). Controlled prospective study on the mental health of women following pregnancy loss. *American Journal of Psychiatry*, *153*(2), 226–230. https://doi.org/10.1176/ajp.153.2.226

Kanes, S. J., Colquhoun, H., Doherty, J., Raines, S., Hoffmann, E., Rubinow, D. R., & Meltzer-Brody, S. (2017). Open-label, proof-of-concept study of brexanolone in the treatment of severe postpartum depression. *Human Psychopharmacology*, *32*(2). https://doi.org/10.1002/hup.2576

Lobel, M., Cannella, D. L., Graham, J. E., DeVincent, C., Schneider, J., & Meyer, B. A. (2008). Pregnancy-specific stress, prenatal health behaviors, and birth outcomes. *Health Psychology*, *27*(5), 604–615. https://doi.org/10.1037/a0013242

McFarland, J., Salisbury, A. L., Battle, C. L., Hawes, K., Halloran, K., & Lester, B. M. (2011). Major depressive disorder during pregnancy and emotional attachment to the fetus. *Archives of Women's Mental Health*, *14*(5), 425–434. https://doi.org/10.1007/s00737-011-0237-z

Meades, R., & Ayers, S. (2011). Anxiety measures validated in perinatal populations: A systematic review. *Journal of Affective Disorders*, *133*(1–2), 1–15. https://doi.org/10.1016/j.jad.2010.10.009

Moog, N. K., Buss, C., Entringer, S., Shahbaba, B., Gillen, D. L., Hobel, C. J., & Wadhwa, P. D. (2016). Maternal exposure to childhood trauma is associated during pregnancy with placental-fetal stress physiology. *Biological Psychiatry*, *79*(10), 831–839. https://doi.org/10.1016/j.biopsych.2015.08.032

Nilsson, C., Hessman, E., Sjoblom, H., Dencker, A., Jangsten, E., Mollberg, M., Patel, H., Sparud-Lundin, C., Wigert, H., & Begley, C. (2018). Definitions, measurements and prevalence of fear of childbirth: A systematic review. *BMC Pregnancy Childbirth*, *18*(1), 28. https://doi.org/10.1186/s12884-018-1659-7

O'Connell, M. A., Khashan, A. S., & Leahy-Warren, P. (2020). Women's experiences of interventions for fear of childbirth in the perinatal period: A meta-synthesis of qualitative research evidence. *Women and Birth*. https://doi.org/10.1016/j.wombi.2020.05.008

O'Connor, T. G., Best, M., Brunner, J., Ciesla, A. A., Cunnings, A., Ntemena, K., Kautz, A., Khoury, L., Macomber, A., Meng, Y., Miller, R. K., Murphy, H. R., Salafia, C., Sefair, A. V., Serrano, J., & Barrett, E. S. (2021). *Cohort profile: Understanding pregnancy signals and infant development (UPSIDE), a pregnancy cohort study on prenatal exposure mechanisms for child health.* [Manuscript submitted for publication].

O'Connor, T. G., Heron, J., Golding, J., Beveridge, M., & Glover, V. (2002). Maternal antenatal anxiety and children's behavioural/emotional problems at 4 years. Report from the Avon Longitudinal Study of Parents and Children. *British Journal of Psychiatry*, *180*, 502–508. https://doi.org/10.1192/bjp.180.6.502

O'Connor, T. G., Monk, C., & Fitelson, E. M. (2014). Practitioner review: Maternal mood in pregnancy and child development – implications for child psychology and psychiatry. *Journal of Child Psychology and Psychiatry, and Allied Disciplines*, *55*(2), 99–111. https://doi.org/10.1111/jcpp.12153

Rini, C. K., Dunkel-Schetter, C., Wadhwa, P. D., & Sandman, C. A. (1999). Psychological adaptation and birth outcomes: The role of personal resources, stress, and sociocultural context in pregnancy. *Health Psychology*, *18*(4), 333–345. https://doi.org/10.1037//0278-6133.18.4.333

Rondung, E., Ternstrom, E., Hildingsson, I., Haines, H. M., Sundin, O., Ekdahl, J., Karlström, A., Larsson, B., Segeblad, B., Baylis, R., & Rubertsson, C. (2018). Comparing internet-based cognitive behavioral therapy with standard care for women with fear of birth: Randomized controlled trial. *JMIR Mental Health*, *5*(3), e10420. https://doi.org/10.2196/10420

Rouhe, H., Salmela-Aro, K., Halmesmaki, E., & Saisto, T. (2009). Fear of childbirth according to parity, gestational age, and obstetric history. *BJOG*, *116*(1), 67–73. https://doi.org/10.1111/j.1471-0528.2008.02002.x

Rouhe, H., Salmela-Aro, K., Toivanen, R., Tokola, M., Halmesmaki, E., Ryding, E. L., & Saisto, T. (2015). Group psychoeducation with relaxation for severe fear of childbirth improves maternal adjustment and childbirth experience – a randomised controlled trial. *Journal of Psychosomatic Obstetrics and Gynaecology*, *36*(1), 1–9. https://doi.org/10.3109/0167482X.2014.980722

Schiller, C. E., Meltzer-Brody, S., & Rubinow, D. R. (2015). The role of reproductive hormones in postpartum depression. *CNS Spectrums, 20*(1), 48–59. https://doi.org/10.1017/S1092852914000480

Sinesi, A., Maxwell, M., O'Carroll, R., & Cheyne, H. (2019). Anxiety scales used in pregnancy: Systematic review. *BJPsych Open, 5*(1), e5. https://doi.org/10.1192/bjo.2018.75

Sit, D., Rothschild, A. J., & Wisner, K. L. (2006). A review of postpartum psychosis. *Journal of Women's Health, 15*(4), 352–368. https://doi.org/10.1089/jwh.2006.15.352

Smith, V., Gallagher, L., Carroll, M., Hannon, K., & Begley, C. (2019). Antenatal and intrapartum interventions for reducing caesarean section, promoting vaginal birth, and reducing fear of childbirth: An overview of systematic reviews. *PLoS One, 14*(10), e0224313. https://doi.org/10.1371/journal.pone.0224313

Somerville, S., Dedman, K., Hagan, R., Oxnam, E., Wettinger, M., Byrne, S., Coo, S., Doherty, D., & Page, A. C. (2014). The perinatal anxiety screening scale: Development and preliminary validation. *Archives of Women's Mental Health, 17*(5), 443–454. https://doi.org/10.1007/s00737-014-0425-8

Stoll, K., Swift, E. M., Fairbrother, N., Nethery, E., & Janssen, P. (2018). A systematic review of nonpharmacological prenatal interventions for pregnancy-specific anxiety and fear of childbirth. *Birth, 45*(1), 7–18. https://doi.org/10.1111/birt.12316

Striebich, S., Mattern, E., & Ayerle, G. M. (2018). Support for pregnant women identified with fear of childbirth (FOC)/tokophobia – A systematic review of approaches and interventions. *Midwifery, 61*, 97–115. https://doi.org/10.1016/j.midw.2018.02.013

Theut, S. K., Pedersen, F. A., Zaslow, M. J., & Rabinovich, B. A. (1988). Pregnancy subsequent to perinatal loss: Parental anxiety and depression. *Journal of the American Academy of Child and Adolescent Psychiatry, 27*(3), 289–292. https://doi.org/10.1097/00004583-198805000-00004

Turton, P., Hughes, P., Evans, C. D., & Fainman, D. (2001). Incidence, correlates and predictors of post-traumatic stress disorder in the pregnancy after stillbirth. *British Journal of Psychiatry, 178*, 556–560. https://doi.org/10.1192/bjp.178.6.556

Van den Bergh, B. (1990). The influence of maternal emotions during pregnancy on fetal and neonatal behavior. *Journal of Prenatal & Perinatal Psychology & Health, 5*, 119–130.

4 Antecedents of pregnancy-related anxiety

Hamideh Bayrampour

Antecedents of pregnancy-related anxiety

Antecedents are events or incidents that must occur before the occurrence of a concept (Walker & Avant, 2011). In 2016, my colleagues and I conducted a concept analysis to clarify the concept of pregnancy-related anxiety and iden-tify its characteristics and dimensions, including antecedents (Bayrampour et al., 2016). We used a modified approach based on Walker and Avant (2011) for this analysis and searched several databases to obtain the relevant evidence, including qualitative and quantitative studies. We found that for the occurrence of preg-nancy-related anxiety, three antecedents are necessary: (1) a real or perceived threat to pregnancy or its outcomes, (2) self-doubt about one's ability to control or cope with the situation or a low perceived control, and (3) excessive thinking and cognitive activity. All of these antecedents can be considered related to ante-cedents of anxiety in general. What makes pregnancy-related anxiety distinct from other general anxieties is that the cognitions and thoughts in pregnancy-related anxiety are mainly focused on and concentrated around pregnancy, baby's health and mother's well-being, labor, and parenting issues (Huizink et al., 2004). The following section provides an overview of these antecedents.

A real or perceived threat to pregnancy or its outcomes

In a mixed methods study to understand perception of pregnancy risk, it was found that pregnancy-related anxiety and perception of pregnancy risk were closely related (Bayrampour et al., 2012a). We found that a high perception of pregnancy risk correlated with pregnancy-related anxiety and this perception might trigger anxiety due to uncertainty about pregnancy or its outcomes. Oth-ers reported similar insights (Dako-Gyeke et al., 2013; Harpel, 2008). On the other hand, in the review of the literature, we noticed that tangible evidence on potential positive outcomes may decrease this anxiety by reducing perceived risk. For example, in a qualitative investigation, Harpel (2008) found that ultrasound examinations relieved anxiety by providing insight about pregnancy and reduc-ing associated uncertainty about fetal health (Harpel, 2008). One study that examined anxiety levels using the State Trait Anxiety Inventory before and after

DOI: 10.4324/9781003014003-6

prenatal diagnostic procedures (ultrasound group, $N = 37$ and amniocentesis group, $N = 37$) found a significant decrease in anxiety level after the ultrasound (Nakić Radoš et al., 2013).

Self-doubt about one's ability to control or cope with the situation: a low perceived control

Original theories of anxiety show that in the experience of anxiety, there is a core sense of uncontrollability over possible future risks, dangers, or potential negative outcomes. In fact, anxiety has been described as a state of helplessness to predict, control, or acquire the desired outcomes (Barlow, 2000). Some people need to feel that they are in control of events/situations in order to manage their emotions. This is true for pregnant women and during pregnancy as well (Schneider, 2002). Evidence shows that not being allowed to retain control over health and medical decisions or feelings of losing control as a result of labor pain can make pregnant women anxious (Sjogren, 1997). On the other hand, feeling that they have control over a potential risk can decrease women's perception of pregnancy risk and subsequently their anxiety levels (Bayrampour et al., 2012b; McCain & Deatrick, 1994). In fact, pregnant women who had chronic health conditions during pregnancy were not anxious if they felt their health conditions were well-controlled and managed. However, when pregnancy complications occurred suddenly and were unpredictable or became uncontrollable, that triggered considerable anxiety for pregnant women (Bayrampour et al., 2012b). For example, in qualitative research (Bayrampour et al., 2012b), one research participant with gestational diabetes did not present elevated pregnancy-related anxiety symptoms. In the interviews, this participant mentioned that her mother also had gestational diabetes when she was pregnant with her brother, so she was expecting to develop a similar complication and it was not unpredictable.

Excessive thinking and cognitive activity

Excessive thinking and the activation of cognitions to evaluate various scenarios resulting from an uncertain outcome or an uncontrolled situation are the third antecedents of pregnancy-related anxiety. When there is a perceived threat and the person does not feel that they are in control of the situation or the adverse outcomes are manageable, they might engage in a cognitive process to predict potential adverse consequences, sometimes to find a solution or to know what to expect in an effort to gain control and feel prepared. However, a perceived uncontrollable threat in conjunction with low perceived control may result in fruitless re-review of potential adverse outcomes. The review of the literature showed that cognitive activity and worry are considered both a trigger and an attribute of anxiety in general (Biehle & Mickelson, 2011; Purdon & Harrington, 2006).

Risk factors

Individual attributes and physical and social environmental characteristics that increase the likelihood of an adverse outcome are risk factors. There are many studies that explored risk factors of general anxiety during pregnancy and more evidence is emerging on risk factors of pregnancy-related anxiety. Our review of the literature showed that there are some common risk factors for general anxiety and pregnancy-related anxiety such as perceived stress, level of social support, and prior history of mental health issues. However, some factors may be associated with pregnancy-related anxiety but not general anxiety such as previous pregnancy loss (Cote-Arsenault, 2003; Tsartsara & Johnson, 2006) or have stronger associations with pregnancy-related anxiety than general anxiety such as pregnancy complications (Da Costa et al., 1999; King et al., 2010). In the following section, risk factors of anxiety during pregnancy and pregnancy-related anxiety, when evidence is available, are discussed.

Obstetric characteristics

A significant relationship between previous pregnancy loss and anxiety, after controlling for demographic variables, including age, current employment status, education, income, and BMI, has been reported in literature. Indeed, in a large study of over 18,000 women, those with previous pregnancy loss were 2.5 times more likely to experience anxiety as measured by self-rating anxiety scale (SAS) in their subsequent pregnancy (Gong et al., 2013). In 2017, Shapiro and colleagues found that the number of previous stillbirths was significantly associated with anxiety (as measured by the four-item pregnancy specific anxiety scale [PSAS]) in the third trimester, after adjusting for income, ethnicity, unplanned pregnancy, and self-reported complications in multiple regression analyses (Shapiro et al., 2017).

Associations between a history of infertility and anxiety have been reported to be inconsistent in the literature (Bayrampour et al., 2018). A subtle but significant association between unplanned pregnancy and pregnancy-related anxiety (measured using Pregnancy-Related Anxiety Questionnaire Revised [PRAQ-R]) have been reported (Westerneng et al., 2017). McMahon et al. (1997) reported no significant associations with general anxiety and having a history of IVF treatment. However, they found that women who conceived through IVF had significantly higher levels of specific anxieties about the survival of the baby and normality of the pregnancy, injuries to the baby during labor, and separation from babies after birth that persisted throughout pregnancy (McMahon et al., 1997).

Medical or pregnancy complications such as gestational diabetes and hyperemesis gravidarum are considered risk factors for anxiety during pregnancy. Several studies have shown that women who had previous live births had lower anxiety during their current pregnancies than nulliparous women (Arch, 2013; Guardino et al., 2014; Mudra et al., 2020; Shapiro et al., 2017; Westerneng et al., 2017).

Westerneng et al. (2017) reported that nulliparous women, in comparison to multiparous women, had two times higher odds for elevated pregnancy-related anxiety, as measured by the PRAQ-R.

Psychological factors

A significant association between personality traits, including self-esteem and perceived control, and anxiety during pregnancy have been reported. Mudra et al. (2020) reported that women with higher self-efficacy had lower levels of pregnancy-related anxiety (assessed using the Pregnancy-Related Anxiety Questionnaire Revised-2 [PRAQ-R2]).

Denial and acceptance coping styles were also significant risk factors of anxiety symptoms among pregnant women (Bergner et al., 2008; Denis et al., 2012; Gourounti et al., 2013; Rychik et al., 2012; van Bussel et al., 2009). The majority of studies that examined the associations between childhood abuse/early diversity and intimate partner violence reported a significant association between any type of abuse and anxiety in general during pregnancy (Bayrampour et al., 2015, 2018; Martini et al., 2015). The indicators of the intimate relationship, such as relationship quality, tension in the relationship, and partner support are shown to have significant associations with anxiety (Bayrampour et al., 2018; Da Costa et al., 1999; Karaçam & Ançel, 2009; Mahenge et al., 2013; Nasreen et al., 2011). A previous history of mental health problems and low social support have been reported to have strong significant associations with anxiety during pregnancy (Bayrampour et al., 2018). Women with comorbid depression had three times higher odds for elevated pregnancy-specific anxiety levels (assessed using the PRAQ-R) than women with no depression (Westerneng et al., 2017).

Health behaviors and demographic factors

Among studies that examined associations between anxiety and smoking/substance abuse, the majority reported significant associations. Persistent users of tobacco while pregnant were 2.5 times more likely than non-users to have any anxiety disorder. In another study, pregnancy-related anxiety was identified as the strongest predictor of alcohol drinking risk during pregnancy. There is also some evidence that immigrant pregnant women have higher odds for elevated pregnancy-related anxiety levels (as measured by the pregnancy-related thoughts [PRT] or the PRAQ-R) than local women (Fleuriet & Sunil, 2014; Westerneng et al., 2017). Two additional studies showed that higher maternal education (measured in years) was associated with lower pregnancy-related anxiety (Arch, 2013; Shapiro et al., 2017).

Implications

The knowledge of antecedents of anxiety can be useful for management strategies of pregnancy-related anxiety by targeting any of its antecedents; decreasing perceived risk, empowering women through increasing their perceived control; and using psychological techniques to manage excessive thinking. Among these, perceived control is especially important. It should be noted that strategies and interventions that could increase perceived control are unique for each person. For example, some women may feel more in control in hospital because they will have access to medical interventions if they need them. However, some women may feel more in control if they give birth at home because they will feel more in control of labor decisions (Cook & Loomis, 2012).

The knowledge of risk factors for pregnancy-related anxiety can inform screening strategies and management interventions. Our review of risk factors of anxiety showed that multiple factors contribute to antenatal anxiety and individual risk factors only explain a small amount of the variance in anxiety. Therefore, a cumulative measure of risk factors as well as resilience factors might be helpful in developing screening strategies. Several risk factors of pregnancy-related anxiety are identifiable prior to pregnancy such as psychosocial factors (e.g., available social support, previous history of poor mental health, coping styles) highlighting the possibility of pre-conception mental health screening. Additionally, there are factors that can be detectable in routine obstetric visits such as previous pregnancy loss and pregnancy complications and there are several factors that are potentially modifiable, including social support, partner factors. Education about effective coping styles, increased social support, and partner counseling and support are some of the examples of such interventions.

References

Arch, J. J. (2013). Pregnancy-specific anxiety: Which women are highest and what are the alcohol-related risks? *Comprehensive Psychiatry*, 54(3), 217–228. https://doi.org/10.1016/j.comppsych.2012.07.010

Barlow, D. H. (2000). Unraveling the mysteries of anxiety and its disorders from the perspective of emotion theory. *The American Psychologist*, 55(11), 1247–1263. https://doi.org/10.1037//0003-066x.55.11.1247.

Bayrampour, H., Ali, E., McNeil, D. A., Benzies, K., MacQueen, G., & Tough, S. (2016). Pregnancy-related anxiety: A concept analysis. *International Journal of Nursing Studies*, 55, 115–130. https://doi.org/10.1016/j.ijnurstu.2015.10.023

Bayrampour, H., Heaman, M., Duncan, K., & Tough, S. (2012a). Predictors of perception of pregnancy risk among nulliparous women. *Journal of Obstetric, Gynecologic & Neonatal Nursing*, 42(4), 416–427. https://doi.org/10.1111/1552-6909.12215.

Bayrampour, H., Heaman, M., Duncan, K. A., & Tough, S. (2012b). Advanced maternal age and risk perception: A qualitative study. *BMC Pregnancy Childbirth*, 12, 100. https://doi.org/10.1186/1471-2393-12-100

Bayrampour, H., McDonald, S., & Tough, S. (2015). Risk factors of transient and persistent anxiety during pregnancy. *Midwifery*, 31(6), 582–589. https://doi.org/10.1016/j.midw.2015.02.009

Bayrampour, H., Vinturache, A., Hetherington, E., Lorenzetti, D. L., & Tough, S. (2018). Risk factors for antenatal anxiety: A systematic review of the literature.

Journal of Reproductive Infant Psychology, 36(5), 476–503. https://doi.org/10.10 80/02646838.2018.1492097

Bergner, A., Beyer, B., Klapp, B. F., & Rauchfuss, M. (2008). Pregnancy after early pregnancy loss: A prospective study of anxiety, depressive symptomatology and coping. *Journal of Psychosomatic Obstetrics & Gynecology, 29*(2), 105–113. https://doi.org/10.1080/01674820701687521

Biehle, S. N., & Mickelson, K. D. (2011). Worries in expectant parents: Its relation with perinatal well-being and relationship satisfaction. *Personal Relationships, 18*(4), 697–713. https://doi.org/10.1111/j.1475-6811.2010.01335.x

Cook, K., & Loomis, C. (2012). The impact of choice and control on women's childbirth experiences. *Journal of Perinatal Education, 21*(3), 158–168. https://doi.org/10.1891/1058-1243.21.3.158

Cote-Arsenault, D. (2003). The influence of perinatal loss on anxiety in muligravidas. *JOGNN, 32*, 623–629. https://doi.org/ 10.1177/0884217503257140

Da Costa, D., Larouche, J., Drista, M., & Brender, W. (1999). Variations in stress levels over the course of pregnancy: Factors associated with elevated hassles, state anxiety and pregnancy-specific stress. *Journal of Psychosomatic Research, 47*(6), 609–621. https://doi.org/10.1016/S0022-3999(99)00064-1

Dako-Gyeke, P., Aikins, M., Aryeetey, R., McCough, L., & Adongo, P. B. (2013). The influence of socio-cultural interpretations of pregnancy threats on health-seeking behavior among pregnant women in urban Accra, Ghana. *BMC Pregnancy Childbirth, 13*, 211. https://doi.org/10.1186/1471-2393-13-211

Denis, A., Michaux, P., & Callahan, S. (2012). Factors implicated in moderating the risk for depression and anxiety in high risk pregnancy. *Journal of Reproductive and Infant Psychology, 30*(2), 124–134. https://doi.org/10.1080/02646838.2012.6 77020

Fleuriet, K. J., & Sunil, T. S. (2014). Perceived social stress, pregnancy-related anxiety, depression and subjective social status among pregnant Mexican and Mexican American women in South Texas. *Journal of Health Care for the Poor and Underserved, 25*(2), 546–561. https://doi.org/10.1353/hpu.2014.0092

Gong, X., Hao, J., Tao, F., Zhang, J., Wang, H., & Xu, R. (2013). Pregnancy loss and anxiety and depression during subsequent pregnancies: Data from the C-ABC study. *European Journal of Obstetrics & Gynecology and Reproductive Biology, 166*, 30–36. https://doi.org/10.1016/j.ejogrb.2012.09.024

Gourounti, K., Anagnostopoulos, F., & Lykeridou, K. (2013). Coping strategies as psychological risk factor for antenatal anxiety, worries, and depression among Greek women. *Archives of Women's Mental Health, 16*(5), 353–361. https://doi.org/10.1007/s00737-013-0338-y

Guardino, C. M., Schetter, C. D., Bower, J. E., Lu, M. C., & Smalley, S. L. (2014). Randomised controlled pilot trial of mindfulness training for stress reduction during pregnancy. *Psychology & Health, 29*(3), 334–349. https://doi.org/10.1080/0 8870446.2013.852670

Harpel, T. S. (2008). Fear of the unknown: Ultrasound and anxiety about fetal health. *Health, 12*(3), 295–312. https://doi.org/10.1177/1363459308090050

Huizink, A. C., Mulder, E. J., Robles de Medina, P. G., Visser, G. H., & Buitelaar, J. K. (2004). Is pregnancy anxiety a distinctive syndrome? *Early Human Development, 79*(2), 81–91. https://doi.org/10.1016/j.earlhumdev.2004.04.014

Karaçam, Z., & Ançel, G. (2009). Depression, anxiety and influencing factors in pregnancy: A study in a Turkish population. *Midwifery, 25*(4), 344–356. https://doi.org/10.1016/j.midw.2007.03.006

King, N. M. A., Chambers, J., O'Donnell, K., Jayaweera, S. R., Williamson, C., & Glover, V. A. (2010). Anxiety, depression and saliva cortisol in women with a medical disorder during pregnancy. *Archives of Women's Mental Health, 13,* 339–345. https://doi.org/10.1007/s00737-009-0139-5

Mahenge, B., Likindikoki, S., Stockl, H., & Mbwambo, J. (2013). Intimate partner violence during pregnancy and associated mental health symptoms among pregnant women in Tanzania: A cross-sectional study. *BJOG, 120*(8), 940–947. https://doi.org/10.1111/1471-0528.12185

Martini, J., Petzoldt, J., Einsle, F., Beesdo-Baum, K., Höfler, M., & Wittchen, H. U. (2015). Risk factors and course patterns of anxiety and depressive disorders during pregnancy and after delivery: A prospective-longitudinal study. *Journal of Affective Disorders, 175,* 385–395. https://doi.org/10.1016/j.jad.2015.01.012

McCain, G. C., & Deatrick, J. A. (1994). The experience of high-risk pregnancy. *Journal of Obstetric, Gynecologic & Neonatal Nursing, 23*(5), 421–427. https://doi.org/10.1111/j.1552-6909.1994.tb01899.x

McMahon, C. A., Ungerer, J. A., Beaurepaire, J., Tennant, C., & Saunders, D. (1997). Anxiety during pregnancy and fetal attachment after in-vitro fertilization conception. *Human Reproduction, 12*(1), 176–182. https://doi.org/10.1093/humrep/12.1.176

Mudra, S., Göbel, A., Barkmann, C., Goletzke, J., Hecher, K., Schulte-Markwort, M., Diemert, A., & Arck, P. (2020). The longitudinal course of pregnancy-related anxiety in parous and nulliparous women and its association with symptoms of social and generalized anxiety. *Journal of Affective Disorders, 260,* 111–118. https://doi.org/10.1016/j.jad.2019.08.033

Nakić Radoš, S., Košec, V., & Gall, V. (2013). The psychological effects of prenatal diagnostic procedures: Maternal anxiety before and after invasive and noninvasive procedures. *Prenatal Diagnosis, 33*(12), 1194–1200. https://doi.org/10.1002/pd.4223

Nasreen, H. E., Kabir, Z. N., Forsell, Y., & Edhborg, M. (2011). Prevalence and associated factors of depressive and anxiety symptoms during pregnancy: A population based study in rural Bangladesh. *BMC Women's Health, 1*(22), e1–e9. https://doi.org/10.1186/1472-6874-11-22

Purdon, C., & Harrington, J. (2006). Worry in psychopathology. In G. C. L. Davey & A. Wells (Eds.), *Worry and its psychological disorders: Theory, assessment and treatment* (pp. 41–50). Wiley Publishing. https://doi.org/10.1002/9780470713143.ch3

Rychik, J., Donaghue, D. D., Levy, S., Fajardo, C., Combs, J., Zhang, X., Szwast, A., & Diamond, G. S. (2012). Maternal psychological stress after prenatal diagnosis of congenital heart disease. *Journal of Pediatrics, 162*(2), 302–307. https://doi.org/10.1016/j.jpeds.2012.07.023

Schneider, Z. (2002). An Australian study of women's experiences of their first pregnancy. *Midwifery, 18*(3), 238–249. https://doi.org/10.1054/midw.2002.0309

Shapiro, G. D., Seguin, J. R., Muckle, G., Monnier, P., & Fraser, W. D. (2017). Previous pregnancy outcomes and subsequent pregnancy anxiety in a Quebec prospective cohort. *Journal of Psychosomatic Obstetrics & Gynaecology, 38*(2), 121–132. https://doi.org/10.1080/0167482x.2016.1271979

Sjogren, B. (1997). Reasons for anxiety about childbirth in 100 pregnant women. *Journal of Psychosomatic Obstetrics & Gynaecology, 18*(4), 266–272. https://doi.org/10.3109/01674829709080698

Tsartsara, E., & Johnson, M. P. (2006). The impact of miscarriage on women's pregnancy-specific anxiety and feelings of prenatal maternal-fetal attachment during the course of a subsequent pregnancy: An exploratory follow-up study. *Journal of Psychosomatic Obstetrics & Gynaecology, 27*(3), 173–182. https://doi.org/10.1080/01674820600646198

van Bussel, J. C. H., Spitz, B., & Demyttenaere, K. (2009). Anxiety in pregnant and postpartum women: An exploratory study of the role of maternal orientations. *Journal of Affective Disorders, 114*, 232–242. https://doi.org/10.1016/j.jad.2008.07.018

Walker, L. O., & Avant, K. C. (2011). *Strategies for theory construction in nursing* (5th ed.). Prentice Hall. https://www.pearson.com/us/higher-education/program/Walker-Strategies-for-Theory-Construction-in-Nursing-5th-Edition/PGM146725.html

Westerneng, M., Witteveen, A. B., Warmelink, J. C., Spelten, E., Honig, A., & de Cock, P. (2017). Pregnancy-specific anxiety and its association with background characteristics and health-related behaviors in a low-risk population. *Comprehensive Psychiatry, 75*, 6–13. https://doi.org/10.1016/j.comppsych.2017.02.002

5 Pregnancy-related anxiety and birth outcomes

Christine Dunkel Schetter, Melissa Julian, and Carolyn Ponting

Pregnancy-related anxiety and birth outcomes

At least one famous obstetrician devoted his entire career to studying stress in pregnancy and its relation to preterm birth. His early observations and evidence emerging over decades (including his own) indicated that stress might be a factor in earlier delivery (Hobel, 2004; Hobel et al., 2008). As research evolved, anxiety emerged as one of the powerful ingredients contributing to pathways to early birth, perhaps even the key factor explaining stress effects (Dunkel Schetter, 1998). We have yet to determine precisely what forms of stress or anxiety most powerfully predict birth outcomes, but a fast-growing body of evidence indicates that pregnancy-related anxiety has effects independent of sociodemographic and medical risk factors. It is within this broader context that we examine research on pregnancy-related anxiety and birth outcomes.

There is a long history of studying maternal anxiety in relation to pregnancy and birth outcomes dating back to at least the 1960s and 1970s (Davids & DeVault, 1962; Davids et al., 1961; Glazer, 1980; Gorsuch & Key, 1974; Lederman et al., 1978). Early research focused on the elevated risk for obstetrical complications and adverse labor and delivery outcomes among women with high trait or state anxiety. These studies have been reviewed many times over the years (e.g., Istvan, 1986; Reading, 1983) and drew attention in the 1980s to prenatal anxiety as a psychosocial risk factor. Later on, studies focused more on preterm birth (PTB) and low birth weight (LBW), along with the continuous variables on which they are based (i.e., weight at birth in grams and gestational length in weeks).

For present purposes, our focus is primarily on PTB defined as birth at less than 37 weeks, although research on LBW is also reviewed where relevant. LBW refers to infant birth weight of 2,500 grams or less, although consideration of growth percentiles and small for gestational age (SGA) is needed. Rates of PTB are relatively low in most Western and industrialized countries, although the United States is an exception with high rates of PTB, especially among low-income and African American women (March of Dimes, 2019; Martin et al., 2018). The highest rates of PTB worldwide occur in Southern Asia and sub-Saharan Africa (Blencowe et al., 2019; WHO, 2014).

DOI: 10.4324/9781003014003-7

PTB and LBW pose several risks for mothers and infants. Most notably, they are associated with higher risk of infant mortality. Additionally, neonatal complications at birth may require extended time in neonatal intensive care, which influences the amount and quality of time infants and mothers spend together in the weeks after birth. Furthermore, a wide range of infant and developmental effects related to adverse birth outcomes are well documented (Behrman et al., 2007; McCormick et al., 2011).

Prevalence of pregnancy-related anxiety

Perinatal anxiety is common. In fact, it is even more prevalent than perinatal depression, although depressive symptoms in pregnancy have received substantially more attention in the maternal health literature. In 2017, Dennis, Falah-Hassani, and Shiri published a systematic review and meta-analysis of 102 studies on the prevalence of antenatal and postnatal anxiety with data from 221,974 women in 34 countries. They report that elevated anxiety symptoms occurred among about 18.2% of the women in first trimester, 19.1% in second trimester, and 24.6% in third trimester.

In addition, the prevalence of a diagnosis of any anxiety disorder at any time in pregnancy was 15.2% and 4.1% for generalized anxiety disorder. These rates are notable, surpassing global prevalence estimates of 7.3% for anxiety disorders in the general population (Baxter et al., 2013). In addition, rates of self-reported anxiety were higher in studies of women residing in low- to middle-income countries than those in high-income countries. These disparities may be driven by methodological differences among studies, including sampling practices and cultural differences in symptom reporting; yet structural determinants of health such as food insecurity or gender bias are also likely contributors to the higher prevalence.

General prenatal anxiety and birth outcomes

One systematic review and meta-analysis that included 15 prospective cohort studies of a total of 22,252 pregnant women reported evidence on associations between maternal anxiety and birth outcomes (Ding et al., 2014). The authors found that maternal anxiety during pregnancy was associated with significant increased risk of PTB (pooled risk ratio = 1.50) and LBW (pooled risk ratio = 1.76). A later systematic review and meta-analysis (Grigoriadis et al., 2018) examined 29 published empirical articles on maternal prenatal anxiety and adverse perinatal outcomes. Relevant studies on prenatal anxiety were included only if the researchers used validated self-report measures that were over a cutoff score for high anxiety such as the Spielberger State Anxiety Inventory (Spielberger, 1989) or clinical diagnoses. They concluded that prenatal anxiety was associated with increased odds for PTB (pooled odds ratio [OR] = 1.54), spontaneous PTB (OR = 1.41), and low birth weight (OR = 1.80), as well as an infant born small for gestational age (SGA, OR = 1.48). Thus, evidence from these two reviews regarding prenatal anxiety indicates effects on both PTB and LBW where high prenatal anxiety elevated risks of these adverse outcomes by 1.4 to 1.8 times; however, both reviews pertain to studies on general anxiety broadly defined, not on anxiety about pregnancy.

Pregnancy-related anxiety

At some point in the study of perinatal anxiety, attention turned to anxiety about the current pregnancy specifically. Qualitative research and measurement development centered on anxiety about the baby being healthy, labor and delivery, the mother's health and possible risks to her, and motherhood (Beaton & Gupton, 1990; Lederman et al., 1985; Pleschette et al., 1956; Rini et al., 1999). Measurement development was extensive across many settings and countries. In fact, there are now five published reviews exclusively on the measurement of pregnancy anxiety (Alderdice et al., 2012; Brunton et al., 2015; Evans et al., 2015; Nast et al., 2013; Sinesi et al., 2019). By best estimate, there are no fewer than 18 measures of prenatal anxiety. We note that many of these are standardized and have at least some validity and reliability data, although others do not. Thus, there appears to be widespread and international agreement that pregnancy-related anxiety is a concept of importance to assess and there are many options for doing so.

With ample availability of measures, many authors have published empirical studies over the past two decades on pregnancy-related anxiety or worries and birth outcomes. Studies indicate that when anxiety is centered on pregnancy – which means concurrently measured and focused on issues evoked by pregnancy – it poses risk of earlier delivery and related adverse outcomes (e.g., McCool et al., 1994; Perkin et al., 1993; Rini et al., 1999; Wadhwa et al., 1993). With time, further studies have been published replicating these findings with more rigorous measures and procedures and larger samples (e.g., Dole et al., 2003; Kramer et al., 2009). As a result, the conclusion emerged that mothers with high pregnancy-related anxiety are at risk of PTB independent of medical risk factors and other confounds (Dunkel-Schetter & Glynn, 2011; Dunkel Schetter, 2011). In addition, the offspring of mothers with prenatal anxiety are at higher risk for motor, psychological, and neurodevelopmental adversities from infancy to adulthood due in part to fetal programming (Rogers et al., 2020; van den Bergh, 1990; van den Bergh & Marcoen, 2004). Please refer to Chapter 2 (Pregnancy-related anxiety as distinct from state/trait anxiety and depression) and Chapter 6 (Examining the relation between maternal pregnancy-related anxiety and child development) for more detailed discussions on fetal programming. With these findings accumulating, reviews and meta-analyses on the evidence linking pregnancy-specific anxiety with birth outcomes have appeared in the literature, and to these we turn for the latest conclusions.

Reviews on pregnancy anxiety and birth outcomes

In 2015, Staneva et al. published a systematic review of 39 studies on PTB and maternal depression, anxiety, and stress. They reported that general anxiety symptoms predicted PTB in three-quarters of the studies, and that five studies showed links between pregnancy-specific anxiety and PTB. They concluded that "pregnancy-specific anxiety is also a powerfully predictive concept when exploring psychosocial determinants of preterm birth" (p. 192).

Littleton et al. (2007) conducted one of the first meta-analyses relevant to pregnancy-related anxiety. Their analysis included 50 studies on anxiety symptoms in pregnancy and perinatal outcomes. The authors concluded that the association of gestational age at birth with pregnancy-related anxiety was significant with an overall small effect size. Moreover, there was no evidence of a relationship between *general* anxiety symptoms and prenatal outcomes, although general symptoms of anxiety were associated with the use of analgesics in labor and 5-minute Apgar scores. Both were small effect sizes.

Bussières et al. (2015) conducted the largest meta-analysis of 88 prospective studies and 5,889,930 women to examine prenatal factors and birth outcomes. They found that pregnancy-related stress and anxiety had greater effect sizes for gestational age at birth and birth weight than did trait-based anxiety assessments, life events, or exposure to disasters. For pregnancy stress and anxiety together, the effect sizes were similar for birth weight and gestational age ($d = -0.25$ for an aggregated outcome of both). The next largest effect was exposure to natural disasters with an effect size of $d = -0.11$. Furthermore, studies that enrolled high-risk women due to psychological or medical predispositions and women living outside of Europe or North America showed larger associations, which suggests that pregnancy-related anxiety may be more or less salient depending on a woman's context.

In summary, prior reviews differ vastly in what concepts and measures they include (general or pregnancy-related anxiety), their criteria for study inclusion, the birth outcomes of interest, the specific studies reviewed, and in other ways. However, their conclusions are somewhat consistent. All the reviews conclude that pregnancy-related anxiety predicts birth outcomes. Most estimate the effect size for length of gestation or PTB as small but statistically significant. Many also find effects on birth weight, although studies on this outcome do not typically examine growth trajectories or SGA, which is necessary to clarify the findings.

Furthermore, these studies and reviews of the literature typically do not take into account whether length of gestation is controlled for in the prediction of birth weight, or whether birth weight is controlled for in predicting length of gestation. Thus, birth weight effects remain largely confounded by length of gestation, and vice versa. This requires attention in future research. Additional issues needing clarification in this literature include whether effects of pregnancy-related anxiety are for spontaneous preterm labor and delivery or all categories of PTBs. Rarely do investigators control for spontaneous onset of labor, nor do reviews consider this in their commentaries. Similarly, control for medical risk is uneven. Women with identified risk conditions may have higher rates of adverse birth outcomes due to greater anxiety, as a result of their medical risk conditions, or a combination of these factors.

A key study by Kramer et al. in 2009 addresses these issues in a large Canadian sample and found that of many psychological distress variables tested (e.g., perceived stress, depression), pregnancy-related anxiety assessed with the four-item pregnancy-specific anxiety scale (Guardino & Dunkel Schetter, 2014; Roesch et al., 2004) was the only one that predicted spontaneous PTB after controlling for medical and obstetric risk, chronic stressors (i.e., socioeconomic hardship), and perceptions of pregnancy risk. This study is a model for research on the topic in its sample size, covariates, and comparative tests of many psychosocial predictors.

Recent studies on pregnancy anxiety and birth outcomes

Next, we turn attention to four methodologically rigorous studies on pregnancy anxiety, published since the most recent reviews. Other studies that have examined general anxiety (rather than pregnancy-related anxiety) are not included (e.g., Khalesi & Bokaie, 2018; Liou et al., 2016; Pesonen et al., 2016). In a well-controlled longitudinal study, Blackmore et al. (2016) examined the association between pregnancy-related anxiety and birth outcomes in 345 diverse low-income women in an urban clinic with oversampling for elevated levels of anxiety and depression. Pregnancy-related anxiety was measured in second and third trimesters using an adapted version of the Pregnancy-related Anxiety Questionnaire (PRAQ; van den Bergh, 1990; later revised as the PRAQ-R and PRAQ-R2 by Huizink et al., 2004, 2016). Pregnancy-related anxiety in both the second and third trimesters was associated with lower gestational age at birth after controlling for maternal education, race/ethnicity, pre-pregnancy BMI, smoking, and Medicaid recipient status. The authors also found that specific components of pregnancy-related anxiety, namely, concerns about the self and the child, were associated with lower birth weight at both trimesters after controlling for mode of birth, obstetric complications, and PTB. Notably, although a diagnosis of generalized anxiety was associated cross-sectionally with pregnancy-related anxiety (both worries about self and child), generalized anxiety did not predict gestational age at birth. However, medical risk factors were not controlled in this study.

In a study of 246 female active duty military members in the United States and wives of military members, Weis et al. (2020) found that increases in pregnancy-related anxiety over the three trimesters were associated with higher risk of PTB and LBW. This study used the Prenatal Self-Evaluation Questionnaire – Short Form (PSEQ-SF, Lederman et al., 1985), which measures seven dimensions of pregnancy-related anxiety. The authors found that pregnancy-related anxiety regarding acceptance of the pregnancy, preparation for labor, fear of pain, and loss of control in labor increased the risk of PTB. On the other hand, pregnancy-related anxiety regarding concerns for well-being of the self and baby in labor increased the risk of LBW after controlling for PTB. This study highlights the value of examining subtypes of pregnancy-related worries and their changes over time in relation to birth outcomes. However, the authors do not report rates of PTB or LBW in the sample.

Ramos et al. (2019) also examined pregnancy-related anxiety at multiple time points over the course of pregnancy in a sample of 337 women who were identified as Latina or non-Latina White utilizing the pregnancy-related anxiety scale in English and Spanish (Guardino & Dunkel Schetter, 2014; Rini et al., 1999) to predict gestational age at delivery. Pregnancy-related anxiety in the second and third trimesters predicted gestational length controlling for medical risk factors, level of education, household income, age, and parity. Effects were stronger for Latinas than non-Latina Whites. These findings replicate prior work and extend it by demonstrating the value of examining ethnic and cultural factors that may contribute to pregnancy-related anxiety and associations with risk for adverse birth outcomes across groups.

Finally, in a large study, Cole-Lewis et al. (2014) examined the effect of changes in pregnancy-specific stress over pregnancy on PTB and gestational length in 920 Black and Latina adolescent and young adult women in the United States. They found that increases in pregnancy-specific stress (Lobel et al., 2008) from the second to third trimester were associated with an increased likelihood of preterm delivery and shortened gestational age. While this is a well-controlled longitudinal study, the measure used does not purport to assess anxiety per se, though some of the items refer to "worries" about pregnancy. This study illustrates the need to study changes in pregnancy stress and anxiety over the course of pregnancy as the results of these studies can help us understand how the trajectory of anxiety across trimesters influence birth outcomes.

In sum, the few studies published since the last meta-analyses vary in sample size (246–920 participants), in the pregnancy-related anxiety measures used (none used a common measure), birth outcome measures, rigor of statistical methods, and sample type (e.g., low-income clinic, military population). Yet these studies all found effects of pregnancy-related anxiety on gestational length at birth, risk of PTB, or LBW. Two of these studies examined changes in pregnancy-related anxiety over the three trimesters, while the others were at single time points in pregnancy. Two of these recent studies also examined the effects of different subcomponents of pregnancy-related anxiety on birth outcomes. Differentiation between subcomponents of this distinct anxiety can contribute to the identification of more specific treatment targets. Although these more recent studies provide additional evidence for the effect of pregnancy-related anxiety on birth outcomes and add to the existing body of empirical research, additional research is still needed. We end by discussing avenues for future inquiry.

Conclusions and future research issues

At this juncture, we clearly have sufficient evidence to conclude that pregnancy-related anxiety increases the risk of adverse birth outcomes. In our view, stronger evidence exists for the effects on length of gestation and PTB, but there is also evidence for LBW, though it needs further study to clarify if there are effects on growth per se, and the mechanisms involved. The effect sizes are of clinical significance when compared to other known risk factors. Nonetheless, many issues confront researchers who embark on the next set of studies to better understand the intergenerational impacts of pregnancy-related anxiety at birth.

First, all researchers must seek methodological rigor of the highest standards. This means large samples, longitudinal designs, and valid and reliable measures that effectively capture the construct of pregnancy-related anxiety. The rationale for large samples is to have the power to detect effects that may be absent in smaller samples. Studies of PTB and other dichotomous birth outcomes need to enroll hundreds or thousands of women to have sufficient power to test effects on adverse outcomes, even in high-risk samples. To this end, power calculations should be done during study planning. Rates of clinically defined adverse outcomes (PTB, LBW, SGA) in the sample must also be reported in publications to allow researchers to interpret and evaluate the study. These descriptive data do not always appear in published articles. Alternatively, researchers can study outcomes continuously (e.g., length of gestation), but at least 200 participants, ideally more, are still needed. It is also important to consider who to target for recruitment. Women with medical and demographic risk factors are valuable to sample because they have higher likelihood of adverse birth outcomes. Although they may be more difficult to recruit and enroll, it is worth the effort in scientific value. One solution is to sample at more than one site. Collaboration with investigators at multiple sites using standard protocols can enable acquisition of a large sample in a reasonable period of time. Low-risk pregnant women are not as likely to have adverse birth outcomes and, therefore, should not be studied exclusively; however, mixed high and low risk samples may be valuable if large enough variability in risk is present.

Prospective studies are the only study design worthwhile at this point in time. Studies in which measures of pregnancy-related anxiety pertain to the current pregnancy and are not retrospective are essential. In addition, longitudinal studies in which researchers can obtain measures at more than one time point during pregnancy are ideal and necessary. Measures in early, mid, and late pregnancy are recommended, and follow-up of mothers and offspring is valuable to provide data on postpartum health and intergenerational effects of pregnancy-related anxiety.

The choice of pregnancy-related anxiety measures is a critical matter for future studies. First and foremost, as in all research designs, the measure selected by researchers should suit the purposes of the study. Some measures focus exclusively on fear of childbirth, whereas others are broader. Among those that are broad in capturing pregnancy concerns, they may or may not yield subscores of components for research purposes. If a study is exploratory, then it may make sense to design a measure. However, if the goal is to test effects on birth outcomes, a valid and reliable published measure is the optimal choice.

The plethora of measures of pregnancy-related anxiety is a hindrance. Greater agreement in the future on a smaller set of measures is recommended. Available measures have not all been thoroughly tested psychometrically with respect to whether they capture anxiety, depression, and stress, and how clear it is that they are specific to pregnancy. A measure should have some convergent validity as well as reliability evidence and strong predictive validity. The most critical issue for present purposes is that measures have clinically meaningful effect sizes when predicting risk of PTB and/or LBW. Without narrowing our measures to those best suited for detecting risk of these clinically significant outcomes, progress on identifying interventions targets is impeded.

Attention by researchers should also be paid to whether a measure is culturally appropriate, of acceptable length, can be administrated optimally, and has valid translations. Given the international nature of this area of research, more attention to translation and reliability and validity of measures in different languages is needed. Anxiety symptoms are universal, but their acceptance and expression are shaped by life contexts and cultural conceptions of distress (Chavira et al., 2020). For example, outside of Europe and North America and among cultures where stigma of mental illness is high, individuals often report somatic complaints instead of emotional distress, a more culturally acceptable manifestation of worry (Ryder et al., 2002). Because many of our diagnostic tools emphasize psychological symptoms and not physical ones (Marques et al., 2011), it is likely that anxiety is underdetected in non-Western cultures. Further, cultural understandings of distress and causal explanations of anxiety – as resulting from biological, supernatural, or social sources – influence how acceptable individuals consider their worries to be, and their likelihood of disclosure (Chavira et al., 2020). Thus, researchers should have an understanding of traditional knowledge and conceptualizations of distress in the communities where they study maternal anxiety.

Researchers must also conduct rigorous statistical analyses. The prediction of length of gestation should include control of birth weight in the statistical model so as to untangle these confounded outcomes. Birth weight as an outcome can be studied with or without length of gestation in the model, but understanding the factors precipitating early birth requires consideration of the possibility that a baby may be born early for many reasons. An infant may be lower birth weight only as a function of time of delivery, not necessarily due to intrauterine growth abnormalities. Some experts believe it is preferable to study growth curves rather than LBW.

Other necessary covariates in prediction of birth outcomes with pregnancy-related anxiety are medical risk factors. If results do not control for maternal medical risk factors such as preeclampsia, it is impossible to know whether medical risk conditions, which contribute to both maternal anxiety and earlier birth, can account for the findings. Both a mother's pregnancy-related anxiety and her medical risk may be independent contributors to adverse birth outcomes, and by different pathways, and we have yet to examine this complexity. Fortunately, many studies have controlled medical risk and report independent effects of pregnancy-related anxiety on birth outcomes (e.g., Lobel et al., 1992, 2008; Rini et al., 1999).

Another issue for data analyses is to control for spontaneous versus medically induced labor and delivery. Anxiety has been linked to earlier birth, but this could mean that anxious women go into labor earlier, or that they are more likely to be induced due to medical risk factors, or both. Clearly, these are very different processes. One large study on women with spontaneous preterm labor and delivery exclusively indicated that pregnancy-related anxiety increased the risk of spontaneous PTB (e.g., Kramer et al., 2009). Other studies have controlled this variable. Future studies must attend to all of these issues to add to existing knowledge.

The nature of future research on pregnancy-related anxiety and birth outcomes will differ in research design, depending on whether the aim is to screen for risk and predict outcomes or to examine pathways or mechanisms. Conceivably, studies can do both, but that is ambitious. Mechanistic studies to date have been concerned mainly with neuroendocrine and immune pathways, both requiring extensive biomarker measurements, ideally collected over time, and on sufficient sample sizes. Studies on behavioral mechanisms are rare, as noted in Dunkel Schetter and Lobel (2011), but there are a few. Despite the difficulty of conducting mechanistic studies, they are critical to help illuminate pathways and potential markers to target in prevention.

Finally, a clinical goal of this work is to design interventions that may reduce early delivery by reducing anxiety in pregnancy. This will most certainly require that we agree on exactly what the concept of pregnancy-related anxiety is (see Chapter 1), develop best practices for what measures to use with what populations and procedures, and design effective interventions. The best guides for doing this are theoretical frameworks that take into account the women at greatest risk (see Chapter 1), their receptivity to interventions of evidence-based foundations, and the ability to deliver them effectively and broadly. The latest methods of clinical research must be utilized with strong methodologists and statisticians on the team in order to test mechanisms and design effective interventions that can inform the next stage of work. Collaboration among nurses, social workers, psychologists, public health experts, physicians, midwives, and communities will be necessary. The challenges are clear, as is the promise in this area of investigation.

References

Alderdice, F., Lynn, F., & Lobel, M. (2012). A review and psychometric evaluation of pregnancy-specific stress measures. *Journal of Psychosomatic Obstetrics & Gynecology*, *33*(2), 62–77. https://doi.org/10.3109/0167482X.2012.673040

Baxter, A. J., Scott, K. M., Vos, T., & Whiteford, H. A. (2013). Global prevalence of anxiety disorders: A systematic review and meta-regression. *Psychological Medicine*, *43*(5), 897. https://doi.org/10.1017/S003329171200147X

Beaton, J., & Gupton, A. (1990). Childbirth expectations: A qualitative analysis. *Midwifery*, *6*(3), 133–139. https://doi.org/10.1016/s0266-6138(05)80170-6

Behrman, R. E., Butler, A. S., & Institute of Medicine (US) Committee on Understanding Premature Birth and Assuring Healthy Outcomes (Eds.). (2007). *Preterm birth: Causes, consequences, and prevention* (pp. 87–123). National Academy Press.

Blackmore, E. R., Gustafsson, H., Gilchrist, M., Wyman, C., & O'Connor, T. G. (2016). Pregnancy-related anxiety: Evidence of distinct clinical significance from a prospective longitudinal study. *Journal of Affective Disorders*, *197*, 251–258. https://doi.org/10.1016/j.jad.2016.03.008

Blencowe, H., Krasevac, J., de Onis, M., Black, R. E., An, X., Stevens, G. A., Borghi, E., Hayashi, C., Estevez, D., Cevolon, L., Shiekh, S., Hardy, V. P., Lawn, J. E., & Cousens, S. (2019). National, regional, and worldwide estimates of low birthweight in 2015, with trends from 2000: A systematic analysis. *The Lancet Global Health,* *7*(7), e849–e860. https://doi.org/10.1016/S2214-109X(18)30565-5

Brunton, R. J., Dryer, R., Saliba, A., & Kohlhoff, J. (2015). Pregnancy anxiety: A systematic review of current scales. *Journal of Affective Disorders, 176,* 24–34. https://doi.org/10.1016/J.JAD.2015.01.039

Bussières, E. L., Tarabulsy, G. M., Pearson, J., Tessier, R., Forest, J. C., & Giguère, Y. (2015). Maternal prenatal stress and infant birth weight and gestational age: A meta-analysis of prospective studies. *Developmental Review, 36,* 179–199. https://doi.org/10.1016/j.dr.2015.04.001

Chavira, D. A., Ponting, C., & Lewis-Fernández, R. (2020). Cultural and social aspects of anxiety disorders. In N. Simon, E. Hollander, D. J. Stein, & B. O. Rothbaum (Eds.), *The American Psychiatric Association Publishing textbook of anxiety, trauma, and OCD-related disorders* (p. 59). American Psychiatric Publishing.

Cole-Lewis, H. J., Kershaw, T. S., Earnshaw, V. A., Yonkers, K. A., Lin, H., & Ickovics, J. R. (2014). Pregnancy-specific stress, preterm birth, and gestational age among high-risk young women. *Health Psychology, 33*(9), 1033–1045. https://doi.org/10.1037/a0034586

Davids, A., & DeVault, S. (1962). Maternal anxiety during pregnancy and childbirth abnormalities. *Psychosomatic Medicine, 24*(5), 464–470. https://doi.org/10.1097/00006842-196209000-00004

Davids, A., DeVault, S., & Talmadge, M. (1961). Anxiety, pregnancy, and childbirth abnormalities. *Journal of Consulting Psychology, 25*(1), 74–77. https://doi.org/10.1037/h0043550

Dennis, C. L., Falah-Hassani, K., & Shiri, R. (2017). Prevalence of antenatal and postnatal anxiety: Systematic review and meta-analysis. *British Journal of Psychiatry, 210*(5), 315–323. https://doi.org/10.1192/bjp.bp.116.187179

Ding, X. X., Wu, Y. L., Xu, S. J., Zhu, R. P., Jia, X. M., Zhang, S. F., Huang, K., Zhu, P., Hao, J., & Tao, F. B. (2014). Maternal anxiety during pregnancy and adverse birth outcomes: A systematic review and meta-analysis of prospective cohort studies. *Journal of Affective Disorders, 159,* 103–110. https://doi.org/10.1016/j.jad.2014.02.027

Dole, N., Savitz, D. A., Hertz-Picciotto, I., Siega-Riz, A. M., McMahon, M. J., & Buekens, P. (2003). Maternal stress and preterm birth. *American Journal of Epidemiology, 157*(1), 14–24. https://doi.org/ 10.1093/aje/kwf176

Dunkel Schetter, C. (1998). Maternal stress and preterm delivery. *Prenatal Neonatal Medicine, 3,* 39–42.

Dunkel Schetter, C. (2011). Psychological science on pregnancy: Stress processes, biopsychosocial models, and emerging research issues. *Annual Review of Psychology, 62*(1), 531–558. https://doi.org/10.1146/annurev.psych.031809.130727

Dunkel-Schetter, C., & Glynn, L. (2011). Stress in pregnancy: Empirical evidence and the theoretical issues to guide interdisciplinary research. In R. J. Contrada & A. Baum (Eds.), *The handbook of stress science* (pp. 321–347). Springer Publishing Company.

Dunkel Schetter, C., & Lobel, M. (2011). Pregnancy and birth: A multi-level analysis of stress and birthweight. In T. Revenson, A. Baum, & J. Singer (Eds.), *Handbook of health psychology* (2nd ed., pp. 427–453). Psychology Press.

Evans, K., Spiby, H., & Morrell, C. J. (2015). A psychometric systematic review of self-report instruments to identify anxiety in pregnancy. *Journal of Advanced Nursing, 71*(9), 1986–2001. https://doi.org/10.1111/jan.12649

Glazer, G. (1980). Anxiety levels and concerns among pregnant women. *Research in Nursing & Health, 3*(3), 107–113. https://doi.org/10.1002/nur.4770030305

Gorsuch, R. L., & Key, M. K. (1974). Abnormalities of pregnancy as a function of anxiety and life stress. *Psychosomatic Medicine, 36*(4), 352–362. https://doi.org/10.1097/00006842-197407000-00009

Grigoriadis, S., Graves, L., Peer, M., Mamisashvili, L., Tomlinson, G., Vigod, S. N., Dennis, C., Steiner, M., Brown, C., Cheung, A., Dawson, H., Rector, N. A., Guenette, M., & Richter, M. (2018). Maternal anxiety during pregnancy and the association with adverse perinatal outcomes. *The Journal of Clinical Psychiatry, 79*(5), 17r12011. https://doi.org/10.4088/JCP.17r12011

Guardino, C. M., & Dunkel Schetter, C. (2014). Understanding pregnancy anxiety: Concepts, correlates, and consequences. *Zero to Three, 34*(4), 12–21.

Hobel, C. J. (2004). Stress and preterm birth. *Clinical Obstetrics and Gynecology, 47*(4), 856–880. https://doi.org/10.1097/01.grf.0000142512.38733.8c

Hobel, C. J., Goldstein, A., & Barrett, E. S. (2008). Psychosocial stress and pregnancy outcome. *Clinical Obstetrics and Gynecology, 51*(2), 333–348. https://doi.org/10.1097/GRF.0b013e31816f270

Huizink, A. C., Delforterie, M. J., Scheinin, N. M., Tolvanen, M., Karlsson, L., & Karlsson, H. (2016). Adaption of pregnancy anxiety questionnaire-revised for all pregnant women regardless of parity: PRAQ-R2. *Archives of Women's Mental Health, 19*(1), 125–132. https://doi.org/10.1007/s00737-015-0531-2

Huizink, A. C., Mulder, E. J., Robles de Medina, P. G., Visser, G. H., & Buitelaar, J. K. (2004). Is pregnancy anxiety a distinctive syndrome? *Early Human Development, 79*(2), 81–91. https://doi.org/10.1016/j.earlhumdev.2004.04.014

Istvan, J. (1986). Stress, anxiety, and birth outcomes. A critical review of the evidence. *Psychological Bulletin, 100*(3), 331–348. https://doi.org/10.1037/0033-2909.100.3.331

Khalesi, Z. B., & Bokaie, M. (2018). The association between pregnancy-specific anxiety and preterm birth: A cohort study. *African Health Sciences, 18*(3), 569–575. https://doi.org/10.4314/ahs.v18i3.14

Kramer, M. S., Lydon, J., Séguin, L., Goulet, L., Kahn, S. R., McNamara, H., Genest, J., Dassa, C., Chen, M. F., Sharma, S., Meaney, M. J., Thomson, S., Uum, S. V., Koren, G., Dahhou, M., Lamoureux, J., & Platt, R. W. (2009). Stress pathways to spontaneous preterm birth: The role of stressors, psychological distress, and stress hormones. *American Journal of Epidemiology, 169*(11), 1319–1326. https://doi.org/10.1093/aje/kwp061

Lederman, R. P., Lederman, E., Work, B., & McCann, D. S. (1985). Anxiety and epinephrine in multiparous women in labor: Relationship to duration of labor and fetal heart rate pattern. *American Journal of Obstetrics and Gynecology, 153*(8), 870–877. https://doi.org/10.1016/0002-9378(85)90692-1

Lederman, R. P., Lederman, E., Work, B. A., Jr., & McCann, D. S. (1978). The relationship of maternal anxiety, plasma catecholamines, and plasma cortisol to progress in labor. *American Journal of Obstetrics and Gynecology, 132*(5), 495–500. https://doi.org/10.1016/0002-9378(78)90742-1

Liou, S. R., Wang, P., & Cheng, C. Y. (2016). Effects of prenatal maternal mental distress on birth outcomes. *Women and Birth: Journal of the Australian College of Midwives, 29*(4), 376–380. https://doi.org/10.1016/j.wombi.2016.03.004

Littleton, H. L., Breitkopf, C. R., & Berenson, A. B. (2007). Correlates of anxiety symptoms during pregnancy and association with perinatal outcomes: A meta-analysis.

American Journal of Obstetrics and Gynecology, 196(5), 424–432. https://doi.org/10.1016/j.ajog.2007.03.042

Lobel, M., Cannella, L., Graham, J. E., DeVinvent, C., Schneider, J., & Meyer, B. A. (2008). Pregnancy-specific stress, prenatal health behaviors, and birth outcomes. *Health Psychology, 27*(5), 604–615. https://doi.org/10.1037/a0013242

Lobel, M., Dunkel-Schetter, C., & Scrimshaw, S. C. (1992). Prenatal maternal stress and prematurity: A prospective study of socioeconomically disadvantaged women. *Health Psychology, 11*(1), 32–40. https://doi.org/10.1037/0278-6133.11.1.32

March of Dimes. (2019). *Report card*. www.marchofdimes.org/materials/US_REPORTCARD_FINAL.pdf

Marques, L., Robinaugh, D. J., LeBlanc, N. J., & Hinton, D. (2011). Cross-cultural variations in the prevalence and presentation of anxiety disorders. *Expert Review of Neurotherapeutics, 11*(2), 313–322. https://doi.org/10.1586/ern.10.122

Martin, J. A., Hamilton, B. E., Osterman, M. J. K., & Driscoll, A. K. (2019). Births: Final data for 2018. *National Vital Statistics Reports, 68*(13). www.cdc.gov/nchs/products/index.htm

McCool, W. F., Dorn, L. D., & Susman, E. J. (1994). The relation of cortisol reactivity and anxiety to perinatal outcome in primiparous adolescents. *Research in Nursing & Health, 17*(6), 411–420. https://doi.org/10.1002/nur.4770170604

McCormick, M. C., Litt, J. S., Smith, V. C., & Zupancic, J. A. (2011). Prematurity: An overview and public health implications. *Annual Review of Public Health, 32*, 367–379. https://doi.org/10.1146/annurev-publhealth-090810-182459

Nast, I., Bolten, M., Meinlschmidt, G., & Hellhammer, D. H. (2013). How to measure prenatal stress? A systematic review of psychometric instruments to assess psychosocial stress during pregnancy. *Paediatric and Perinatal Epidemiology, 27*(4), 313–322. https://doi.org/10.1111/ppe.12051

Perkin, M. R., Bland, J. M., Peacock, J. L., & Anderson, H. R. (1993). The effect of anxiety and depression during pregnancy on obstetric complications. *BJOG: An International Journal of Obstetrics and Gynaecology, 100*(7), 629–634. https://doi.org/10.1111/j.1471-0528.1993.tb14228.x

Pesonen, A. K., Lahti, M., Kuusinen, T., Tuovinen, S., Villa, P., Hämäläinen, E., . . . Räikkönen, K. (2016). Maternal prenatal positive affect, depressive and anxiety symptoms and birth outcomes: The PREDO study. *PLoS One, 11*(2), e0150058. https://doi.org/10.1371/journal.pone.0150058

Pleshette, N., Asch, S. S., & Chase, J. (1956). A study of anxieties during pregnancy, labor, the early and late puerperium. *Bulletin of the New York Academy of Medicine, 32*(6), 436–455.

Ramos, I. F., Guardino, C. M., Mansolf, M., Glynn, L. M., Sandman, C. A., Hobel, C. J., & Dunkel Schetter, C. (2019). Pregnancy anxiety predicts shorter gestation in Latina and non-Latina white women: The role of placental corticotrophin-releasing hormone. *Psychoneuroendocrinology, 99*, 166–173. https://doi.org/10.1016/j.psyneuen.2018.09.008

Reading, A. E. (1983). The influence of maternal anxiety on the course and outcome of pregnancy: A review. *Health Psychology, 2*(2), 187–202. https://doi.org/10.1037/0278-6133.2.2.187

Rini, C. K., Dunkel-Schetter, C., Wadhwa, P. D., & Sandman, C. A. (1999). Psychological adaptation and birth outcomes: The role of personal resources, stress, and sociocultural context in pregnancy. *Health Psychology, 18*(4), 333–345. https://doi.org/10.1037/0278-6133.18.4.333

Roesch, S. C., Dunkel-Schetter, C., Woo, G., & Hobel, C. J. (2004). Modeling the types and timing of stress in pregnancy. *Anxiety, Stress, and Coping, 17*(1), 87–102. https://doi.org/10.1080/1061580031000123667

Rogers, A., Obst, S., Teague, S. J., Rossen, L., Spry, E. A., MacDonald, J. A., Sunderland, M., Olsson, C. A., Youssef, G., & Hutchinson, D. (2020). Association between maternal perinatal depression and anxiety and child and adolescent development: A meta-analysis. *JAMA Pediatrics.* https://doi.org/10.1001/jamapediatrics.2020.2910

Ryder, A. G., Yang, J., & Heine, S. J. (2002). Somatization vs. psychologization of emotional distress: A paradigmatic example for cultural psychopathology. *Online Readings in Psychology and Culture, 10*(2). https://doi.org/10.9707/2307-0919.1080

Sinesi, A., Maxwell, M., O'Carroll, R., & Cheyne, H. (2019). Anxiety scales used in pregnancy: Systematic review. *BJPsych Open, 5*(1), e5. https://doi.org/10.1192/bjo.2018.75

Spielberger, C. D. (1989). *State-trait anxiety inventory: Bibliography* (2nd ed.). Consulting Psychologists Press.

Staneva, A., Bogossian, F., Pritchard, M., & Wittkowski, A. (2015). The effects of maternal depression, anxiety, and perceived stress during pregnancy on preterm birth: A systematic review. *Women and Birth, 28*(3), 179–193. https://doi.org/10.1016/j.wombi.2015.02.003

Van den Bergh, B. R. (1990). The influence of maternal emotions during pregnancy on fetal and neonatal behavior. *Journal of Prenatal & Perinatal Psychology & Health, 5*(2), 119–130.

Van Den Bergh, B. R. H., & Marcoen, A. (2004). High antenatal maternal anxiety is related to ADHD symptoms, externalizing problems, and anxiety in 8- and 9-year-olds. *Child Development, 75*(4), 1085–1097. https://doi.org/10.1111/j.1467-8624.2004.00727.x

Wadhwa, P. D., Sandman, C. A., Porto, M., Dunkel-Schetter, C., & Garite, T. J. (1993). The association between prenatal stress and infant birth weight and gestational age at birth: A prospective investigation. *American Journal of Obstetrics and Gynecology, 169*(4), 858–865. https://doi.org/10.1016/0002-9378(93)90016-C

Weis, K. L., Walker, K. C., Chan, W., Yuan, T. T., & Lederman, R. P. (2020). Risk of preterm birth and newborn low birthweight in military women with increased pregnancy-specific anxiety. *Military Medicine, 185*(5–6), E678–E685. https://doi.org/10.1093/milmed/usz399

World Health Organization (WHO). (2014). *Global nutrition targets 2025: Low birth weight policy brief.* World Health Organization.

6 Examining the relation between maternal pregnancy-related anxiety and child development

Sarah E. Garcia, Sarah E. D. Perzow,
Ella-Marie P. Hennessey, Laura M. Glynn,
and Elysia Poggi Davis

Examining the relation between maternal pregnancy-related anxiety and child development

Maternal psychopathology is a well-established contributor to offspring develop-ment and psychopathology (for reviews, see Goodman & Gotlib, 1999; Good-man et al., 2011; Madigan et al., 2018). This contribution to risk is thought to occur through multiple pathways, including genetics (shared genes as well as gene-environment interactions), parenting, and exposure to maternal mental health problems during critical stages of infant and child socio-emotional devel-opment (Goodman & Gotlib, 1999). The impact of maternal psychopathology and psychological distress during the prenatal period on fetal development has been explored as an additional pathway through which transmission of risk may occur (for reviews see Davis et al., 2018; Korja et al., 2017; Van den Bergh et al., 2017). Indeed, the fetal programming hypothesis or developmental origins of health and disease hypothesis posit that the prenatal period is a window of sensi-tivity during which the intrauterine environment profoundly impacts the devel-opment of fetal systems with lasting impacts on offspring functioning, including psychological health.

Fetal brain development occurs at a rapid rate compared to other stages of life. For example, 200 billion neurons are generated by the end of the second trimester (Bourgeois, 2001). This accelerated pace of development renders the fetus more susceptible to environmental influences, including maternal psychological and biological stress signals. Through this sensitive period of development, mater-nal prenatal depression and general anxiety can impact offspring neurodevelop-ment, temperament, stress reactivity, and cognitive function (Davis et al., 2018; Entringer et al., 2015). Among indicators of maternal psychological distress, pregnancy-related anxiety is emerging as a particularly potent predictor, with studies showing it is more strongly associated with infant and child developmen-tal outcomes as compared to other aspects of maternal distress (Blair et al., 2011; Lobel et al., 2008). Although beyond the scope of this chapter, it is important to note that pregnancy-related anxiety may impact fetal development through

DOI: 10.4324/9781003014003-8

a variety of mechanisms, including the hypothalamic-pituitary-adrenocortical (HPA) axis (Kane et al., 2014; Peterson et al., 2020), epigenetic (Nugent & Bale, 2015), vascular, and inflammatory pathways (Bolton & Bilbo, 2014).

In this chapter, we summarize evidence of links between pregnancy-related anxiety and infant and child socio-emotional, cognitive, motor, and brain development, and HPA axis regulation. We include details of sample demographics and factors considered in analyses, such as pre- and postnatal psychological symptoms and birth phenotype, in Table 6.1. Cultural considerations such as race, ethnicity, and acculturation are related to social support and interactions with the medical profession (e.g., McLemore et al., 2018), and may be implicated in pregnancy-related anxiety and its link to child development (Mahrer et al., 2020). Therefore, we highlight studies that use diverse samples in the text and in Table 6.1. When studies have included measures of postnatal distress, we provide summary comments regarding whether associations between pregnancy-related anxiety and infant and child outcomes persist after accounting for postnatal distress. Next, we consider the strength of evidence for the unique associations between pregnancy-related anxiety and offspring outcomes compared to associations with other types of prenatal maternal psychological distress. We also consider factors that may modify associations between pregnancy-related anxiety and infant and child outcomes, such as timing of fetal exposure and child sex. Finally, we suggest directions for future research and highlight potential avenues for intervention to benefit both mother and child.

Measurement of pregnancy-related anxiety

During pregnancy, women may experience a unique form of anxiety termed pregnancy-related anxiety. Pregnancy-related anxiety is a multidimensional construct that encompasses fear or distress associated with pregnancy, including concerns about labor and delivery, changes in physical appearance, the health of the developing child, future motherhood and parenting, experience with the health care system, and social and financial issues in the context of pregnancy, and is accompanied by affective, cognitive, and somatic symptoms (Bayrampour et al., 2016; Guardino & Dunkel Schetter, 2014). The context in which pregnancy-related anxiety is experienced is likely influenced by culture, prior experiences, and pregnancy-specific considerations, including method of conception (e.g., pregnancy-related anxiety is higher in women who have conceived through assisted reproductive technology; Gourounti, 2016) and history of miscarriage, stillbirth, or infant death.

Versions of the pregnancy-related anxiety scale (PAS; Rini et al., 1999) and the Pregnancy-related Anxiety Questionnaire (PRAQ; PRAQ-R; PRAQ-R2; Huizink et al., 2016) are used most often in studies examining associations between pregnancy-related anxiety and infant and child development. Other measures that have been used to examine pregnancy-related anxiety include the five-item anxiety concerning health and defects in the child scale from the BABY Schema questionnaire (AHDC; Gloger-Tippelt, 1983); the four-item pregnancy-specific

Table 6.1 Pregnancy-related anxiety and offspring outcomes (arranged by age at infant or child assessment within developmental area)

Citation	N	PRA measure	Outcome Measure	Association between PRA and outcome	Prenatal psychological symptoms covaried?	Postnatal psychological symptoms covaried?	GA at birth covaried?	Birth weight covaried?	Medical/ Obstetric factors covaried?	Sample	Country and maternal race and/or ethnicity	Socioeconomic status	Socio-demographic factors covaried?
Emotional Development - Negative Affectivity													
Thomas et al., 2017	254	PAS	IBQ-R: Negative Affectivity scale at 3 months	Y	Y: depression (EPDS)	Y: depression (EPDS), anxiety (SCL-90)	C	N	N	AProN cohort: community sample recruited from OB clinics	Canada White: 81% Asian: 6% Latina: 4% Chinese: 3%	55% > $100,000 annual household income	C
McMahon et al., 2013	501	AHDC	STSI: Difficulty scale at 4 months	N	Y: state and trait anxiety (STAI) C: depression (EPDS)	Y: depression (EPDS), state anxiety (STAI)	C	C	Y	PATPA cohort: ART clinics; private + public clinics	Australia Race/ethnicity not reported	Not reported	Y
Nolvi et al., 2016	282	PRAQ-R2	IBQ-R: Negative Affectivity scale at 6 months	Y	Y: depression (EPDS), anxiety (SCL-90)	Y: depression (EPDS), anxiety (SCL-90)	N	N	N	FinnBrain Birth Cohort Study: community sample recruited from OB clinics	Finland Race/ethnicity not reported	49% = €1000-2000; 25% > €2000 monthly household income	Y
Henrichs et al., 2009	2997	POQ	IBQ-R: Distress to Limitations, Fearfulness, Recovery from Distress, Sadness subscales at 6 months	M: Only Fearfulness and Sadness remain significant with covariates	Y: anxiety (BSI)	Y: depression (EPDS), anxiety (BSI)	Y	Y	Y	Population-based Generation R cohort	The Netherlands Dutch: 66% Other Western: 10% Non-Western: 24%	90% > €1200 monthly household income	Y
Blair et al., 2011	120	PAS	ECBQ: Negative Affectivity scale at 2 years	Y	N	Y: state anxiety (STAI)	C	N	C	Community sample recruited from OB clinics	USA White: 48% Latina: 30% Asian: 18%	53% > $60,000 annual household income	Y

Gutteling et al., 2005b	119	PRAQ-R: FoGB and FoBHC subscales	ICQ: Restless-Disruptive and Irritability factor-analyzed scales at 27 months	M: FoBHC scale—Restless-Disruptive but not Irritability	N	N	Y	Y	Community sample recruited from OB clinics	The Netherlands Race/ethnicity not reported	73% classified as middle-high SES	Y
Mahrer et al., 2020	95	PSAS	CBQ-Very Brief version: Negative Affectivity scale at 4 years	Y	N	Y: depression (CES-D)	C	N	CHRN cohort	USA White: 33% Latina: 45%	Mean per capita annual household income: $17,520	Y
Emotional Development - Psychopathology												
Ali et al., 2019	182	PAS	CBCL: internalizing, externalizing scales at 2 years	Y	Y: depression (EPDS), anxiety (SCL-90)	Y: depression (EDPS), anxiety (SCL-90)	N	N	AProN cohort: community sample recruited from OB clinics	Canada White: 85%	58% ≥ $100,000 annual household income	Y
Gutteling et al., 2005b	119	PRAQ-R: FoGB and FoBHC subscales	CBCL: total, internalizing, externalizing scales at 27 months	N	N	N	Y	Y	Community sample recruited from OB clinics	The Netherlands Race/ethnicity not reported	73% classified as middle-high SES	Y
Pickles et al., 2017	81	PAS	CBCL: Anxious/depressed, aggression, attentional subscales; internalizing, externalizing scales at 3.5 years	M: Externalizing + Aggression; Internalizing + Anxious/depressed do not remain significant with covariates	N	Y: depression (EPDS), state anxiety (STAI)	Y[c]	Y	WCHD cohort: community sample recruited from OB clinic	United Kingdom White British: 76%	41% in "most deprived" quintile of UK neighborhoods[b]	Y
Acosta et al., 2019[a]	27	PRAQ-R2	SDQ: emotional symptoms; conduct problems; hyperactivity/inattention; peer relationship problems; total difficulties scales at 4 years	M: Only total problems and emotional symptoms; neither remain significant with covariates	Y: depression (EPDS), anxiety (SCL-90)	Y: depression (EPDS), anxiety (SCL-90)	Y	Y	FinnBrain Birth Cohort Study: community sample recruited from OB clinics	Finland Race/ethnicity not reported	Not reported	Y
Davis et al., 2012	178	PAS	CBCL: anxiety problems subscale at 6-9 years	Y	Y: depression (CES-D-SF), state anxiety (STAI)	Y: depression (CES-D-SF), state anxiety (STAI)	N	C	Community sample recruited from OB clinics	USA White: 49% Latina: 18% Asian: 13% Black: 10%	78% > $60,000 annual household income	Y

(Continued)

Table 6.1 (Continued)

Citation	N	PRA measure	Outcome Measure	Association between PRA and outcome	Prenatal psychological symptoms covaried?	Postnatal psychological symptoms covaried?	GA at birth covaried?	Birth weight covaried?	Medical/Obstetric factors covaried?	Sample	Country and maternal race and/or ethnicity	Socioeconomic status	Socio-demographic factors covaried?
Cognitive Development													
Davis & Sandman, 2010	125	PAS	BSID-II: MDI scale at 3, 6, and 12 months	Y	N	Y: depression (CES-D-SF), state anxiety (STAI)	Y	N	Y	Community sample recruited from OB clinics	USA White: 50% Latina: 30% Asian: 10%	57% > $60,000 annual household income	Y
Buitelaar et al., 2003	170	PRAQ-R: FoGB and FoBHC subscales	BSID: MDI scale at 3 and 8 months	Y: FoGB scale (8-month-olds but not 3-month-olds)	N	Y: depression (EPDS)	Y	Y	N	Community sample recruited from OB clinics	The Netherlands Race/ethnicity not reported	Not reported	N
Huizink et al., 2003	170	PRAQ-R: FoGB and FoBHC subscales	BSID: MDI scale at 3 and 8 months	Y: FoGB scale (8-month-olds but not 3-month-olds)	N	Y: depression (EPDS)	Y	Y	C	Community sample recruited from OB clinics	The Netherlands White: 96%	92% classified as middle-high SES	C
Huizink et al., 2002	170	PRAQ-R: FoGB and FoBHC subscales	BSID: MDI scale at 3 and 8 months	Y: FoGB scale (8-month-olds but not 3-month-olds)	N	Y: depression (EPDS)	Y	Y	C	Community sample recruited from OB clinics	The Netherlands Race/ethnicity not reported	Not reported	C
Nolvi et al., 2018	214	PRAQ-R2	Executive functioning (modified A-not-B task) at 8 months	N	C: depression (EPDS), anxiety (SCL-90)	C: depression (EPDS), anxiety (SCL-90)	C	N	C	FinnBrain Birth Cohort Study: community sample recruited from OB clinics	Finland Race/ethnicity not reported	48% €1000-2000; 19% < €1000 monthly household income	C
Gutteling et al., 2005b	119	PRAQ-R: FoGB and FoBHC subscales	Attention regulation problems (researcher rated during BSID) at 27 months	Y: FoBHC scale	N	N	Y	Y	Y	Community sample recruited from OB clinics	The Netherlands Race/ethnicity not reported	73% classified as middle-high SES	Y

Study	N	Prenatal anxiety measure	Outcome measure	Findings						Sample	Country, race/ethnicity	Income	
Buss et al., 2011	89	PAS	Working memory, inhibitory control at 6-9 years	Y: working memory; inhibitory control in girls	Y: depression (CES-D), anxiety (STAI)	Y: depression (CES-D), anxiety (STAI)	C (CES-D)	N	Y	Community sample recruited from OB clinics	USA White: 55% Latina: 22% Black: 7% Asian: 14%	68% > $60,000 annual household income	Y
Motor Development													
Davis & Sandman, 2010	125	PAS	BSID-II: PDI scale at 3, 6, and 12 months	N	N	Y: depression (CES-D-SF), state anxiety (STAI)	Y: depression (CES-D-SF), state anxiety (STAI)	N	C	Community sample recruited from OB clinics	USA White: 50% Latina: 30% Asian: 10%	57% > $60,000 annual household income	Y
Buitelaar et al., 2003	170	PRAQ-R: FoGB and FoBHC subscales	BSID: PDI scale at 3 and 8 months	Y: FoGB scale (8-month-olds but not 3-month-olds)	N	Y: depression (EPDS)	Y	Y	N	Community sample recruited from OB clinics	The Netherlands Race/ethnicity not reported	Not reported	N
Huizink et al., 2003	170	PRAQ-R: FoGB and FoBHC subscales	BSID: PDI scale at 3 and 8 months	Y: FoGB scale (8-month-olds but not 3-month-olds)	N	Y: depression (EPDS)	Y	Y	C	Community sample recruited from OB clinics	The Netherlands White: 96%	92% classified as middle-high SES	C
Brain Development													
Maria et al., 2020a	19	PRAQ-R2	Functional DOT during emotional speech at 2 months	Y: activity to sad speech in left temporoparietal junction	Y: depression (EPDS), anxiety (SCL-90)	Y: depression (EPDS), anxiety (SCL-90)	N	N	N	FinnBrain Birth Cohort Study: community sample recruited from OB clinics	Finland White: 100%	Mean income = €2000-2500	N
Acosta et al., 2019a	27	PRAQ-R2	Structural MRI scans: gray matter volume at 4 years	M: Left relative amygdala volume, but not other areas	Y: depression (EPDS), anxiety (SCL-90)	Y: depression (EPDS), anxiety (SCL-90)	Y	Y	Y	FinnBrain Birth Cohort Study: community sample recruited from OB clinics	Finland Race/ethnicity not reported	Not reported	Y

(Continued)

Table 6.1 (Continued)

Citation	N	PRA measure	Outcome Measure	Association between PRA and outcome	Prenatal psychological symptoms covaried?	Postnatal psychological symptoms covaried?	GA at birth covaried?	Birth weight covaried?	Medical/ Obstetric factors covaried?	Sample	Country and maternal race and/or ethnicity	Socioeconomic status	Socio-demographic factors covaried?
Buss et al., 2010	35	PAS	Structural MRI scans: gray matter volume and density at 6-9 years	Y	N	N	Y	N	C	Community sample recruited from OB clinics	USA White: 37% Latina: 20% Black: 9% Asian: 31%	56% > $60,000 annual household income	C
Hypothalamic-Pituitary-Adrenocortical Axis Regulation													
Tollenaar et al., 2011	173	PRAQ-R: FoGB and FoBHC subscales	Cortisol response to bathing session, vaccination, Still Face, and Strange Situation tasks at 5 weeks, 8 weeks, 5 months, and 12 months	M: FoBHC--bathing session; vaccination; Strange Situation	C: state anxiety (STAI)	C: state anxiety (STAI)	N	C	C	Community sample recruited from midwife clinics	The Netherlands Race/ethnicity not reported	Not reported	C
Gutteling et al., 2005a	29	PRAQ-R: FoGB and FoBHC subscales	Cortisol slopes 1st day of school year at 5 years	Y: FoBHC subscale	N	N	N	N	N	Community sample recruited from OB clinic	The Netherlands Race/ethnicity not reported	Not reported	N

Note. Columns indicating association between pregnancy-related anxiety and offspring outcome: Y indicates significant finding, N indicates null finding, M indicates mixed evidence for association. Columns indicating covariates: Y indicates the factor was covaried in models, N indicates the factor was not considered as a covariate in any way, C indicates the factor was considered as a covariate but not included in models because it did not meet certain conditions (e.g., not significantly correlated with the outcome variable). PRA = pregnancy-related anxiety; PAS = Pregnancy-related Anxiety Scale; AHDC = Anxiety concerning Health and Defects in the Child scale; PRAQ/PRAQ-R/PRAQ-R2 = Pregnancy Related Anxiety Questionnaire; POQ = Pregnancy Outcome Questionnaire; FoGB = Fear of Giving Birth subscale of the PRAQ; FoBHC = Fear of Birthing a Handicapped Child subscale of the PRAQ; PSAS = Pregnancy-Specific Anxiety Scale; IBQ-R = Infant Behavior Questionnaire-Revised (Gartstein & Rothbart, 2003); STSI = Short Temperament Scale for Infants (Sanson et al., 1987); ECBQ = Early Childhood Behavior Questionnaire (Putnam et al., 2006); ICQ = Infant Characteristics Questionnaire (Bates et al., 1979); CBQ-VB = Children's Behavior Questionnaire-Very Brief version (Putnam & Rothbart, 2006); CBCL = Child Behavior Checklist (Achenbach & Rescorla, 2000); SDQ = Strengths and Difficulties Questionnaire (Goodman, 1997); BSID/BSID-II = Bayley Scales of Infant Development (Bayley, 1993); MDI = Mental Development Index; PDI = Psychomotor Development Index; DOT = diffuse optical tomography; EPDS = Edinburgh Postnatal Depression Scale; SCL-90 = Symptom Checklist-90; BSI = Brief Symptom Inventory; STAI = State-Trait Anxiety Inventory; CES-D = Center for Epidemiological Studies Depression Scale; GA = gestational age; OB = Obstetric; PATPA = Parental Age and Transition to Parenthood Australia; ART = Assisted Reproductive Technology; CHRN = Child Health Research Network; AProN = Alberta Pregnancy and Nutrition Study; WCHD = Wirral Child Health and Development; SES = socioeconomic status.

[a] Each covariate was tested separately.
[b] IMD ranks assigned based on neighborhood deprivation in 7 domains: income, employment, health, education and training, barriers to housing and services, living environment, crime.
[c] Calculated a birth weight to gestational age ratio.

anxiety scale (PSAS; Roesch et al., 2004); and the Pregnancy Outcome Questionnaire (POQ; Theut et al., 1988). To allow for comparison throughout this chapter, we include the abbreviation of the measure used to assess pregnancy-related anxiety in each study discussed.

Pregnancy-related anxiety and child emotional development

Early childhood temperament and indices of behavioral and psychological symptoms are associated with subsequent negative outcomes, including psychopathology (Finsaas et al., 2018). There is evidence of continuity between infant temperament and later psychopathology (e.g., Buss & Kiel, 2013; Kagan et al., 1999). Further, behavioral problems during the preschool years are associated with later impairment in global, academic, and social functioning (Belden et al., 2012; Danzig et al., 2013; Keenan et al., 2011). Altering risk trajectories that lead to the development of psychopathology requires an understanding of contributors to individual differences in early-life socio-emotional development, such as pregnancy-related anxiety.

Negative affectivity

Negative affectivity is a temperamental tendency to experience negative emotions more quickly and intensely and to react more easily to stressful life events (Gartstein et al., 2012; Rothbart & Sheese, 2007). Though moderated by environmental factors (Shiner et al., 2012), negative affectivity is a moderate yet robust predictor of psychopathology in later childhood, adolescence, and adulthood (Kagan et al., 2007; Kostyrka-Allchorne et al., 2020; Wichstrøm et al., 2018).

Accumulating evidence links pregnancy-related anxiety to maternal report of infant negative affectivity during the first postnatal year. For example, higher levels of pregnancy-related anxiety predicted greater infant negative affectivity in 3-month-old (Thomas et al., 2017) and 6-month-old infants (Nolvi et al., 2016). Greater pregnancy-related anxiety was associated with higher levels of infant fearfulness and sadness, but not distress to limitations (fussiness, crying, or showing distress while in a confined place or position), or recovery from distress, at 6 months of age (Henrichs et al., 2009).

There is evidence that the association between pregnancy-related anxiety and negative affectivity observed in infancy persists into toddlerhood and early childhood. In two racially and ethnically diverse samples, higher levels of pregnancy-related anxiety were associated with greater mother-reported negative affectivity in 2-year-olds (Blair et al., 2011), and 4-year-olds (Mahrer et al., 2020; CBQ-VB).

Although links between pregnancy-related anxiety and infant and child negative affectivity are robust, findings are mixed when assessing other aspects of temperament. For example, pregnancy-related anxiety was not related to maternal report of 4-month-olds' difficult temperament (comprising approach, cooperation, and irritability scales) (McMahon et al., 2013). In another set of studies, pregnancy-related anxiety was not related to difficult behavior or inadaptability at 3 or 8 months (Huizink et al., 2002). When this sample was assessed again at 2 years of age, higher scores on one subscale of the PRAQ predicted restless/disruptive temperament, but neither subscale predicted irritable temperament (Gutteling et al., 2005b).

Overall, as shown in Table 6.1, there is compelling evidence of an association of small magnitude between pregnancy-related anxiety and offspring negative affectivity from infancy into early childhood. This relation persists after covarying other prenatally experienced distress (Henrichs et al., 2009; Nolvi et al., 2016; Thomas et al., 2017) as well as postnatal maternal distress (Blair et al., 2011; Henrichs et al., 2009; Mahrer et al., 2020; Nolvi et al., 2016; Thomas et al., 2017). Null effects tend to result when subscales, rather than whole scales, of pregnancy-related anxiety measures were used and aspects of temperament other than negative affectivity were measured.

Psychopathology

Research on the association between pregnancy-related anxiety and child psycho-pathology or socio-emotional problems indicates that children whose mothers reported elevated pregnancy-related anxiety are at increased risk for internalizing and externalizing problems and clinical anxiety (see Table 6.1). Two studies in early childhood found that higher levels of pregnancy-related anxiety were associated with greater child internalizing and externalizing problems at 2 years of age (Ali et al., 2020) and 3.5 years of age (Pickles et al., 2017). The study by Pickles et al. (2017) is notable for its large sample size and socioeconomic variability. Similarly, greater pregnancy-related anxiety was associated with more emotional symptoms and behavioral difficulties at 4 years of age (Acosta et al., 2019). Six-to nine-year-old children who were exposed to higher levels of pregnancy-related anxiety had higher levels of anxiety symptoms and were more likely to fall within the clinical or borderline-clinical range on anxiety as compared to children who were exposed to lower levels of pregnancy-related anxiety (Davis & Sandman, 2012). In contrast, no associations between pregnancy-related anxiety and inter-nalizing, externalizing, or total problem behaviors were found in a sample of 2-year-olds (Gutteling et al., 2005b). In sum, there appears to be growing sup-port for links between pregnancy-related anxiety and psychopathology during early and middle childhood, with most studies having covaried effects of addi-tional types of pre- and postnatal psychological distress. There is some evidence that these effects persist beyond other types of prenatal (Ali et al., 2020; Davis & Sandman, 2012) and postnatal maternal distress (Ali et al., 2020; Davis & Sand-man, 2012; Pickles et al., 2017), but other studies find that the association is reduced and/or becomes non-significant after covarying other types of prena-tal and/or postnatal maternal psychological distress (Pickles et al., 2017; Acosta et al., 2019). Studies have yet to explore whether these associations persist into adolescence.

Pregnancy-related anxiety and child cognitive development

Aspects of infant cognitive development, such as attention regulation, predict cognitive performance later in childhood (Lemelin et al., 2006; Sajaniemi et al., 2001). Childhood executive function is associated with cognitive and academic competency in adolescence (Ahmed et al., 2019; Chung et al., 2017). Therefore, it is important to understand factors, such as pregnancy-related anxiety, that may inform infant and child cognitive development.

Evidence suggests that greater pregnancy-related anxiety is related to poorer cognitive functioning (see Table 6.1). Greater pregnancy-related anxiety predicted poorer infant cognitive performance on an index that measures sensory-perception, knowledge, memory, problem-solving, and early language, at 3, 6, and 12 months (Davis & Sandman, 2010). Higher levels of pregnancy-related anxiety predicted poorer cognitive performance at 8 months (Buitelaar et al., 2003; Huizink et al., 2003). Additionally, greater pregnancy-related anxiety predicted lower attention regulation, measured by evaluator-rated test-affectivity and goal-directedness, in 3-month-olds and 8-month-olds (Buitelaar et al., 2003). This association persisted into toddlerhood such that when offspring were 2 years old, higher pregnancy-related anxiety scores on one of the PRAQ subscales predicted poorer researcher-rated attention regulation (Gutteling et al., 2005b).

Pregnancy-related anxiety may also relate to child executive function, which encompasses cognitive processes such as inhibition, decision-making, planning, working memory, and problem-solving. In a sample of 6- to 9-year-olds, pregnancy-related anxiety was associated with poorer visuospatial working memory performance in boys and girls, and poorer inhibitory control in girls (Buss et al., 2011). However, Nolvi et al. (2018) found no relation between pregnancy-related anxiety and performance on a modified AB task at 8 months of age, which requires the infant to hold and update information about the location of an object while inhibiting a prepotent response. This may be due to challenges in measuring executive function reliably during infancy (Pushina et al., 2005). In sum, pregnancy-related anxiety is consistently associated with poorer cognitive performance in infancy, and these associations continue into toddlerhood and middle childhood. The majority of studies have covaried for important infant and maternal psychological factors, which provides some evidence that these effects may persist after accounting for gestational age at birth and birth weight, other forms of prenatal maternal psychological distress (Davis & Sandman, 2010), and postnatal maternal psychological distress (Buitelaar et al., 2003; Buss et al., 2011; Davis & Sandman, 2010; Huizink et al., 2003).

Pregnancy-related anxiety and child motor development

Although research examining the associations between pregnancy-related anxiety and psychomotor development is sparse, a few studies have identified an association (see Table 6.1). Pregnancy-related anxiety is related to motor development, including fine and gross motor skills. Greater pregnancy-related anxiety predicted poorer infant motor development at both 3 months (Buitelaar et al., 2003) and 8 months (Buitelaar et al., 2003; Huizink et al., 2003). These studies covaried infant gestational age at birth, birth weight, and postnatal psychological distress, but not other types of prenatal maternal psychological distress. In contrast, in another cohort of children, infant motor development at 3, 6, and 12 months was not associated with pregnancy-related anxiety (Davis & Sandman, 2010). Reasons for this discrepancy are not clear; further research is necessary to elucidate the association between pregnancy-related anxiety and infant motor development.

Pregnancy-related anxiety and child brain development

The neural mechanisms underlying the link between pregnancy-related anxiety and child outcomes are not well understood. There is evidence that other aspects of prenatal maternal distress impact child brain development, but only a handful of studies have considered pregnancy-related anxiety (see Demers et al., 2021, for review), indicating the importance of further research in this area. Greater pregnancy-related anxiety was associated with reduced gray matter volume in the prefrontal cortex, premotor cortex, medial temporal lobe, lateral temporal cortex, postcentral gyrus, and cerebellar region in 6- to 9-year-old children (Buss et al., 2010). Regions associated with pregnancy-related anxiety are associated with a variety of functions, including language processing, executive function, memory, and social and emotional processing. In a study evaluating the link between pregnancy-related anxiety and the amygdala, a brain structure implicated in emotion reactivity and known to be impacted by early life adversity (e.g., McEwen et al., 2016; Van Tieghem & Tottenham, 2018), higher levels of pregnancy-related anxiety were related to greater left amygdala volume at 4 years in girls but not in boys (Acosta et al. (2019). It is plausible that altered amygdala development contributes to the link between fetal exposure to pregnancy-related anxiety and child psychopathology. Finally, one functional imaging study using diffuse optical tomography provides evidence that pregnancy-related anxiety is related to infants' neural responses to sad stimuli, even after covarying pre- and postnatal maternal general anxiety and depressive symptoms (Maria et al., 2020). In sum, the extant literature examining links between pregnancy-related anxiety and infant and child brain development is sparse and has relied on small samples, with few studies covarying additional prenatal and postnatal psychological distress (see Table 6.1). Thus, only tentative evidence exists that the association persists beyond the contributions of other types of prenatal (Acosta et al., 2019; Maria et al., 2020) and postnatal maternal distress (Maria et al., 2020).

Pregnancy-related anxiety and child HPA axis regulation

The HPA axis is one of the body's major stress response systems. Activation of the HPA axis stimulates the release of a cascade of hormones, including the production of cortisol, a primary glucocorticoid in humans. Observational human research (Davis et al., 2011; Howland et al., 2017; Noroña-Zhou et al., 2020) and experimental animal research (Abe et al., 2007; Kapoor et al., 2008; Thayer et al., 2018) provide strong evidence that prenatal experiences influence the development of the HPA axis. Consistent with this literature, a small body of literature supports the possibility that pregnancy-related anxiety may be associated with offspring HPA axis development. For example, higher levels of pregnancy-related anxiety (fear of bearing a handicapped child subscale of the PRAQ but not the fear of giving birth subscale) was associated with infant salivary cortisol reactivity to a variety of normative stressors at multiple time points during the first year of life, although the direction of the association was not consistent and perhaps dependent on infant age and nature of stressor (Tollenaar et al., 2011). In a small sample, greater pregnancy-related anxiety (subscale of the PRAQ) was also associated with higher cortisol levels in 5-year-old children sampled four times over the course of two schooldays during the first 2 weeks of the school year (Gutteling et al., 2005a). These studies provide preliminary evidence that pregnancy-related anxiety may contribute to HPA axis development in offspring such that children whose mothers experience more pregnancy-related anxiety produce altered cortisol responses to normative challenges such as receiving a vaccine or returning to school. However, there is a clear need for additional research considering other types of prenatal and postnatal psychological distress (see Table 6.1).

Unique effects: pregnancy-related anxiety versus other types of prenatal distress

There is conceptual overlap between pregnancy-related anxiety and other measures of prenatal distress such as depression, state and trait anxiety, and perceived stress. There are affective, cognitive, and physical symptoms common among these types of distress that may be experienced during the prenatal period, and the prenatal maternal biological profile of these various types of distress may be similar.

In studies investigating links between pregnancy-related anxiety and child outcomes, the most common outcome examined has been infant and toddler temperament. In this literature, there is robust evidence of unique associations between pregnancy-related anxiety and infant and child negative affectivity over and above the contributions of prenatal depression and general anxiety (Henrichs et al., 2009; Mahrer et al., 2020; Nolvi et al., 2016; Thomas et al., 2017). Few studies have examined other child outcomes or investigated unique pregnancy-related anxiety effects. Among studies that have assessed independent contributions, support is evident for unique associations between pregnancy-related anxiety and infant and child outcomes such as preadolescent anxiety (Davis & Sandman, 2012), infant attention regulation (Huizink et al., 2002), child executive functioning (Buss et al., 2011), and amygdala volume (Acosta et al., 2019), over and above other forms of prenatal distress such as general anxiety and depression (with the exception of Nolvi et al., 2016). This evidence highlights the need for specific attention to screening for and monitoring of pregnancy-related anxiety and ensuring that interventions target pregnancy-related anxiety in a focused manner in order to potentially improve offspring outcomes.

Timing of fetal exposure to pregnancy-related anxiety

Pregnancy-related anxiety and its specific components such as concern of one's physical appearance and fears related to the health of the unborn baby may decrease over the course of pregnancy (Blackmore et al., 2016; Mudra et al., 2020), while fears related to childbirth may increase (Mudra et al., 2020). The timing of fetal exposure to pregnancy-related anxiety may be particularly important for understanding mechanisms through which this distinct type of anxiety influence offspring development. Specific fetal systems (e.g., brain, HPA axis) undergo more or less rapid development at different stages of pregnancy, which may render them more or less vulnerable to the effects of pregnancy-related anxiety that may peak in the first half of pregnancy and then decline.

Studies that have examined fetal exposure to pregnancy-related anxiety at different gestational stages have generally found that earlier exposure (late first trimester or early second trimester) versus later exposure (typically late second trimester and beyond) is more strongly associated with developmental outcomes (Acosta et al., 2019; Blair et al., 2011; Buss et al., 2011; Davis & Sandman, 2010; Huizink et al., 2002; Mahrer et al., 2020). Exposure to pregnancy-related anxiety even earlier during the first trimester may be most detrimental, but studies have yet to investigate this. Available findings do highlight the importance of early screening and intervention in order to mitigate effects of pregnancy-related anxiety on infant and child development.

Potential moderators of pregnancy-related anxiety – child development association

Sex differences

Sex differences in the rates of mental health disorders are well documented throughout the lifespan (e.g., Bale & Epperson, 2015). The etiology of sex differences is not well understood (Rutter et al., 2003); however, there is increasing evidence to suggest that sex differences may originate during the prenatal period (Davis & Pfaff, 2014; Glover & Hill, 2012; Sandman et al., 2013). There is evidence of sex differences in fetal vulnerability to maternal distress, and these differences may contribute to sexually dimorphic rates of adult psychopathology (Hicks et al., 2019; Sandman et al., 2013). Research shows that males may be more susceptible to the effects of early adversity in terms of viability, but females may be more vulnerable to effects of prenatal adversity on risk for internalizing psychopathology (see Sandman et al., 2013). Consistent with this possibility, there is some evidence that females may be more susceptible to the impact of pregnancy-related anxiety on cognitive and emotional function. Associations between higher levels of pregnancy-related anxiety and poorer inhibitory control (Buss et al., 2011), greater left amygdala volume (Acosta et al., 2019), and smaller gray matter volume in specific regions, including the prefrontal cortex, premotor cortex, medial temporal lobe, lateral temporal cortex, postcentral gyrus, and cerebellum (Sandman et al., 2013), were found only in female offspring. However, Henrichs et al. (2009) showed no evidence of sex differences in the relation between pregnancy-related anxiety and infant temperament (activity, fearfulness, and sadness). Additional studies testing the moderating effects of offspring sex on associations between pregnancy-related anxiety and infant and child outcomes are needed to determine whether developmental risk posed by this anxiety impacts females and males differently.

Potentiating and ameliorating factors

There is important emerging work considering environmental factors that may potentiate or ameliorate the association between pregnancy-related anxiety and infant and child development. In addition to increasing understanding of how pregnancy-related anxiety may impact offspring outcomes, this work highlights possible avenues for altering negative developmental trajectories of children of mothers who experienced elevated pregnancy-related anxiety. Mahrer et al. (2020) tested whether relations between pregnancy-related anxiety and negative affectivity in 4-year-olds differed according to language preference, a proxy for acculturation. Spanish-preference Latina women reported significantly higher levels of pregnancy-related anxiety than English-preference Latina women and non-Hispanic White women. The association between pregnancy-related anxiety and negative affectivity was strongest in Spanish-preference Latina women and was not present in English-preference Latina and non-Hispanic White women. Sociocultural considerations such as acculturation, experiences of discrimination, and poverty may exacerbate or buffer the consequences of pregnancy-related anxiety. Further research is needed to better understand these complex relations.

Another recent study found that the association between pregnancy-related anxiety and childhood psychosocial problems was ameliorated by postnatal maternal behavior. Pickles et al. (2017) demonstrated that maternal report of how frequently she stroked her infant at 5- and 9-weeks postpartum moderated associations between pregnancy-related anxiety and maternal report of child symptoms at 3.5 years of age. Specifically, pregnancy-related anxiety was positively associated with child internalizing, externalizing, and aggressive symptoms, but this association was reduced for children whose mothers reported more frequent stroking behavior. The risk posed by pregnancy-related anxiety may thus be mitigated by positive postnatal environmental factors, including the early parent-child relationship. Although evidence in human samples is still modest, there is strong evidence from experimental animal models that high-quality maternal care can compensate for exposure to prenatal maternal stress (Lemaire et al., 2006; Raineki et al., 2014; Wakshlak & Weinstock, 1990).

Future directions

There is growing evidence that pregnancy-related anxiety is associated with aspects of infant and child development that are, in turn, associated with greater risk or resilience across the lifespan. Several methodological issues should be considered moving forward to further refine understanding of the link between pregnancy-related anxiety and infant and child outcomes. First, many of the robust associations observed have been in studies using versions of the PRAQ and the PAS, but some studies have used subscales of the PRAQ-R in isolation or combination. Future studies should report associations with the full scales as well as subscales in order to systematically examine whether specific components or the broad construct of pregnancy-related anxiety better predict offspring outcomes. Second, future studies should consistently account for other types of prenatal distress such as general anxiety or depression experienced during the prenatal period. Third, psychological distress experienced during the prenatal period may continue into the postnatal period. Thus, it is important to consistently account for postnatal distress to determine whether pregnancy-related anxiety exerts a unique effect on child development during the prenatal period or is better conceptualized as an early indicator of developmental consequences associated with maternal distress in the postnatal period. Fourth, to date, many study samples have been relatively homogeneous with respect to racial and ethnic composition and indicators of socioeconomic status; the majority of published studies include samples that are predominantly White and of higher socioeconomic status. Few studies have investigated critical questions about how racial/ethnic identity and socioeconomic factors may affect associations between pregnancy-related anxiety and child development (see Mahrer et al., 2020 for an exception). It will be important for future studies to consider social and contextual factors because evidence suggests that these factors may relate to prenatal maternal distress, including pregnancy-related anxiety as well as infant and child developmental outcomes (Katz et al., 2018; Koleva et al., 2011). Fifth, studies should account for birth phenotype (e.g., gestational age at birth and birth weight), which may be impacted by pregnancy-related anxiety and contribute to the offspring outcomes reviewed in this chapter. Although a number of studies restricted their samples to infants born at 37 weeks or later or covaried for other indicators of birth phenotype, not all studies have done so, and birth outcomes should be consistently considered in future research. Finally, pregnancy-related anxiety is, by definition, confined to the prenatal period. Thus, although we can consider postnatal maternal distress, such as postnatal depression and general anxiety, we cannot adjust for postnatal effects of pregnancy-related anxiety. Inclusion of measures of postnatal constructs that may be related to this specific anxiety such as parental precaution would enhance our understanding of the unique impact of pregnancy-related anxiety.

Future directions to explore include potential links between pregnancy-related anxiety and additional aspects of infant and child socio-emotional development as well as physical indicators such as body mass index that are related to later disease. To date, only one study (Nolvi et al., 2016) has reported on the association between pregnancy-related anxiety and aspects of infant temperament related to positive affect. Additional research into relations between pregnancy-related anxiety and infant and child physiological functioning, such as HPA axis reactivity and regulation and heart-rate variability, will enrich understanding of the pathways through which pregnancy-related anxiety may influence offspring functioning later in life. Another promising direction is investigation of prior pregnancy and birth-related experiences, such as assisted reproductive technology (ART) conception methods and history of recurrent miscarriage, stillbirth, or infant death that may strengthen the association between pregnancy-related anxiety and offspring outcomes. Women with these histories might be identified to receive psychological support early in their pregnancies. In addition, obstetric complications, which could influence both elevated levels of pregnancy-related anxiety and child outcomes, have not been consistently considered. Finally, little is known about how much shared genetics may explain links between pregnancy-related anxiety and infant and child outcomes. Epigenetics may play a role in how pregnancy-related anxiety may impact the developing fetus. Indeed, the prenatal environment is the first environment encountered by the fetus and gene-environment interactions that begin here may have significant and persisting implications for offspring health and development.

Pregnancy-related anxiety may prove a highly fruitful target for intervention given its time-limited specificity and focus and its clear and consistent associations with child developmental outcomes. Early intervention during pregnancy may be imminently beneficial to mothers and ultimately prove a promising avenue for supporting physical and cognitive development and preventing the potential development of psychopathology among their children. Studies that isolate mechanisms through which pregnancy-related anxiety may exert an effect on offspring outcomes, with specific attention to those mechanisms that may prove amenable to intervention, are exciting avenues of future research.

References

Abe, H., Hidaka, N., Kawagoe, C., Odagiri, K., Watanabe, Y., Ikeda, T., Ishizuka, Y., Hashiguchi, H., Takeda, R., Nishimori, T., & Ishida, Y. (2007). Prenatal psychological stress causes higher emotionality, depression-like behavior, and elevated activity in the hypothalamo-pituitary-adrenal axis. *Neuroscience Research, 59*(2), 145–151. https://doi.org/10.1016/j.neures.2007.06.1465

Achenbach, T. M., & Rescorla, L. A. (2000). *Manual for the ASEBA preschool forms and profiles* (Vol. 30). University of Vermont, Research Center for Children, Youth & Families.

Acosta, H., Tuulari, J. J., Scheinin, N. M., Hashempour, N., Rajasilta, O., Lavonius, T. I., Pelto, J., Saunavaara, V., Parkkola, R., & Lähdesmäki, T. (2019). Maternal pregnancy-related anxiety is associated with sexually dimorphic alterations in amygdala volume in four-year-old children. *Frontiers in Behavioral Neuroscience, 13*, 175. https://doi.org/10.3389/fnbeh.2019.00175

Ahmed, S. F., Tang, S., Waters, N. E., & Davis-Kean, P. (2019). Executive function and academic achievement: Longitudinal relations from early childhood to adolescence. *Journal of Educational Psychology, 111*(3), 446. https://doi.org/10.1037/edu0000296

Ali, E., Letourneau, N., Benzies, K., Ntanda, H., Dewey, D., Campbell, T., & Giesbrecht, G. (2020). Maternal prenatal anxiety and children's externalizing and internalizing behavioral problems: The moderating roles of maternal-child attachment security and child sex. *Canadian Journal of Nursing Research, 52*(2), 88–99. https://doi.org/10.1177%2F0844562119894184

Bale, T. L., & Epperson, C. N. (2015). Sex differences and stress across the lifespan. *Nature Neuroscience, 18*(10), 1413–1420. https://doi.org/10.1038%2Fnn.4112

Bates, J., Freeland, C., & Lounsbury, M. (1979). The infant characteristics questionnaire. *Child Development, 48*, 195–203.

Bayley, N. (1993). *Bayley scales of infant development* (2nd ed.). Psychological Corporation. https://doi.org/10.1177%2F073428290001800208

Bayrampour, H., Ali, E., McNeil, D. A., Benzies, K., MacQueen, G., & Tough, S. (2016). Pregnancy-related anxiety: A concept analysis. *International Journal of Nursing Studies, 55*, 115–130. https://doi.org/10.1016/j.ijnurstu.2015.10.023

Belden, A. C., Gaffrey, M. S., & Luby, J. L. (2012). Relational aggression in children with preschool-onset psychiatric disorders. *Journal of the American Academy of Child & Adolescent Psychiatry, 51*(9), 889–901. https://doi.org/10.1016/j.jaac.2012.06.018

Blackmore, E. R., Gustafsson, H., Gilchrist, M., Wyman, C., & O'Connor, T. G. (2016). Pregnancy-related anxiety: Evidence of distinct clinical significance from a prospective longitudinal study. *Journal of Affective Disorders, 197*, 251–258. https://doi.org/10.1016/j.jad.2016.03.008

Blair, M. M., Glynn, L. M., Sandman, C. A., & Davis, E. P. (2011). Prenatal maternal anxiety and early childhood temperament. *Stress, 14*(6), 644–651. https://doi.org/10.3109/10253890.2011.594121

Bolton, J. L., & Bilbo, S. D. (2014). Developmental programming of brain and behavior by perinatal diet: Focus on inflammatory mechanisms. *Dialogues in Clinical Neuroscience, 16*(3), 307–320. www.ncbi.nlm.nih.gov/pmc/articles/PMC4214174/

Bourgeois, J. (2001). Synaptogenesis in the neocortex of the newborn: The ultimate frontier for individuation? In C. A. Nelson & M. Luciana (Eds.), *Handbook of developmental cognitive neuroscience* (pp. 23–34). MIT Press.

Buitelaar, J. K., Huizink, A. C., Mulder, E. J., de Medina, P. G. R., & Visser, G. H. (2003). Prenatal stress and cognitive development and temperament in infants. *Neurobiology of Aging, 24*, S53–S60. https://doi.org/10.1016/S0197-4580(03)00050-2

Buss, C., Davis, E., Hobel, C., & Sandman, C. (2011). Maternal pregnancy-specific anxiety is associated with child executive function at 6–9 years age. *Stress, 14*(6), 665–676. https://doi.org/ 10.3109/10253890.2011.623250

Buss, C., Davis, E. P., Muftuler, L. T., Head, K., & Sandman, C. A. (2010). High pregnancy anxiety during mid-gestation is associated with decreased gray matter density in 6–9-year-old children. *Psychoneuroendocrinology, 35*(1), 141–153. http://doi.org/10.1016/j.psyneuen.2009.07.010

Buss, K. A., & Kiel, E. J. (2013). Temperamental risk factors for pediatric anxiety disorders. In R. A. Vasa & A. K. Roy (Eds.), *Current clinical psychiatry. Pediatric anxiety disorders: A clinical guide* (pp. 47–68). Humana Press. https://doi/10.1007/978-1-4614-6599-7_3

Chung, K. K., Liu, H., McBride, C., Wong, A. M. Y., & Lo, J. C. (2017). How socioeconomic status, executive functioning and verbal interactions contribute to early academic achievement in Chinese children. *Educational Psychology*, *37*(4), 402–420. https://doi.org/10.1080/01443410.2016.1179264

Danzig, A. P., Bufferd, S. J., Dougherty, L. R., Carlson, G. A., Olino, T. M., & Klein, D. N. (2013). Longitudinal associations between preschool psychopathology and school-age peer functioning. *Child Psychiatry & Human Development*, *44*(5), 621–632. https:///doi.org/10.1007/s10578-012-0356-4

Davis, E. P., Glynn, L. M., Waffarn, F., & Sandman, C. A. (2011). Prenatal maternal stress programs infant stress regulation. *Journal of Child Psychology and Psychiatry*, *52*(2), 119–129. https://doi.org/10.1111%2Fj.1469-7610.2010.02314.x

Davis, E. P., Hankin, B. L., Swales, D. A., & Hoffman, M. C. (2018). An experimental test of the fetal programming hypothesis: Can we reduce child ontogenetic vulnerability to psychopathology by decreasing maternal depression? *Development and Psychopathology*, *30*(3), 787–806. https://doi.org/10.1017/S0954579418000470

Davis, E. P., & Pfaff, D. (2014). Sexually dimorphic responses to early adversity: Implications for affective problems and autism spectrum disorder. *Psychoneuroendocrinology*, *49*, 11–25. https://doi.org/10.1016/j.psyneuen.2014.06.014

Davis, E. P., & Sandman, C. A. (2010). The timing of prenatal exposure to maternal cortisol and psychosocial stress is associated with human infant cognitive development. *Child Development*, *81*(1), 131–148. https://doi.org/10.1111/j.1467-8624.2009.01385.x

Davis, E. P., & Sandman, C. A. (2012). Prenatal psychobiological predictors of anxiety risk in preadolescent children. *Psychoneuroendocrinology*, *37*(8), 1224–1233. https://doi.org/10.1016/j.psyneuen.2011.12.016

Demers, C. H., Aran, Ö., Glynn, L. M., & Davis, E. P. (2021). Prenatal programming of neurodevelopment: Imaging and structural changes. In A. Wazana, E. Székely, & T. F. Oberlander (Eds.), *Prenatal stress and child development*. Springer International Publishing. [in press]

Entringer, S., Buss, C., & Wadhwa, P. D. (2015). Prenatal stress, development, health and disease risk: A psychobiological perspective-2015 Curt Richter Award Winner. *Psychoneuroendocrinology*, *62*, 366–375. https://doi.org/10.1016%2Fj.psyneuen.2015.08.019

Finsaas, M. C., Bufferd, S. J., Dougherty, L. R., Carlson, G. A., & Klein, D. N. (2018). Preschool psychiatric disorders: Homotypic and heterotypic continuity through middle childhood and early adolescence. *Psychological Medicine*, *48*(13), 2159–2168. https://doi.org/10.1017/S0033291717003646

Gartstein, M. A., Putnam, S. P., & Rothbart, M. K. (2012). Etiology of preschool behavior problems: Contributions of temperament attributes in early childhood. *Infant Mental Health Journal*, *33*(2), 197–211. https://doi.org/10.1002/imhj.21312

Gartstein, M. A., & Rothbart, M. K. (2003). Studying infant temperament via the revised infant behavior questionnaire. *Infant Behavior and Development*, *26*(1), 64–86. https://doi.org/10.1016/S0163-6383(02)00169-8

Gloger-Tippelt, G. (1983). A process model of the pregnancy course. *Human Development*, *26*(3), 134–148. https://doi.org/10.1159/000272877

Glover, V., & Hill, J. (2012). Sex differences in the programming effects of prenatal stress on psychopathology and stress responses: An evolutionary perspective. *Physiology & Behavior*, *106*(5), 736–740. https://doi.org/10.1016/j.physbeh.2012.02.011

Goodman, R. (1997). The strengths and difficulties questionnaire: A research note. *Journal of Child Psychology and Psychiatry*, *38*(5), 581–586. https://doi.org/10.1111/j.1469-7610.1997.tb01545.x

Goodman, S. H., & Gotlib, I. H. (1999). Risk for psychopathology in the children of depressed mothers: A developmental model for understanding mechanisms of transmission. *Psychological Review*, *106*(3), 458. https://doi.org/10.1037/0033-295x.106.3.458

Goodman, S. H., Rouse, M. H., Connell, A. M., Broth, M. R., Hall, C. M., & Heyward, D. (2011). Maternal depression and child psychopathology: A meta-analytic review. *Clinical Child and Family Psychology Review*, *14*(1), 1–27. https://doi.org/10.1007/s10567-010-0080-1

Gourounti, K. (2016). Psychological stress and adjustment in pregnancy following assisted reproductive technology and spontaneous conception: A systematic review. *Women & Health*, *56*(1), 98–118. https://doi.org/10.1080/03630242.2015.1074642

Guardino, C. M., & Dunkel Schetter, C. (2014). Understanding pregnancy anxiety: Concepts, correlates, and consequences. *Zero to Three*, *34*(4), 12–21. www.zerotothree.org

Gutteling, B. M., de Weerth, C., & Buitelaar, J. K. (2005a). Prenatal stress and children's cortisol reaction to the first day of school. *Psychoneuroendocrinology*, *30*(6), 541–549. https://doi.org/10.1016/j.psyneuen.2005.01.002

Gutteling, B. M., de Weerth, C., Willemsen-Swinkels, S. H., Huizink, A. C., Mulder, E. J., Visser, G. H., & Buitelaar, J. K. (2005b). The effects of prenatal stress on temperament and problem behavior of 27-month-old toddlers. *European Child & Adolescent Psychiatry*, *14*(1), 41–51. https://doi.org/10.1007/s00787-005-0435-1

Henrichs, J., Schenk, J. J., Schmidt, H. G., Velders, F. P., Hofman, A., Jaddoe, V. W., Verhulst, F. C., & Tiemeier, H. (2009). Maternal pre-and postnatal anxiety and infant temperament. The generation R study. *Infant and Child Development*, *18*(6), 556–572. https://doi.org/10.1002/Icd.639

Hicks, L. M., Swales, D. A., Garcia, S. E., Driver, C., & Davis, E. P. (2019). Does prenatal maternal distress contribute to sex differences in child psychopathology? *Current Psychiatry Reports*, *21*(2), 7. https://doi.org/10.1007/s11920-019-0992-5

Howland, M. A., Sandman, C. A., & Glynn, L. M. (2017). Developmental origins of the human hypothalamic-pituitary-adrenal axis. *Expert Review of Endocrinology & Metabolism*, *12*(5), 321–339. https://doi.org/10.1080/17446651.2017.1356222

Huizink, A., Delforterie, M., Scheinin, N., Tolvanen, M., Karlsson, L., & Karlsson, H. (2016). Adaption of pregnancy anxiety questionnaire – revised for all pregnant women regardless of parity: PRAQ-R2. *Archives of Women's Mental Health*, *19*(1), 125–132. https://doi.org/ 10.1007/s00737-015-0531-2

Huizink, A. C., De Medina, P. G. R., Mulder, E. J., Visser, G. H., & Buitelaar, J. K. (2002). Psychological measures of prenatal stress as predictors of infant temperament. *Journal of the American Academy of Child & Adolescent Psychiatry*, *41*(9), 1078–1085. http://doi.org/10.1097/00004583-200209000-00008

Huizink, A. C., Robles de Medina, P. G., Mulder, E. J., Visser, G. H., & Buitelaar, J. K. (2003). Stress during pregnancy is associated with developmental outcome in infancy. *Journal of Child Psychology and Psychiatry*, *44*(6), 810–818. https://doi.org/10.1111/1469-7610.00166.

Kagan, J., Snidman, N., Kahn, V., Towsley, S., Steinberg, L., & Fox, N. A. (2007). The preservation of two infant temperaments into adolescence. *Monographs of the*

Society for Research in Child Development, *72*(2), 61–76. https://doi.org/10.1111/j.1540-5834.2007.00437.x

Kagan, J., Snidman, N., Zentner, M., & Peterson, E. (1999). Infant temperament and anxious symptoms in school age children. *Development and Psychopathology*, *11*(2), 209–224. https://doi.org/10.1017/S0954579499002023

Kane, H. S., Schetter, C. D., Glynn, L. M., Hobel, C. J., & Sandman, C. A. (2014). Pregnancy anxiety and prenatal cortisol trajectories. *Biological Psychology*, *100*, 13–19. http://doi.org/10.1016/j.biopsycho.2014.04.003

Kapoor, A., Petropoulos, S., & Matthews, S. G. (2008). Fetal programming of hypothalamic – pituitary – adrenal (HPA) axis function and behavior by synthetic glucocorticoids. *Brain Research Reviews*, *57*(2), 586–595. https://doi.org/10.1016/j.brainresrev.2007.06.013

Katz, J., Crean, H. F., Cerulli, C., & Poleshuck, E. L. (2018). Material hardship and mental health symptoms among a predominantly low income sample of pregnant women seeking prenatal care. *Maternal and Child Health Journal*, *22*(9), 1360–1367. https/doi.org/10.1007/s10995-018-2518-x.

Keenan, K., Boeldt, D., Chen, D., Coyne, C., Donald, R., Duax, J., Hart, K., Perrott, J., Strickland, J., & Danis, B., Hill, C., Davis, S., Kampani, S., & Humphries, M. (2011). Predictive validity of DSM-IV oppositional defiant and conduct disorders in clinically referred preschoolers. *Journal of Child Psychology and Psychiatry*, *52*(1), 47–55. https://doi.org/10.1111/j.1469-7610.2010.02290.x

Koleva, H., Stuart, S., O'Hara, M. W., & Bowman-Reif, J. (2011). Risk factors for depressive symptoms during pregnancy. *Archives of Women's Mental Health*, *14*(2), 99–105. https://doi.org/10.1007%2Fs00737-010-0184-0

Korja, R., Nolvi, S., Grant, K. A., & McMahon, C. (2017). The relations between maternal prenatal anxiety or stress and child's early negative reactivity or self-regulation: A systematic review. *Child Psychiatry & Human Development*, *48*(6), 851–869. https://doi.org/10.1007/s10578-017-0709-0

Kostyrka-Allchorne, K., Wass, S. V., & Sonuga-Barke, E. J. (2020). Research review: Do parent ratings of infant negative emotionality and self-regulation predict psychopathology in childhood and adolescence? A systematic review and meta-analysis of prospective longitudinal studies. *Journal of Child Psychology and Psychiatry*, *61*(4), 401–416. https://doi.org/10.1111/jcpp.13144

Lemaire, V., Lamarque, S., Le Moal, M., Piazza, P. V., & Abrous, D. N. (2006). Postnatal stimulation of the pups counteracts prenatal stress-induced deficits in hippocampal neurogenesis. *Biological Psychiatry*, *59*(9), 786–792. https://doi.org/10.1016/j.biopsych.2005.11.009

Lemelin, J.-P., Tarabulsy, G. M., & Provost, M. A. (2006). Predicting preschool cognitive development from infant temperament, maternal sensitivity, and psychosocial risk. *Merrill-Palmer Quarterly*, *52*(4), 779–806. https://doi.org/10.1353/mpq.2006.0038

Lobel, M., Cannella, D. L., Graham, J. E., DeVincent, C., Schneider, J., & Meyer, B. A. (2008). Pregnancy-specific stress, prenatal health behaviors, and birth outcomes. *Health Psychology*, *27*(5), 604. https://doi.org/10.1037/a0013242

Madigan, S., Oatley, H., Racine, N., Fearon, R. P., Schumacher, L., Akbari, E., Cooke, J. E., & Tarabulsy, G. M. (2018). A meta-analysis of maternal prenatal depression and anxiety on child socioemotional development. *Journal of the American Academy of Child & Adolescent Psychiatry*, *57*(9), 645–657. https://doi.org/10.1016/j.jaac.2018.06.012

Mahrer, N. E., Ramos, I. F., Guardino, C., Davis, E. P., Ramey, S. L., Shalowitz, M., & Schetter, C. D. (2020). Pregnancy anxiety in expectant mothers predicts off-spring negative affect: The moderating role of acculturation. *Early Human Development, 141,* 104932. https://doi.org/10.1016/j.earlhumdev.2019.104932

Maria, A., Nissilä, I., Shekhar, S., Kotilahti, K., Tuulari, J. J., Hirvi, P., Huotilainen, M., Heiskala, J., Karlsson, L., & Karlsson, H. (2020). Relationship between mater-nal pregnancy-related anxiety and infant brain responses to emotional speech-a pilot study. *Journal of Affective Disorders, 262,* 62–70. https://doi.org/10.1016/j.jad.2019.10.047

McEwen, B. S., Nasca, C., & Gray, J. D. (2016). Stress effects on neuronal structure: Hippocampus, amygdala, and prefrontal cortex. *Neuropsychopharmacology, 41*(1), 3–23. https://doi.org/10.1038/npp.2015.171

McLemore, M. R., Altman, M. R., Cooper, N., Williams, S., Rand, L., & Franck, L. (2018). Health care experiences of pregnant, birthing and postnatal women of color at risk for preterm birth. *Social Science & Medicine, 201,* 127–135. https://doi.org/10.1016/j.socscimed.2018.02.013

McMahon, C., Boivin, J., Gibson, F., Hammarberg, K., Wynter, K., Saunders, D., & Fisher, J. (2013). Pregnancy-specific anxiety, ART conception and infant tempera-ment at 4 months post-partum. *Human Reproduction, 28*(4), 997–1005. https://doi.org/10.1093/humrep/det029

Mudra, S., Göbel, A., Barkmann, C., Goletzke, J., Hecher, K., Schulte-Markwort, M., Diemert, A., & Arck, P. (2020). The longitudinal course of pregnancy-related anxi-ety in parous and nulliparous women and its association with symptoms of social and generalized anxiety. *Journal of Affective Disorders, 260,* 111–118. https://doi.org/10.1016/j.jad.2019.08.033

Nolvi, S., Karlsson, L., Bridgett, D. J., Korja, R., Huizink, A. C., Kataja, E.-L., & Karlsson, H. (2016). Maternal prenatal stress and infant emotional reactivity six months postpartum. *Journal of Affective Disorders, 199,* 163–170. https://doi.org/10.1016/j.jad.2016.04.020

Nolvi, S., Pesonen, H., Bridgett, D. J., Korja, R., Kataja, E. L., Karlsson, H., & Karls-son, L. (2018). Infant sex moderates the effects of maternal pre-and postnatal stress on executive functioning at 8 months of age. *Infancy, 23*(2), 194–210. https://doi.org/10.1111/infa.12206

Noroña-Zhou, A. N., Morgan, A., Glynn, L. M., Sandman, C. A., Baram, T. Z., Stern, H. S., & Davis, E. P. (2020). Unpredictable maternal behavior is associ-ated with a blunted infant cortisol response. *Developmental Psychobiology, 62*(6), 882–888. https://doi.org/10.1002/dev.21964

Nugent, B. M., & Bale, T. L. (2015). The omniscient placenta: Metabolic and epige-netic regulation of fetal programming. *Frontiers in Neuroendocrinology, 39,* 28–37. https://doi.org/10.1016%2Fj.yfrne.2015.09.001

Peterson, G. F., Espel, E. V., Davis, E. P., Sandman, C. A., & Glynn, L. M. (2020). Characterizing prenatal maternal distress with unique prenatal cortisol trajectories. *Health Psychology, 39*(11), 1013–1019. https://doi.org/10.1037/hea0001018

Pickles, A., Sharp, H., Hellier, J., & Hill, J. (2017). Prenatal anxiety, maternal strok-ing in infancy, and symptoms of emotional and behavioral disorders at 3.5 years. *European Child & Adolescent Psychiatry, 26*(3), 325–334. https://doi.org/10.1007%2Fs00787-016-0886-6

Pushina, N., Orekhova, E., & Stroganova, T. (2005). Age-related and individual dif-ferences in the performance of a delayed response task (the A-not-B task) in infant twins aged 7–12 months. *Neuroscience and Behavioral Physiology, 35*(5), 481–490. https://doi.org/10.1007/s11055-005-0083-4

Putnam, S. P., Gartstein, M. A., & Rothbart, M. K. (2006). Measurement of fine-grained aspects of toddler temperament: The early childhood behavior questionnaire. *Infant Behavior and Development, 29*(3), 386–401. https://doi.org/10.1016%2Fj.infbeh.2006.01.004

Putnam, S. P., & Rothbart, M. K. (2006). Development of short and very short forms of the children's behavior questionnaire. *Journal of Personality Assessment, 87*(1), 102–112. https://doi.org/10.1207/s15327752jpa8701_09

Raineki, C., Lucion, A. B., & Weinberg, J. (2014). Neonatal handling: An overview of the positive and negative effects. *Developmental Psychobiology, 56*(8), 1613–1625. https://dx.doi.org/10.1002%2Fdev.21241

Rini, C. K., Dunkel-Schetter, C., Wadhwa, P. D., & Sandman, C. A. (1999). Psychological adaptation and birth outcomes: The role of personal resources, stress, and sociocultural context in pregnancy. *Health Psychology, 18*(4), 333–345. https://doi.org/10.1037//0278-6133.18.4.333

Roesch, S. C., Schetter, C. D., Woo, G., & Hobel, C. J. (2004). Modeling the types and timing of stress in pregnancy. *Anxiety, Stress & Coping, 17*(1), 87–102. https://doi.org/10.1080/1061580031000123667

Rothbart, M. K., & Sheese, B. E. (2007). Temperament and emotion regulation. In J. J. Gross (Ed.), *Handbook of emotion regulation* (pp. 331–350). The Guildford Press.

Rutter, M., Caspi, A., & Moffitt, T. E. (2003). Using sex differences in psychopathology to study causal mechanisms: Unifying issues and research strategies. *Journal of Child Psychology and Psychiatry, 44*(8), 1092–1115. https://doi.org/10.1111/1469-7610.00194

Sajaniemi, N., Hakamies-Blomqvist, L., Katainen, S., & von Wendt, L. (2001). Early cognitive and behavioral predictors of later performance: A follow-up study of ELBW children from ages 2 to 4. *Early Childhood Research Quarterly, 16*(3), 343–361. https://doi.org/10.1016/S0885-2006(01)00107-7

Sandman, C. A., Glynn, L. M., & Davis, E. P. (2013). Is there a viability – vulnerability tradeoff? Sex differences in fetal programming. *Journal of Psychosomatic Research, 75*(4), 327–335. https://doi.org/10.1016/j.jpsychores.2013.07.009

Sanson, A., Prior, M., Garino, E., Oberklaid, F., & Sewell, J. (1987). The structure of infant temperament: Factor analysis of the revised infant temperament questionnaire. *Infant Behavior & Development, 10*(1), 97–104. https://doi.org/10.1016/0163-6383(87)90009-9

Shiner, R. L., Buss, K. A., McClowry, S. G., Putnam, S. P., Saudino, K. J., & Zentner, M. (2012). What is temperament now? Assessing progress in temperament research on the twenty-fifth Anniversary of Goldsmith et al. (1987). *Child Development Perspectives, 6*(4), 436–444. https://doi.org/10.1111/j.1750-8606.2012.00254.x

Thayer, Z. M., Wilson, M. A., Kim, A. W., & Jaeggi, A. V. (2018). Impact of prenatal stress on offspring glucocorticoid levels: A phylogenetic meta-analysis across 14 vertebrate species. *Scientific Reports, 8*(1), 1–9. https://doi.org/10.1038%2Fs41598-018-23169-w

Theut, S. K., Pedersen, F. A., Zaslow, M. J., & Rabinovich, B. A. (1988). Pregnancy subsequent to perinatal loss: Parental anxiety and depression. *Journal of the American Academy of Child & Adolescent Psychiatry, 27*(3), 289–292. https://doi.org/10.1097/00004583-198805000-00004

Thomas, J. C., Letourneau, N., Campbell, T. S., Tomfohr-Madsen, L., & Giesbrecht, G. F. (2017). Developmental origins of infant emotion regulation: Mediation by temperamental negativity and moderation by maternal sensitivity. *Developmental Psychology, 53*(4), 611–628. https://doi.org/10.1037/dev0000279

Tollenaar, M., Beijers, R., Jansen, J., Riksen-Walraven, J., & de Weerth, C. (2011). Maternal prenatal stress and cortisol reactivity to stressors in human infants. *Stress, 14*(1), 53–65. https://doi.org/10.3109/10253890.2010.499485

Van den Bergh, B. R., van den Heuvel, M. I., Lahti, M., Braeken, M., de Rooij, S. R., Entringer, S., Hoyer, D., Roseboom, T., Räikkönen, K., King, S., & Schwab, M. (2017). Prenatal developmental origins of behavior and mental health: The influence of maternal stress in pregnancy. *Neuroscience & Biobehavioral Reviews, 16*, 30734–30735. https://doi.org/10.1016/j.neubiorev.2017.07.003

Van Tieghem, M. R., & Tottenham, N. (2018). Neurobiological programming of early life stress: Functional development of amygdala-prefrontal circuitry and vulnerability for stress-related psychopathology. *Current Topics in Behavioral Neurosciences, 38*, 117–136. https://doi.org/10.1007/7854_2016_42

Wakshlak, A., & Weinstock, M. (1990). Neonatal handling reverses behavioral abnormalities induced in rats by prenatal stress. *Physiology & Behavior, 48*(2), 289–292. https://doi.org/10.1016/0031-9384(90)90315-u

Wichstrøm, L., Penelo, E., Rensvik Viddal, K., de la Osa, N., & Ezpeleta, L. (2018). Explaining the relationship between temperament and symptoms of psychiatric disorders from preschool to middle childhood: Hybrid fixed and random effects models of Norwegian and Spanish children. *Journal of Child Psychology and Psychiatry, 59*(3), 285–295. https://doi.org/10.1111/jcpp.12772

Part II
Implications for practice

7   Current diagnostic practices and their limitations

Jane Kohlhoff

Current diagnostic practices and their limitations

Pregnancy-related anxiety

The term pregnancy-related anxiety refers to anxiety related specifically to pregnancy and childbirth, the health and well-being of the fetus, infant or mother, accessibility and parenting/newborn care (Bayrampour et al., 2016; Dunkel Schetter, 2011; Orr et al., 2007; Rini et al., 1999). Pregnancy-related anxiety is often preceded by real or anticipated threat to pregnancy or its outcomes, low perceived control, or excessive cognitive activity (Bayrampour et al., 2016). Symptom presentation can span affective, cognitive, and somatic domains; and it is often associated with range of negative behaviors and cognitive patterns, including negative attitudes, difficulty concentrating, rumination, excessive reassurance-seeking, and avoidance (Bayrampour et al., 2016).

Pregnancy-related anxiety's status as a type of anxiety discrete from general anxiety or depression in pregnancy was initially suggested in light of evidence that only a small amount (8–27%) of the variation in pregnancy-related concerns was explained by generalized anxiety or depression (Huizink et al., 2004; Orr et al., 2007). The notion that pregnancy-related anxiety is a distinct phenomenon has been further strengthened by evidence of unique associations between pregnancy-related anxiety (independent of general anxiety and stress) and a range of adverse maternal and child outcomes, including delivery via caesarean section (Koelewijn et al., 2017; Madhavanprabhakaran et al., 2013), preterm labor and low infant birth weight (Kramer et al., 2009; Madhavanprabhakaran et al., 2013; Orr et al., 2007; Robertson-Blackmore et al., 2016), complications during pregnancy and delivery (Fertl et al., 2009), postnatal mood disturbance (Robertson-Blackmore et al., 2016), and child cognitive functioning and negative affectivity (Blair et al., 2011; Buss et al., 2011). For further details, see Chapters 5 and 6.

Diagnosing pregnancy-related anxiety

The process of developing specific diagnostic measures for pregnancy-related anxiety is still at a preliminary stage. Pregnancy-related anxiety has not been

DOI: 10.4324/9781003014003-10

formally acknowledged in the Diagnostic and Statistical Manual version 5 (DSM V; American Psychiatric Association, 2013) or the International Classification of Diseases version 10 (ICD-10; World Health Organization, 2004). There are some opportunities to classify pregnancy-related anxiety using these classification systems, but ultimately these are inadequate as they fail to acknowledge the unique status and clinical implications of the condition.

The diagnostic and statistical manual version 5 (DSM-V; American Psychiatric Association, 2013)

The DSM-V is the taxonomic and diagnostic tool published by the American Psychiatric Association. Clinicians and researchers in the United States and many other countries of the world use it as their diagnostic authority, relying on it to make psychiatric diagnoses and inform treatment plans.

The "Anxiety Disorders" section of DSM-V, located within Section II, groups together disorders that share the central features of cognitive and physical symptoms related to the experience of fear and anxiety, with associated behavioral disturbances, including avoidance (social anxiety disorder; generalized anxiety disorder, panic disorder with/without agoraphobia). While the DSM-V anxiety disorders can be differentiated from one another by different mean ages of onset, different precipitants, and different types of cognitive ideation, they are grouped together given their shared underlying pathology (Shang et al., 2014).

The anxiety disorders section of the DSM-V does not contain a pregnancy-related anxiety classification. There is, however, opportunity to capture pregnancy-related anxiety through the classification of "other specified anxiety disorder," a classification used in instances where symptoms characteristic of an anxiety disorder are present but do not meet the full criteria of any of the anxiety disorders, and the clinician wishes to specify the reason that the criteria are not met. For example, a pregnant woman who presents with excessive anxiety and worry and who meets all of the criteria for generalized anxiety disorder except that the worry is confined to the one general topic (i.e., pregnancy and motherhood), a classification of "generalized anxiety focused on pregnancy and parenthood" may be appropriate.

Another way of capturing pregnancy-related anxiety within the DSM-V classification system is to use the "adjustment disorder" classification. Adjustment disorder, also in Section II, falls within the "trauma- and stress-related disorders," a group of conditions for which one of the explicit criteria is exposure to a traumatic or stressful event. Adjustment disorder is phenomenologically nonspecific (Strain et al., 2011) and diagnosis requires the presence of emotional or behavioral symptoms occurring within 3 months of an identifiable stressor(s), causing marked distress or functional impairment and with symptoms resolving within 6 months of the removal of the stressor or its consequences. For a pregnant woman who presents with pregnancy-related anxiety, the stressor could have been the start of the pregnancy, or some other relevant event that occurred in the 6 months prior to the onset of symptoms. The diagnosis of adjustment disorder is also accompanied by a symptom-based specifier ("with depressed mood," "with anxiety," "with mixed anxiety and depression," "with disturbance of conduct," "unspecified"), any one of which may be relevant in the case of pregnancy-related anxiety.

International classification of diseases version 10 (ICD-10)[1]
(World Health Organization, 1992)

ICD is the World Health Organization's (WHO) health information standard for mortality and morbidity statistics. By providing definitions of diseases, it facilitates the study of disease patterns and the management of health care, outcome monitoring, and resource allocation (World Health Organization, 2020).

The ICD-10 disorder most appropriate for the diagnosis of pregnancy-related anxiety is "adjustment disorder" (F43.2). This disorder, located within the "reaction to severe stress, and adjustment disorders" (F43) section, is defined as "states of subjective distress and emotional disturbance, usually interfering with social functioning and performance, arising in the period of adaptation to a significant life change or a stressful life event." According to the ICD-10, the stressor may have been a major developmental transition or crisis, including "becoming a parent." The symptoms described for this disorder also align with many of those described in the literature for pregnancy-related anxiety, namely, anxiety, worry, low mood (or a mixture of these), feelings of inability to cope, plan ahead, or continue in the present situation, with an impact on daily functioning.

Chapter V of ICD-10 ("mental and behavioral disorders") lists the "neurotic, stress-related and somatoform disorders" (F40-F48). Within this broad category, there are various classifications that may be appropriate for the classification of pregnancy-related anxiety, depending on the individual's particular symptom presentation. Of particular note are the "other anxiety disorders" (F41), a group that includes codes for presentations not severe enough to justify a diagnosis of other anxiety disorders. Examples include "mixed anxiety and depression" (F41.2; used when symptoms of anxiety and depression are both present, but neither predominates or is present to the extent that separate diagnoses are considered), "other mixed anxiety disorders" (F41.3; used when symptoms of anxiety are mixed with features of other disorders in F42–F48, but neither type of symptom is severe enough to justify a diagnosis if considered separately), "other specified anxiety disorders" (F41.8; used in cases of anxiety hysteria); and "anxiety disorder, unspecified" (F41.9). While some of the classification codes within the "other anxiety disorders" section may be relevant for an individual suffering from pregnancy-related anxiety, this section of the ICD-10 still has limited utility for describing this anxiety as there are no codes that specifically refer to anxiety about pregnancy, and no specifiers available to indicate onset during pregnancy.

Screening for antenatal anxiety in clinical practice

In recent years, governments and peak bodies from around the world have acknowledged the prevalence and negative impacts of anxiety during pregnancy. Many countries have released policy statements recommending that anxiety screening be implemented as a routine part of antenatal clinical practice. As described earlier, due to a lack of a diagnostic category for pregnancy-related anxiety, there are currently no screening measures for this anxiety with validated cutoffs for caseness. Thus, while individual clinicians may be assessing pregnant women for pregnancy-related anxiety, due to a lack of validated screening tools, routine screening for pregnancy-related anxiety does not typically take place in clinical practice. Limitations in this area, however, are not confined to pregnancy-related anxiety. At a broader level, there is also a lack of brief, user-friendly, validated screening tools for antenatal anxiety in general. This means that in many places, screening does not take place at all, and where it does, there are differences with regard to screening tools utilized. To illustrate this, the following section describes the antenatal screening approaches recommended by three prominent English-speaking countries (the United Kingdom, the United States, and Australia) and discusses the likelihood that each of these approaches would be able to identify women who are suffering from pregnancy-related anxiety. For a summary of the approaches recommended by each country, see Table 7.1.

Table 7.1 *Recommended antenatal anxiety screening tools in Australia*

Country	Recommend antenatal anxiety screening tool	Relevant guideline/policy
UK	• GAD-2, with follow-up using the GAD-7 if required	National Institute for Health and Care Excellence. (2020). Antenatal and postnatal mental health: clinical management and service guidance (CG192). www.nice.org.uk/guidance/cg192/resources/antenatal-and-postnatal-mental-health-clinical-management-and-service-guidance-pdf-35109869806789.
US	• EPDS items 3, 4, and 5; OR • Postpartum Depression Screening Scale; OR • Patient Health Questionnaire – 9; OR • Beck Depression Inventory; OR • Beck Depression Inventory-II; OR • Center for Epidemiological Studies Depression Scale; OR • Zung Self-Rating Depression Scale	ACOG Committee. (2018). ACOG Committee opinion: screening for perinatal depression. *Obstetrics and Gynecology, 132*(5), e208–e212.
Australia	• EPDS items 3, 4, and 5; OR • DASS anxiety items; OR • K-10 items 2, 3, 5, and 6; AND • Relevant items in structured psychosocial assessment tools	Austin, M. P., Highet, N., & Expert Working Group. (2017). Mental health care in the perinatal period: Australian clinical practice guideline. Melbourne.

The United Kingdom

The United Kingdom National Institute for Health and Clinical Excellence guidelines (National Institute for Health and Care Excellence [NICE], 2020) state that "the range and prevalence of anxiety disorders . . . and depression are under-recognized throughout pregnancy and the postnatal period" and recommends that questions about mental health be asked of all women at the "first contact with primary care or her booking visit, and during the early postnatal period" (NICE, 2020, pp. 28–29). The NICE guidelines then suggest that on a woman's first contact with primary care or her booking visit, the clinician should consider asking about anxiety using the 2-item Generalized Anxiety Disorder scale (GAD-2) (items: *"Over the last 2 weeks, how often have you been bothered by feeling nervous, anxious or on edge?"* and *"Over the last 2 weeks, how often have you been bothered by not being able to stop or control worrying?"*) If a woman scores 3 or more on the GAD-2 scale, the guidelines suggest that the clinician consider using the GAD-7 scale for further assessment or referring the woman to her General Practitioner (GP) or a mental health professional. If a woman scores less than 3 on the GAD-2 scale, but the clinician is still concerned, a follow-up question is recommended (*"Do you find yourself avoiding places or activities and does this cause you problems?"*) If she responds positively, further assessment with the GAD-7 or referral to GP or a mental health professional is recommended.

The United States

The American College of Obstetricians and Gynecologists (ACOG) recommends that all obstetricians – gynecologists and other obstetric care providers complete a "full assessment of mood and emotional well-being (including screening for postpartum depression and anxiety with a validated instrument)" for each patient during the comprehensive postpartum visit (ACOG Committee, 2018, p. e208). A list of possible validated tools is provided, including the Edinburgh Postnatal Depression Scale (EPDS, Cox et al., 1987). The ACOG statement mentions that the EPDS contains anxiety items but provides no other specific recommendations regarding validated tools to be used when screening for anxiety.

Australia

The Australian national clinical practice guidelines (Austin et al., 2017) warn that "anxiety disorder is very common in the perinatal period and should be considered in the broader clinical assessment" (p. 30) and suggest that "accurately identifying women experiencing symptoms of depression and anxiety enables referral for more formal mental health assessment and suitable follow-up, with a view to improving outcomes for women" (Austin et al., 2017, p. 27). The guidelines note the absence of free, practical, and validated anxiety screening tools for use in the perinatal period and advise clinicians to use anxiety items from other screening tools, namely, items 3, 4 and 5 from the EPDS (Cox et al., 1987); anxiety items from the DASS (Lovibond & Lovibond, 1995), items 2, 3, 5, and

6 from the Kessler Psychological Distress Scale (K-10, Spies et al., 2009), and relevant items in structured psychosocial assessment tools such as the Antenatal Risk Questionnaire (ANRQ, Austin et al., 2013; Reilly et al., 2015).

Australia is the only country to have legislated the requirement for perinatal mental health screening. In 2017, new billing items were introduced through the national Medicare scheme for the planning and management of pregnancy, and for postnatal consultations between 4 and 8 weeks of the birth – with an expectation that a mental health assessment be offered by the obstetrician or another suitably qualified health professional. The Medicare Billing Scheme does not prescribe the method by which health professionals undertake mental health assessments for obstetric patients. While it is recommended that the National Clinical Guidelines (Austin et al., 2017) be followed, this is not a requirement and so given the lack of an easily administered and validated tool for pregnancy-related anxiety (and similarly for anxiety more generally), many time-poor clinicians may be using informal assessment methods.

Identifying pregnancy-related anxiety using generalist anxiety screening tools

As discussed earlier, antenatal anxiety screening programs tend to focus on general anxiety symptoms rather than specific anxiety disorders (including pregnancy-related anxiety). This approach maximizes the possibility of identifying as many sufferers as possible, and it also reduces the time taken to complete the screening questions, thus minimizing the burden on pregnant women and busy health professionals/systems. Given the evidence of a unique set of adverse outcomes arising from pregnancy-related anxiety, there could clearly be benefits in screening specifically for this anxiety. However, given the symptom overlap between pregnancy-related anxiety and other forms of anxiety, the generalist antenatal anxiety screening approach is still likely to be effective in identifying women who are suffering from pregnancy-related anxiety. Importantly, all antenatal anxiety screening guidelines recommend that positive responses to screening questions are followed up by a clinician with further questioning and discussion. If such an approach is taken, women with pregnancy-related anxiety are likely to be identified. This is, however, an area of clinical practice that would benefit from further research investigation.

Summary and conclusions

This chapter discussed options available to clinicians wishing to assign DSM-V or ICD-10 diagnoses to women suffering from pregnancy-related anxiety. It was concluded that while no precise classification exists, opportunities are available in the DSM-V classifications of "other specified anxiety disorder" or "adjustment disorder," or the ICD-10 classifications of "adjustment disorder" or "other anxiety disorders." Ultimately, however, these diagnoses fail to do justice to the condition of pregnancy-related anxiety due to their lack of specificity, and this highlights the need for consideration of specifiers that are more specific and descriptive of pregnancy-related anxiety, prior to subsequent DSM and ICD revisions. The chapter also provided an overview of current antenatal anxiety screening policy recommendations in the United States, United Kingdom, and Australia, and concluded that while routine screening for pregnancy-related anxiety does not take place, women with this anxiety are likely to screen positive on generalist anxiety screening measures. The precise nature and impacts of their pregnancy-related anxiety should be identified through further clinical assessment by a health professional.

To conclude, while understanding and recognition of pregnancy-related anxiety has come a long way in recent years, further research should be conducted to explore the validity of currently available diagnostic and screening practices for this type of anxiety, and to gather a clearer understanding of the tools and methods that health professionals are currently using in clinical practice, both in the public and private sectors. Pregnancy-related anxiety is an important health condition to understand and treat and so it is vital that diagnostic categories and psychometrically sound symptom severity screening measures are developed and used, to enable accurate identification of individuals suffering from the condition. This will ensure the provision of effective clinical interventions to those who most need them.

Note

1 The ICD-10 is currently in use, but an 11th version has been released and will come into usage in 2022.

References

ACOG Committee. (2018). ACOG Committee opinion: Screening for perinatal depression. *Obstetrics and Gynecology*, *132*(5), e208–e212. https://doi.org/10.1097/AOG.0000000000002927

American Psychiatric Association. (2013). *Diagnostic and statistical manual of mental disorders* (5th ed.). American Psychiatric Publishing.

Austin, M. P., Colton, J., & Priest, S. (2013). The antenatal risk questionnaire (ANRQ): Acceptability and use for psychosocial risk assessment in the maternity setting. *Women Birth*, *26*(1), 17–25. https://doi.org/10.1016/j.wombi.2011.06.002

Austin, M. P., Highet, N., & Expert Working Group. (2017). *Mental health care in the perinatal period: Australian clinical practice guideline*. Centre for Perinatal Excellence.

Bayrampour, H., Ali, E., McNeil, D. A., Benzies, K., MacQueen, G., & Tough, S. (2016). Pregnancy-related anxiety: A concept analysis. *International Journal of Nursing Studies*, *55*, 115–130. https://doi.org/10.1016/j.ijnurstu.2015.10.023

Blair, M. M., Glynn, L. M., Sandman, C. A., & Davis, E. P. (2011). Prenatal maternal anxiety and early childhood temperament. *Stress*, *14*(6), 644–651. https://doi.org/10.3109/10253890.2011.594121

Buss, C., Davis, E. P., Hobel, C. J., & Sandman, C. A. (2011). Maternal pregnancy-specific anxiety is associated with child executive function at 6–9 years age. *Stress*, *14*(6), 665–676. https://doi.org/10.3109/10253890.2011.623250

Cox, J. L., Holden, J. M., & Sagovsky, R. (1987). Detection of postnatal depression: Development of the 10-item Edinburgh Postnatal Depression Scale. *British Journal of Psychiatry, 150*, 782–786. https://doi.org/10.1192/bjp.150.6.782

Dunkel Schetter, C. (2011). Psychological science on pregnancy: Stress processes, biopsychosocial models, and emerging research issues. *Annual Review of Psychology, 62*, 531–558. https://doi.org/10.1146/annurev.psych.031809.130727

Fertl, K. I., Bergner, A., Beyer, R., Klapp, B. F., & Rauchfuss, M. (2009). Levels and effects of different forms of anxiety during pregnancy after a prior miscarriage. *European Journal of Obstetrics & Gynecology and Reproductive Biology, 142*, 23–29. https://doi.org/10.1016/j.ejogrb.2008.09.009

Huizink, A. C., Mulder, E. J. H., Robles de Medina, P. G., Visser, G. H. A., & Buitelaar, J. K. (2004). Is pregnancy anxiety a distinctive syndrome? *Early Human Develeopment, 79*, 81–91. https://doi.org/10.1016/j.earlhumdev.2004.04.014

Koelewijn, J. M., Sluijs, A. M., & Vrijkotte, T. G. M. (2017). Possible relationship between general and pregnancy-related anxiety during the first half of pregnancy and the birth process: A prospective cohort study. *BMJ Open, 7*(e013413). https://doi.org/10.1136/bmjopen2016-013413

Kramer, M. S., Lydon, J., Seguin, L., Goulet, L., Kahn, S. R., & McNamara, H. (2009). Stress pathways to spontaneous preterm birth: The role of stressors, psychological distress, and stress hormones. *American Journal of Epidemiology, 169*(11), 1319–1326. https://doi.org/10.1093/aje/kwp061

Lovibond, S. H., & Lovibond, P. F. (1995). *Manual for the depression anxiety stress scales* (2nd ed.). Psychology Foundation. Sydney: Psychology Foundation

Madhavanprabhakaran, G. K., Kumar, K. A., Ramasubramaniam, S., & Akintola, A. A. (2013). Effects of pregnancy related anxiety on labour outcomes: A prospective cohort study. *Journal of Research in Nursing and Midwifery, 2*(7), 96–103. http:/dx.doi.org/10.14303/JRNM.2013.061

National Institute for Health and Care Excellence. (2020). *Antenatal and postnatal mental health: Clinical management and service guidance (CG192)*. Retrieved July 8, 2021, from www.nice.org.uk/guidance/cg192/resources/antenatal-and-postnatal-mental-health-clinical-management-and-service-guidance-pdf-35109869806789

Orr, S. T., Reiter, J. P., Blazer, D. G., & James, S. A. (2007). Maternal prenatal pregnancy-related anxiety and spontaneous preterm birth in Baltimore, Maryland. *Psychosomatic Medicine, 69*(6), 566–570. https://doi.org/10.1097/PSY.0b013e3180cac25d

Reilly, N., Yin, C., Monterosso, L., Bradshaw, S. N. K., Harrison, B., & Austin, M.-P. (2015). Identifying psychosocial risk among mothers in an Australian private maternity setting: A pilot study. *Australian and New Zealand Journal of Obstetrics and Gynaecology, 55*(5), 453–458. https://doi.org/10.1111/ajo.12370

Rini, C. K., Dunkel-Schetter, C., Wadhwa, P. D., & Sandman, C. A. (1999). Psychological adaptation and birth outcomes: The role of personal resources, stress, and sociocultural context in pregnancy. *Health Psychology, 18*(4), 333–345. https://doi.org/10.1037//0278-6133.18.4.333

Robertson-Blackmore, E., Gustafsson, H., Gilchrist, M., Wymand, C., & O'Connor, T. G. (2016). Pregnancy-related anxiety: Evidence of distinct clinical significance from a prospective longitudinal study. *Journal of Affective Disorders, 197*, 251–258. https://doi.org/10.1016/j.jad.2016.03.008

Shang, J., Fu, Y., Ren, Z., Zhang, T., Du, M., Gong, Q., Lui, S., & Zhang, W. (2014). The common traits of the ACC and PFC in anxiety disorders in the DSM-5: Meta-analysis of voxel-based morphometry studies. *PLoS One, 9*(3), e93432. https://doi.org/10.1371/journal.pone.0093432

Spies, G., Stein, D. J., & Roos, A. (2009). Validity of the Kessler 10 (K-10) in detecting DSM-IV defined mood and anxiety disorders among pregnant women. *Archives of Women's Mental Health, 12*(2), 69–74. https://doi.org/10.1007/s00737-009-0050-0

Strain, J. J., & Friedman, M. J. (2011). Considering adjustment disorders as stress response syndromes for DSM-5. *Depression and Anxiety, 28*, 818–823. https://doi.org/10.1002/da.20782

World Health Organisation. (2004). ICD-10: *International statistical classification of diseases and related health problems, 10th revision* (2nd ed.). World Health Organization. Retrieved from https://apps.who.int/iris/handle/10665/42980

World Health Organisation. (2020). *Classifications*. Retrieved from https://www.who.int/standards/classifications

8 Review of current scales and their psychometric properties

Andrea Sinesi, Margaret Maxwell, and Helen Cheyne

Review of current scales and their psychometric properties

As other chapters attend to, the problem of antenatal anxiety and its impact is significant and warrants early detection and intervention. This chapter looks at the concept of pregnancy-related anxiety and how it can be assessed. Pregnancy-related anxiety is a relatively recent psychological construct, which has emerged over the course of the last few decades in the research literature on perinatal mental health (Blackmore et al., 2016; Huizink et al., 2004; Levin, 1991). Dimensions of pregnancy-related anxiety, commonly described as components of this psychological construct, include fear of childbirth, concerns about the safety and health of the fetus and fetal loss, health-care-related worries, concerns about body image, as well as other pregnancy-specific fears and persistent worries (Bayrampour et al., 2016; Brunton et al., 2015) The assessment and measurement of pregnancy-related anxiety in antenatal care is of critical importance for a number of reasons. First, women experiencing this specific type of anxiety are unlikely to meet formal diagnostic criteria for an anxiety disorder (Ayers et al., 2015; Matthey & Ross-Hamid, 2011), and may thus not be identified using scales to assess anxiety symptoms developed for the general population. Second, the increased risk of a range of negative maternal and child health outcomes such as preterm birth or postnatal depression, as detailed in Chapters 5 and 6, is also of considerable importance, and evidence of the specific role played by pregnancy-related anxiety in predicting poorer health outcomes for mother and child has been documented in numerous studies (e.g., Buss et al., 2011; Orr et al., 2007). A third reason refers to the increased rates of elective cesarean sections (Klabbers et al., 2016; Koelewijn et al., 2017; Ryding et al., 1998) generally found in women experiencing fear of childbirth, a specific component of pregnancy-related anxiety also known as tokophobia (Hofberg & Ward, 2003). It can thus be argued that if women experiencing pregnancy-related anxiety or fear of childbirth were identified and offered support as early as possible in the antenatal period, this could potentially lead to a smaller number of women opting for elective cesarean section, as well as to improved birth and postnatal outcomes for mother and child. The opportunities for preventative

DOI: 10.4324/9781003014003-11

interventions are thus particularly significant in this specific area of maternity care (Sinesi et al., 2019).

While the reasons briefly outlined earlier and discussed in more detail in previous chapters would suggest that it is particularly important to identify women experiencing pregnancy-related anxiety, its assessment in clinical practice has been generally neglected and is not widely recommended in national clinical guidelines for perinatal mental health (Centre Of Perinatal Excellence [COPE], 2017; National Institute for Health and Care Excellence [NICE], 2014; Office on Women's Health, 2014;). In the UK, for instance, NICE has only recommended introduction of a brief screening tool (GAD-2 – Generalized Anxiety Disorder-2: Spitzer et al., 2006) to screen for general anxiety symptoms during pregnancy in its most recent guidelines (2014), while the use of a screening scale for pregnancy-related anxiety is not considered. There is thus currently a significant gap in the identification of pregnancy-related anxiety symptoms in the antenatal period, with potentially negative consequences for maternal and child health outcomes, both in the short and long term.

The prevalence of pregnancy-related anxiety

A number of studies have been published in recent years that have estimated the prevalence of problematic anxiety symptoms during pregnancy. It has been observed, however, that the majority of these studies have focused on the prevalence of anxiety disorders or clinically significant anxiety symptoms as determined by anxiety scales developed for the general population (Sinesi et al., 2019), such as the State-Trait Anxiety Inventory (STAI, Spielberger et al., 1983) or the Hospital Anxiety and Depression Scale (HADS, Zigmond & Snaith, 1983). A comprehensive systematic review and meta-analysis by Dennis and colleagues (2017) has recently provided estimates of the prevalence of anxiety disorders and self-reported anxiety symptoms in the antenatal period. The pooled prevalence of pregnant women meeting diagnostic criteria for an anxiety disorder was 15.2% (95% CI: 9.0%–21.4%), while self-reported anxiety symptoms (i.e., as measured by a scale) were estimated to affect 18.2% of women in the first trimester, increasing to 24.6% in the third trimester.

On the other hand, prevalence estimates specifically for pregnancy-related anxiety tend to vary considerably depending on the method of assessment used (i.e., different scales), specific timing of screening, and characteristics of the population under investigation (Leach et al., 2015). Studies on the prevalence of pregnancy-related anxiety are also somewhat scarce compared to those estimating the prevalence of general anxiety symptoms or anxiety disorders during pregnancy. Furthermore, in the context of pregnancy-related anxiety, some assessment measures were developed to include different dimensions of this construct, while others focus specifically on one of its domains (e.g., fear of childbirth; pregnancy-specific worries).

Notwithstanding the previous considerations, a small number of studies have attempted to provide an overall estimate of the prevalence of pregnancy-related anxiety or fear of childbirth. Koelewijn and colleagues (2017) estimated the prevalence of women experiencing significant symptoms of pregnancy-related anxiety to be approximately 11.0%, when measured with the Pregnancy-related Anxiety Questionnaire – Revised (PRAQ-R: Huizink et al., 2004), a scale specific to pregnancy-related anxiety and discussed later in the chapter. This study, however, simply used scores above the 90th percentile to categorize women experiencing significant pregnancy-related anxiety, with the limitation that a cutoff score was determined post hoc rather than established by validation against predefined criteria. Other studies have specifically focused on the prevalence of fear of childbirth, which is estimated to affect approximately 10.0% of pregnant women (Wijma et al., 1998). It has also been documented that at least 5.5%–6.0% of all pregnant women experience fear related to childbirth that is severe or disabling (Heimstad et al., 2006; Lukasse et al., 2014). In particular, Lukasse and colleagues (2014) conducted a large study that aimed to examine the prevalence of fear of childbirth in six European countries and found that severe fear of childbirth affected between 4.5% and 15.2% of women (respectively in Belgium and Sweden). These studies would thus appear to indicate that pregnancy-related anxiety and fear of childbirth both are relatively common in antenatal populations. The focus on these specific types of anxiety symptoms, however, has remained limited in routine antenatal care, with the consequence of missed important opportunities for early identification and support.

Current issues and perspectives in the measurement of pregnancy-related anxiety

Psychological constructs such as depression, anxiety, or pregnancy-related anxiety are intangible and consequently cannot be directly observed and measured (DeVellis, 2012). Over the course of the last century, the field of psychometric research has emerged to provide objective and standardized ways of assessing a range of psychological constructs. Self-report rating instruments (i.e., scales) typically consist of a number of effect indicators (i.e., symptoms) and can be used to measure levels of a psychological construct in an individual (Rattray & Jones, 2007). Rating scales, also known as Likert scales, have thus become increasingly popular in the assessment of psychological symptoms, for both clinical and research purposes. In rating scales, respondents are typically asked to score each item or question (i.e., assign a numerical value based on a specific characteristic such as frequency or severity) and a total score is obtained by summing the scores of all items as a measure of the overall level of the target construct in an individual (Simms, 2008). The psychometric properties of a scale can be examined in order to evaluate its overall quality and accuracy, as they indicate the extent to which a scale measures what it purports to measure (validity) in a way that is consistent and reproducible (reliability).

The assessment of pregnancy-related anxiety is potentially problematic for a number of reasons. One of the key issues is that a conceptual overlap is often found in the research literature between general symptoms of anxiety or stress during pregnancy and pregnancy-related anxiety (Ayers et al., 2015). If the target construct of a scale is not defined accurately, this may lead to assessment measures with poor psychometric properties with regard to their screening accuracy, and more generally to their content and construct validity (Sinesi et al., 2019). The accurate screening and identification of women experiencing pregnancy-related anxiety is further complicated by the fact that, unlike anxiety disorders, there is not an objective "reference standard" that can be used to compare scale scores measuring this anxiety to a standard criterion. It follows that the majority of pregnancy-related anxiety scales do not have a validated cutoff score that can be used to distinguish "positive" cases. This is a significant challenge that needs to be considered to provide an accurate assessment that would enable implementation of standardized screening procedures for women experiencing significant pregnancy-related anxiety symptoms.

With regard to psychometric properties, a number of forms of reliability and validity testing exist, and their examination can be used to evaluate the psychometric robustness of a scale. The remainder of this section provides a brief overview of the most commonly evaluated psychometric properties of scales assessing pregnancy-related anxiety. Only forms of scale reliability and validity that are relevant to the evaluation of pregnancy-related anxiety scales and to the review of the scales presented in the following section are discussed here.

Internal consistency reliability. This is the most commonly examined and reported form of scale reliability. A scale can be considered internally consistent when inter-item correlations within a scale are robust, indicating that all items are measuring the same underlying construct. This is typically determined by calculating Cronbach's alpha (Cronbach, 1951), expressed as a value between 0 and 1 with 1 indicating perfect internal consistency. The most commonly cited value of alpha that can be considered to suggest adequate internal consistency is the one indicated by Nunnally of 0.70 (1978).

Content validity. This type of validity is concerned with evaluating whether a set of items composing a scale collectively reflect the target construct and are all relevant to its measurement.

Construct validity. Two forms of validity are often considered to inform the evaluation of construct validity. Convergent or concurrent validity is based on the assumption that correlations of a scale with other scales measuring theoretically related constructs will be found to be moderately large to large. Discriminant or divergent validity is based on the assumption that the degree of correlation between a scale and other scales measuring relatively unrelated constructs will be small to moderate. Both forms of validity are typically measured by using correlation indexes such as Pearson's *r* or Spearman's rho. The widely used recommendations proposed by Cohen (1988) to evaluate the strength of correlations were used as follows: small correlation (0.10–0.29), medium correlation (0.30–0.49), and large correlation (≥0.50).

Criterion validity. This is arguably the most important indicator of scale validity, as it refers to the correlation of the scale under investigation with a criterion measure or "reference standard" of the target construct. In the psychometric literature, 70% is often cited as a minimally acceptable value for both sensitivity (i.e., proportion of true positives) and specificity (i.e., proportion of true negatives), with values over 70% considered good, ≥80% very good, and ≥90% excellent (Furr, 2011).

Structural validity. This type of validity is concerned with the factor structure of a scale and is determined by conducting principal component analysis, exploratory factor analysis, or confirmatory factor analysis on scale scores. Factors can be described as set of variables (i.e., scale items) that share common variance. Structural validity thus provides evidence of whether a scale measures a single construct or is multidimensional.

Overview of scales used for the assessment of pregnancy-related anxiety

In the following section, scales that have been or are currently used in research studies for the assessment and measurement of pregnancy-related anxiety are presented. Scales were selected based on their use in research studies or for their potential as screening tools in research and clinical settings for this specific type of anxiety. When evidence regarding their psychometric properties is available, this is also briefly discussed. The order of presentation of the scales was based on the quantity and quality of current evidence regarding their psychometric properties. This review does not include general anxiety measures used in studies with pregnant women. A detailed discussion of general anxiety measures can be found in several systematic reviews published in the last decade (Evans et al., 2015; Meades & Ayers, 2011; Sinesi et al., 2019).

Pregnancy-related Anxiety Questionnaire – Revised (PRAQ-R; PRAQ-R2)

In the context of pregnancy-related anxiety, a seminal study by Huizink and colleagues (2004) indicated that this specific psychological construct can be differentiated from general symptoms of anxiety, with only 8.0%–27.0% of pregnancy-related anxiety symptoms explained by general anxiety or depression in pregnancy as measured by scales developed for the general population (e.g., STAI, Spielberger et al., 1983). This paper has been highly cited in the literature as evidence of the clinical distinctiveness of this specific anxiety type (e.g., Bayrampour et al., 2016; Blackmore et al., 2016; Sinesi et al., 2019). The authors of this influential study used the Pregnancy Related Anxiety – Revised (PRAQ-R) to assess pregnancy-related anxiety in a sample of 230 nulliparous women at three time points during pregnancy. Study participants completed a shortened version of the PRAQ developed by Van den Bergh (1990) consisting of 34 items. The resulting PRAQ-R (Huizink et al., 2004) was obtained by conducting exploratory factor analysis on the original PRAQ, which resulted in the removal of various items due to high error variance. The PRAQ-R consists of 10-items and includes three pregnancy-related anxiety domains, namely, "Fear of giving birth,"

"Worries about bearing a physically or mentally handicapped child," and "Concern about own appearance," which were identified through confirmatory factor analysis. The internal consistency of the three factors was found to vary between $\alpha = 0.76$ and $\alpha = 0.88$. Items in the PRAQ-R are scored on a 5-point Likert scale ranging from "*Definitely not true*" to "*Definitely true.*" The scale enquires about current feelings related to these specific aspects of pregnancy (e.g., 'I am worried about the pain of contractions and the pain during delivery').

One item in the PRAQ-R (item 8: "I am anxious about the delivery, because I have never experienced one before") is only applicable to women at their first pregnancy (i.e., nulliparous). In a subsequent study, the scale developers of the PRAQ-R altered the problematic item (item 8) to make it relevant to all women regardless of parity, with the item reworded to "I am anxious about the delivery." This modification resulted in the scale's factorial and metric invariance. This further revised version of the scale was named the PRAQ-R2 and the authors indicated that it can be used with all pregnant women regardless of parity (Huizink et al., 2016). Both Westerneng and colleagues (2015) and Huizink and colleagues (2016) also confirmed a three-factor solution, as described earlier, for the scale to provide the best fit to the data. Finally, although a validated cutoff score was not indicated in the original paper (Huizink et al., 2004), a subsequent study (Matthey et al., 2013) found that the top 15% of women with higher scores were identified using a cutoff of 26 or more. In this study, the internal consistency of the scale was $\alpha = 0.82$.

Pregnancy-related Anxiety Scale (PrAS)

The PrAS was recently developed with the aim to address the gap in psychometrically robust scales for the assessment of this specific anxiety type and provide a comprehensive screening measure for use in both research and clinical settings (Brunton et al., 2018, 2019). The development of the PrAS was based on the combination of a rigorous process of conceptualization of the target construct, in order to maximize its substantive validity, and a number of statistical procedures aimed to refine the scale and discard items that did not significantly contribute to its psychometric robustness (Brunton et al., 2019). Specifically, a systematic review and input from an expert review panel were used in the initial phase of scale development to formulate a definition of the target construct that included eight pregnancy-related anxiety domains, and to formulate a preliminary item pool consisting of 217 items. This initial pool of items was subsequently reviewed by experts, who removed or revised items and endorsed a response format consisting of a 4-point Likert scale (ranging from 1 = *not at all* to 4 = *very often*). All items were also revised to check their clarity and to ensure that different domains were represented proportionally to their theoretical relevance to the construct of pregnancy-related anxiety.

In a second phase, both principal component analysis and confirmatory factor analysis were carried out on two distinct samples recruited online to further reduce the number of items and examine the factor structure of the scale.

The revised, final version of the PrAS (Brunton et al., 2018) includes 32 items, with eight identified factors (childbirth concerns, body image concerns, attitudes toward childbirth, worry about motherhood, acceptance of pregnancy, anxiety indicators, attitudes toward medical staff, avoidance and baby concerns). Cronbach's alpha for the eight domains ranged from 0.77 to 0.90. Consistently with the construct definition, specific domains considered to be central to the construct were represented with a larger number of items (e.g., childbirth concerns and anxiety indicators). Subsequently, different samples of pregnant women were recruited to test a range of psychometric properties of the scale. The PrAS' construct validity was evaluated through its concurrent and divergent validity, by examining correlations between the scale and several other scales, either theoretically related or unrelated to the target construct of the PrAS. The resulting correlations provided good evidence of both convergent and divergent validity of the scale. Furthermore, the PrAS showed an ability to discriminate between an anxious group of women (i.e., women who disclosed a current diagnosis of an anxiety disorder) and a non-anxious group. The optimal cutoff score for the scale was found to be 75.5, with an Area Under the Receiver Operating Characteristic Curve (AUROC) of 0.70 [CI (95) = 0.65–0.75] indicating a moderately accurate screening performance of the scale (Brunton et al., 2019).

These overall findings suggest that the PrAS shows promise as a screening tool for the identification of pregnancy-related anxiety, which includes domains (e.g., physical indicators of anxiety) ensuring a comprehensive assessment of the target construct and previously overlooked in other pregnancy-related anxiety scales. A potential limitation of the PrAS for applications in clinical practice is its length, as with 32 items it might be considered excessively time-consuming for screening use in routine antenatal care. While the scale developers do not advocate for a distinct interpretation of the eight subscales (Brunton et al., 2018), a key strength of the PrAS appears to lie in its ability to identify particular areas of concern, which may in turn provide health professionals with opportunities for targeted support in clinical settings.

Stirling Antenatal Anxiety Scale (SAAS)

The SAAS (Sinesi et al., 2020) is a clinically derived self-report measure that was recently developed for the identification of a range of problematic anxiety symptoms in pregnant women. It thus includes both general and pregnancy-specific anxiety items unlike other scales for the assessment of clinically significant anxiety in pregnant populations. Its development was based on a systematic review of the psychometric properties and content of existing anxiety scales used with antenatal populations (Sinesi et al., 2019) and qualitative interviews with women with experience of anxiety during pregnancy. An initial pool of items was formulated based on these two sources. The wording and clarity of items was reviewed by women with lived experience of perinatal mental health problems and their feedback used to modify and refine the wording and improve its overall clarity. The initial pool of items was subsequently reviewed, through a Delphi study, by clinicians with expertise in perinatal mental health who indicated which items they considered to be the most reliable and valid clinical indicators for the assessment of the target construct of antenatal anxiety. The SAAS includes a relatively small number of items (ten), in order to be applicable to both clinical and research settings (NICE, 2014), with three items specifically aimed to assess pregnancy-related anxiety. Examples of items included in the SAAS are "My anxiety stopped me from doing things" and "I have had negative thoughts about childbirth."

The SAAS is scored on a 5-point scale with response options ranging from "*Never*" to "*Always.*" The screening accuracy of the SAAS and its other psychometric properties were evaluated on a sample of 174 women in their second and third trimester of pregnancy. The scale showed an internal consistency reliability close to excellent (α = 0.88) and exhibited a single-factor structure. Its convergent validity was supported by a moderately large correlation with the Generalized Anxiety Disorder-7 scale (GAD-7: Spitzer et al., 2006), a measure of generalized anxiety, with a correlation coefficient of r = 0.70. The screening accuracy of the SAAS was tested against a diagnostic interview and compared to the scale currently recommended by the UK National Institute for Health and Care Excellence to screen for antenatal anxiety (i.e., GAD-2/7). The SAAS was found to have excellent sensitivity (91.0%) and very good specificity (85.0%) at its optimal cutoff score of ≥8. The SAAS also showed a superior screening performance when compared to both the GAD-2 and the GAD-7 at their NICE-recommended cutoff scores. Furthermore, in this preliminary psychometric validation of the scale, the SAAS was found to be highly acceptable to pregnant women (mean score = 9.48; range 1–10) and easy to complete (mean score = 8.93; range 1–10). The potential suitability of the SAAS for the assessment and identification of problematic antenatal anxiety, including pregnancy-related anxiety symptoms, is that it is a clinically derived measure developed specifically for this purpose on the basis of evidence from the research literature, the target population, and experts in the field. It is also one of a limited number of measures currently available that includes both general and pregnancy-specific anxiety items, thus ensuring a comprehensive assessment of problematic anxiety symptoms in the antenatal period.

Cambridge Worry Scale (CWS)

The CWS was originally developed specifically to investigate the content and extent of worries that pregnant women may experience in relation to the health of their baby, as well as other pregnancy-related concerns and more general worries (Statham & Green, 1994). Within the context of pregnancy-related anxiety, the scale developers decided to focus specifically on the construct of worry because of the connotation that it is less pathological than the construct of anxiety, and based on evidence of the significant correlation between worry and trait anxiety (Green et al., 2003). The 16 items comprising the CWS are scored on a Likert scale consisting of six response options, with the extremes being 0 ("*Not a worry*") and 5 ("*Major worry*"). Psychometric data from the Cambridge Prenatal

Screening study (see, for example, Green et al., 1993; Statham & Green, 1994), in which the scale was originally validated on a sample of over 1,200 women at three time points during pregnancy, indicated satisfactory reliability, in terms of both the scale's internal consistency reliability (Cronbach's Alpha ranging from 0.76 to 0.79 across trimesters) and test-retest reliability. The authors also evaluated the convergent validity of the CWS by examining its covariation with STAI scores and found moderate to large correlations (Pearson's $r = 0.44$–0.54). A number of studies have also explored the factor structure of the CWS (Green et al., 2003) and translated versions of the scale (e.g., Carmona Monge et al., 2012; Gourounti et al., 2012; Petersen et al., 2009) and all identified a four-factor solution, consisting of the following subscales: (i) socio-medical; (ii) health of mother and baby; (iii) socioeconomic issues; (iv) relationships with partner, family, and friends. Sinesi and colleagues (2019) in a recent systematic review compared four studies examining the factor structure of the scale and identified a small number of specific items ("The possibility of something being wrong with the baby"; and "The possibility of miscarriage" for the "Health of mother and baby" subscale, and "Giving birth" for the "Socio-medical" subscale) that were consistently found to exhibit high factor loadings in all reviewed studies, and may thus be considered robust indicators of significant pregnancy-related worries.

Pregnancy-related thoughts

This scale was originally called the Pregnancy-related Anxiety Questionnaire and was developed in the late 1990s by Rini and colleagues (1999) as a brief screening measure for pregnancy-related anxiety symptoms. Since its first use, a number of authors (e.g., Brunton et al., 2015; Matthey et al., 2013) have referred to the scale as the Pregnancy-Related Thoughts (PRT) scale to avoid confusion with other measures with the same acronym (e.g., PRAQ-R: Huizink et al., 2004). This name is also used here to distinguish it from the PRAQ-R, also reviewed earlier in the chapter. The PRT is a unidimensional measure of pregnancy-related anxiety that includes ten items, derived from previous psychometric work on this form of anxiety (Wadhwa et al., 1993), and consists of four domains (concerns about a woman's health, labor and childbirth, health of the baby, and care of the infant). Items enquire about the frequency of worries and are scored on a 4-point scale (ranging from 1 = *never* or *not at all* to 4 = *a lot of the time* or *very much*), with the total score ranging from 10 to 40. Despite its relatively frequent use in the last two decades (Bayrampour et al., 2016), very little information on its psychometric performance is available in the research literature (Brunton et al., 2015). The internal consistency reliability of the scale was originally found to be $\alpha = 0.78$ (Rini et al., 1999), and was subsequently confirmed to be acceptable in other studies ($\alpha = 0.79$ in Matthey et al., 2013; $\alpha = 0.81$ in Oliva-Pérez et al., 2019). Oliva-Pérez and colleagues (2019) also confirmed the unidimensional nature of the scale and additionally found good evidence of the scale's construct validity as indicated by moderately large correlations with theoretically related constructs and differences in scores between groups known to differ in anxiety scores.

Pregnancy-Specific Anxiety Scale (PSAS)

This pregnancy-related anxiety measure was developed in 2004 as part of a study on the effect of maternal antenatal stress and anxiety on gestational age (Roesch et al., 2004). The authors of this study derived a 4-item scale specific to pregnancy anxiety from factor analysis conducted on other pregnancy-related anxiety items, although the origin of this broader pool of items is unclear in the original paper by Roesch and colleagues (2004). The four items of the PSAS all refer to the question: "How have you felt about being pregnant in the past week, including today?" and women are asked to indicate the frequency of feeling anxious, afraid, concerned, and panicky, with response options on a 5-point scale ranging from "*Not at all*" to "*Very much*." A single score related to pregnancy-related anxiety is obtained by summing responses to the individual items. Only a limited number of studies have utilized the PSAS since its development, including an investigation from the group that originally developed the scale (Mancuso et al., 2004) and other studies that have not reported any psychometric data on the scale (e.g., Gurung et al., 2005). The internal consistency reliability of the PSAS was shown to be in the satisfactory range from Roesch and colleagues (2004) with $\alpha = 0.65–0.72$ across all trimesters of pregnancy. There is some limited evidence of the construct validity of the PSAS, as indicated by higher pregnancy-related anxiety scores correlating with shorter gestational age and preterm birth (Kramer et al., 2009; Mancuso et al., 2004; Roesch et al., 2004).

Conclusions and recommendations for future research and clinical practice

In sum, the research literature briefly discussed in the introduction and explored in more detail in other chapters of this book clearly indicates that the accurate assessment of women experiencing pregnancy-related anxiety should be considered a priority in maternity care services. Prevalence estimates of pregnancy-related anxiety have varied considerably depending on a number of factors, including the heterogeneity of scales used, the differences in the conceptualization of the target construct, and timing of assessment. It appears, however, that significant symptoms of pregnancy-related anxiety are common in the antenatal period and there is robust evidence that, if untreated, they can result in negative health outcomes for mother and child. Clinical guidelines for health professionals in a number of countries have recommended screening procedures for perinatal depression and, more recently, for perinatal anxiety (COPE, 2017; NICE, 2014). The identification of pregnancy-related anxiety, however, remains a largely overlooked area. Additional work on an accurate definition of the construct of pregnancy-related anxiety, and further psychometric investigations on the screening accuracy, as well as the acceptability, of existing pregnancy-related anxiety measures would provide the necessary evidence base for the implementation of rigorous screening in clinical practice. Timely detection and early support may be particularly beneficial for specific groups of women, including those who have experienced obstetric complications, traumatic births, or other adverse events in previous pregnancies (Dunkel-Schetter et al., 2016). Among the scales reviewed in this chapter, the choice of a specific measure is likely to depend on the purpose and setting for screening (i.e., research versus use in clinical practice by non-mental health professionals) and on further evidence regarding their psychometric robustness that may become available in the future. The PRAQ-R2 and the SAAS hold promise as brief screening tools for use in routine antenatal care or research, while the PrAS with its 32 items would appear to be best suited for research purposes.

Women's views on the use of screening scales to identify problematic anxiety symptoms in routine antenatal care were recently examined by Evans and colleagues (2017). In this qualitative study, the authors found that pregnant women were largely supportive of the use of assessment measures focusing on general anxiety and pregnancy-related anxiety, which were perceived as instrumental in facilitating conversation with health professionals and enabling women to recognize and reflect on emotional difficulties they may experience throughout pregnancy. This and other qualitative work (e.g., Furber et al., 2009) strongly suggest that the systematic use of screening procedures for mental health difficulties in the antenatal period, including pregnancy-related anxiety, is likely to be well received by women and can provide opportunities for timely monitoring and identification of psychological symptoms, so that the appropriate support or treatment can be offered when required. In this regard, screening scales for pregnancy-related anxiety such as those reviewed in this chapter can play an important role in improving the early identification and support of women, and consequently improve maternal, birth, and child outcomes.

References

Ayers, S., Coates, R., & Matthey, S. (2015). Identifying perinatal anxiety. In J. Milgrom & A. W. Gemmill (Eds.), *Identifying perinatal depression and anxiety: Evidence-based practice in screening, psychosocial assessment, and management*. Wiley-Blackwell.

Bayrampour, H., Ali, E., McNeil, D., Benzies, K., MacQueen, G., & Tough, S. (2016). Pregnancy-related anxiety: A concept analysis. *International Journal of Nursing Studies, 55*, 115–130. https://doi.org/10.1016/j.ijnurstu.2015.10.023

Blackmore, E. R., Gustafsson, H., Gilchrist, M., Wyman, C., & O'Connor, T. G. (2016). Pregnancy-related anxiety: Evidence of distinct clinical significance from a prospective longitudinal study. *Journal of Affective Disorders, 197*, 251–258. https://doi.org/10.1016/j.jad.2016.03.008

Brunton, R. J., Dryer, R., Krägeloh, C., Saliba, A., Kohlhoff, J., & Medvedev, O. (2018). The pregnancy-related anxiety scale: A validity examination using Rasch analysis. *Journal of Affective Disorders, 236*, 127–135. https://doi.org/10.1016/j.jad.2018.04.116

Brunton, R. J., Dryer, R., Saliba, A., & Kohlhoff, J. (2015). Pregnancy anxiety: A systematic review of current scales. *Journal of Affective Disorders, 176*, 24–34. https://doi.org/10.1016/j.jad.2015.01.039

Brunton, R. J., Dryer, R., Saliba, A., & Kohlhoff, J. (2019). The initial development of the pregnancy-related anxiety scale. *Women and Birth, 32*, e118–e130. https://doi.org/10.1016/j.wombi.2018.05.004

Buss, C., Davis, E. P., Hobel, C. J., & Sandman, C. A. (2011). Maternal pregnancy-specific anxiety is associated with child executive function at 6–9 years age. *Stress*, *14*, 665–676. https://doi.org/10.3109/10253890.2011.623250

Carmona Monge, F. J., Peñacoba-Puente, C., Marín Morales, D., & Carretero Abellán, I. (2012). Factor structure, validity and reliability of the Spanish version of the Cambridge Worry Scale. *Midwifery*, *28*(1), 112–119. https://doi.org/10.1016/j.midw.2010.11.006

Centre Of Perinatal Excellence. (2017). *Effective mental health care in the perinatal period: Australian COPE clinical practice guideline*. Centre of Perinatal Excellence [COPE].

Cohen, J. (1988). *Statistical power analysis for the behavioral sciences* (2nd ed.). Lawrence Erlbaum Associates.

Cronbach, L. J. (1951). Coefficient alpha and the internal structure of tests. *Psychometrika*, *16*, 297–334.

Dennis, C. L., Falah-Hassani, K., & Shiri, R. (2017). Prevalence of antenatal and postnatal anxiety: Systematic review and meta-analysis. *British Journal of Psychiatry*, *210*(5), 315–323. https://doi.org/10.1192/bjp.bp.116.187179

DeVellis, R. F. (2012). *Scale development: Theory and applications*. Sage Publications, Inc.

Dunkel-Schetter, C., Niles, A. N., Guardino, C. M., Khaled, M., & Kramer, M. S. (2016). Demographic, medical, and psychosocial predictors of pregnancy anxiety. *Paediatric and Perinatal Epidemiology*, *30*, 421–429. https://doi.org/10.1111/ppe.12300

Evans, K., Morrell, C. J., & Spiby, H. (2017). Women's views on anxiety in pregnancy and the use of anxiety instruments: A qualitative study. *Journal of Reproductive and Infant Psychology*, *35*, 77–90. https://doi.org/10.1080/02646838.2016.1245413

Evans, K., Spiby, H., & Morrell, C. J. (2015). A psychometric systematic review of self-report instruments to identify anxiety in pregnancy. *Journal of Advanced Nursing*, *71*(9), 1986–2001. https://doi.org/10.1111/jan.12649

Furber, C. M., Garrod, D., Maloney, E., Lovell, K., & McGowan, L. (2009). A qualitative study of mild to moderate psychological distress during pregnancy. *International Journal of Nursing Studies*, *46*, 669–677. https://doi.org/10.1016/j.ijnurstu.2008.12.003

Furr, R. M. (2011). *Scale construction and psychometrics for social and personality psychology*. Sage Publications, Inc.

Gourounti, K., Lykeridou, K., Taskou, C., Kafetsios, K., & Sandall, J. (2012). A survey of worries of pregnant women: Reliability and validity of the Greek version of the Cambridge Worry Scale. *Midwifery*, *28*(6), 746–753. https://doi.org/10.1016/j.midw.2011.09.004

Green, J. M., Kafetsios, K., Statham, H. E., & Snowdon, C. M. (2003). Factor structure, validity and reliability of the Cambridge Worry Scale in a pregnant population. *Journal of Health Psychology*, *8*(6), 753–764. https://doi.org/10.1177/13591053030086008

Green, J. M., Snowdon, C., & Statham, H. (1993). Pregnant women's attitudes to abortion and prenatal screening. *Journal of Reproductive and Infant Psychology*, *11*, 31–39. https://doi.org/10.1080/02646839308403192

Gurung, R. A., Dunkel-Schetter, C., Collins, N., Rini, C. K., & Hobel, C. J. (2005). Psychosocial predictors of prenatal anxiety. *Journal of Social and Clinical Psychology*, *24*, 497–519. https://doi.org/10.1521/jscp.2005.24.4.497

Heimstad, R., Dahloe, R., Laache, I., Skogvoll, E., & Schei, B. (2006). Fear of childbirth and history of abuse: Implications for pregnancy and delivery. *Acta Obstetricia et Gynecologica Scandinavica, 85*(4), 435–440. https://doi.org/10.1080/00016340500432507

Hofberg, K., & Ward, M. R. (2003). Fear of pregnancy and childbirth. *Postgraduate Medical Journal, 79*, 505–510. https://doi.org/10.1136/pmj.79.935.505

Huizink, A. C., Delforterie, M. J., Scheinin, N. M., Tolvanen, M., Karlsson, L., & Karlsson, H. (2016). Adaption of pregnancy anxiety questionnaire – revised for all pregnant women regardless of parity: PRAQ-R2. *Archives of Women's Mental Health, 19*(1), 125–132. https://doi.org/10.1007/s00737-015-0531-2

Huizink, A. C., Mulder, E. J. H., Robles De Medina, P. G., Visser, G. H. A., & Buitelaar, J. K. (2004). Is pregnancy anxiety a distinctive syndrome? *Early Human Development, 79*(2), 81–91. https://doi.org/10.1016/j.earlhumdev.2004.04.014

Klabbers, G. A., Van Bakel, H. J. A., Van den Heuvel, M. A., & Marit, M. A., & Vingerhoets, J. J. M. (2016). Severe fear of childbirth: Its features, assessment, prevalence, determinants, consequences and possible treatments. *Psychological Topics, 25*, 107–127. https://hrcak.srce.hr/156335

Koelewijn, J. M., Sluijs, A. M., & Vrijkotte, T. G. M. (2017). Possible relationship between general and pregnancy-related anxiety during the first half of pregnancy and the birth process: A prospective cohort study. *BMJ Open, 7*, e013413. https://doi.org/10.1136/10.1136/bmjopen2016-013413

Kramer, M. S., Lydon, J., Seguin, L., Goulet, L., Kahn, S. R., & McNamara, H. (2009). Stress pathways to spontaneous preterm birth: The role of stressors, psychological distress, and stress hormones. *American Journal of Epidemiology, 169*, 67–71. https://doi.org/10.1093/aje/kwp061

Leach, L. S., Poyser, C., & Fairweather-Schmidt, K. (2015). Maternal perinatal anxiety: A review of prevalence and correlates. *Clinical Psychologist, 21*(1), 4–19. https://doi.org/10.1111/cp.12058

Levin, J. S. (1991). The factor structure of the pregnancy anxiety scale. *Journal of Health and Social Behavior, 32*(4), 368–381. https://doi.org/10.2307/2137104

Lukasse, M., Schei, B., Ryding, E. L., & Group, B. S. (2014). Prevalence and associated factors of fear of childbirth in six European countries. *Sexual & Reproductive Healthcare, 5*(3), 99–106. https://doi.org/10.1016/j.srhc.2014.06.007

Mancuso, R. A., Dunkel-Schetter, C., Rini, C. M., Roesch, S. C., & Hobel, C. J. (2004). Maternal prenatal anxiety and corticotropin-releasing hormone associated with timing of delivery. *Psychosomatic Medicine, 66*, 762–769. https://doi.org/10.1097/01.psy.0000138284.70670.d5

Matthey, S., & Ross-Hamid, C. (2011). The validity of DSM symptoms for depression and anxiety disorders during pregnancy. *Journal of Affective Disorders, 133*, 546–552. https://doi.org/10.1016/j.jad.2011.05.004

Matthey, S., Valenti, B., Souter, K., & Ross-Hamid, C. (2013). Comparison of four self-report measures and a generic mood question to screen for anxiety during pregnancy in English-speaking women. *Journal of Affective Disorders, 148*(2–3), 347–351. http://dx.doi.org/10.1016/j.jad.2012.12.022

Meades, R., & Ayers, S. (2011). Anxiety measures validated in perinatal populations: A systematic review. *Journal of Affective Disorders, 133*(1–2), 1–15. https://doi.org/10.1016/j.jad.2010.10.009

National Institute for Health and Care Excellence. (2014). *Antenatal and postnatal mental health: Clinical management and service guidance (CG192)*. National Institute for Health and Clinical Excellence.

Nunnally, J. C. (1978). *Psychometric theory* (2nd ed.). McGraw-Hill.

Office on Women's Health. (2014). *U.S. Department of Health and Human Services, womenshealth.gov.* www.womenshealth.gov.

Oliva-Pérez, J., Cabrero-García, J., Cabañero-Martínez, M. J., Richart-Martínez, M., & Oliver-Roig, A. (2019). Validity and reliability of the Spanish version of the pregnancy-related thoughts scale. *Journal of Obstetric, Gynecologic, & Neonatal Nursing, 48*(5), 526–537. https://doi.org/10.1016/j.jogn.2019.07.006

Orr, S. T., Reiter, J. P., Blazer, D. G., & James, S. A. (2007). Maternal prenatal pregnancy-related anxiety and spontaneous preterm birth in Baltimore, Maryland. *Psychosomatic Medicine, 69,* 566–570. https://doi.org/10.1097/PSY.0b013e3180cac25d

Petersen, J. J., Paulitsch, M. A., Guethlin, C., Gensichen, J., & Jahn, A. (2009). A survey on worries of pregnant women – testing the German version of the Cambridge Worry Scale. *BMC Public Health, 9,* 490–498. http://doi.org/10.1186/1471-2458-9-490

Rattray, J., & Jones, M. C. (2007). Essential elements of questionnaire design and development. *Journal of Clinical Nursing, 16*(2), 234–243. https://doi.org/10.1111/j.1365-2702.2006.01573.x

Rini, C. K., Dunkel-Schetter, C., Wadhwa, P. D., & Sandman, C. (1999). Psychological adaptation and birth outcomes: The role of personal resources, stress, and sociocultural context in pregnancy. *Health Psychology, 18,* 333–345. https://doi.org/10.1037/0278-6133.18.4.333

Roesch, S. C., Dunkel-Schetter, C., Woo, G., & Hobel, C. J. (2004). Modeling the types and timing of stress in pregnancy. *Anxiety Stress and Coping, 17,* 87–102. https://doi.org/10.1080/1061580031000123667

Ryding, E. L., Wijma, B., Wijma, K., & Rydhstrom, H. (1998). Fear of childbirth during pregnancy may increase the risk of emergency cesarean section. *Acta Obstetricia et Gynecologica Scandinavica, 77,* 542–547. https://doi.org/10.1034/j.1600-0412.1998.770512.x

Simms, L. J. (2008). Classical and modern methods of psychological scale construction. *Social and Personality Psychology Compass, 2*(1), 414–433. https://doi.org/10.1111/j.1751-9004.2007.00044.x

Sinesi, A., Cheyne, H., Maxwell, M., & O' Carroll, R. O. (2020). *The development and initial psychometric validation of the Stirling Antenatal Anxiety Scale (SAAS).* NMAHP Research Unit, University of Stirling. [Manuscript in preparation].

Sinesi, A., Maxwell, M., Carroll, R., & Cheyne, H. (2019). Anxiety scales used in pregnancy: Systematic review. *BJPsych Open, 5,* 1–13. https://doi.org/10.1192/bjo.2018.75

Spielberger, C. D., Gorsuch, R. L., Lushene, R., Vagge, P. R., & Jacobs, G. A. (1983). *Manual for the state-trait anxiety inventory.* Consulting Psychologists Press.

Spitzer, R. L., Kroenke, K., Williams, J. B., & Löwe, B. (2006). A brief measure for assessing generalized anxiety disorder: The GAD-7. *Archives Internal Medicine, 166*(10), 1092–1097. https://doi.org/10.1001/archinte.166.10.1092

Statham, H., & Green, J. M. (1994). The effects of miscarriage and other 'unsuccessful' pregnancies on feelings early in a subsequent pregnancy. *Journal of Reproductive and Infant Psychology, 12,* 45–54. https://doi.org/10.1080/02646839408408867

Van den Bergh, B. (1990). The influence of maternal emotions during pregnancy on fetal and neonatal behavior. *The Journal of Prenatal and Perinatal Psychology and Health, 5,* 119–130.

Wadhwa, P. D., Sandman, C. A., Porto, M., Dunkel-Schetter, C., & Garite, T. J. (1993). The association between prenatal stress and infant birth weight and gestational age at birth: A prospective investigation. *American Journal of Obstetrics and Gynecology, 169*, 858–865. https://doi.org/10.1016/0002-9378(93)90016-c

Westerneng, M., de Cock, P., Spelten, E. R., Honig, A., & Hutton, E. K. (2015). Factorial invariance of pregnancy-specific anxiety dimensions across nulliparous and parous pregnant women. *Journal of Health Psychology, 20*(2), 164–172. https://doi.org/10.1177%2F1359105313500684

Wijma, K., Wijma, B., & Zar, M. (1998). Psychometric aspects of the W-DEQ; a new questionnaire for the measurement of fear of childbirth. *Journal of Psychosomatic Obstetrics & Gynecology, 19*(2), 84–97. https://doi.org/10.3109/01674829809048501

Zigmond, A. S., & Snaith, R. P. (1983). The hospital anxiety and depression scale. *Acta Psychiatrica Scandinavica, 67*, 361–370. https://doi.org/10.1111/j.1600-0447.1983.tb09716.x

9 Current psychological and psychosocial treatments for anxiety during pregnancy

Bronwyn Leigh and Robyn Brunton

Current psychological and psychosocial treatments for anxiety during pregnancy

One does not "become" a mother by giving birth. *Becoming* is a process that requires a psychological reorganization of one's identity, relationships, and place in the world. This process called *the motherhood mindset* is an overarching frame incorporating the numerous psychosocial adaptations required in becoming a mother (Stern & Bruschweiler-Stern, 1998).

When an expectant mother has significant pregnancy-related anxiety,[1] it may interfere with normative maternal psychological development. This interference can come from anxiety preoccupying and diminishing a woman's capacity to reflect on motherhood, a necessary developmental step in becoming a mother (Harpel, 2008; Lederman & Weiss, 2009). Anxiety may create a need for excessive reassurance behaviors that the unborn baby is well (Hart & McMahon, 2006; Lederman & Weiss, 2009) and stifle the ability of the woman to envisage the baby with personhood as the woman's mind is focused on perceived fears. Women may also psychologically distance themselves from the pregnancy (e.g., avoiding discussing it) or withhold bonding with the baby (Stern & Bruschweiler-Stern, 1998). Thus, anxiety can interfere with the developmental trajectory of becoming a mother and may make her vulnerable to psychopathology. Given this, the primary goal of any psychological or psychosocial pregnancy-related anxiety intervention should be symptom reduction *and* reconnection with the developmental processes of pregnancy.

Current interventions for anxiety in pregnancy

It has taken some years for the perinatal research lens to widen to include anxiety as a legitimate area of endeavor. Research and treatment interventions for pregnancy have tended to focus on the prevalence and development of depression (Leach et al., 2017). As a result, empirical evidence for the treatment of both non-specific anxiety in pregnancy (i.e., general anxiety that does not reference specific events, e.g., I found it difficult to relax) and specific anxiety that refers

DOI: 10.4324/9781003014003-12

to specific pregnancy-related events (Matthey & Souter, 2019) is limited. More-over, given that pregnancy-related anxiety is a "relatively new" recognized type of anxiety (Sinesi et al., 2019), few studies have examined interventions for this specific anxiety. Systematic reviews provide some confirmation that psychological and psychosocial interventions are effective for non-specific anxiety in pregnancy (e.g., Loughnan et al., 2018; Nillni et al., 2018), but few have considered pregnancy-related anxiety and further clinical trials are needed.

Therefore, this chapter aims to provide an overview of the current treatments for anxiety in pregnancy. While this review is not inclusive of all available therapies, it does present interventions that have available evidence as to their efficacy for pregnant women with anxiety. We provide tentative conclusions on these treatments as they pertain to pregnancy-related anxiety and recommendations for future directions.

First, it should be noted that while first-line treatments for mild-moderate pregnancy anxiety are usually psychological, pharmacological treatment may be recommended for moderate to severe presentations (Austin et al., 2017). However, many expectant mothers are reluctant to take psychotropic medications due to concerns for the unborn baby (Goodman et al., 2014); therefore, in this chapter, we explore only non-pharmacological treatments. For further information on pharmacological treatments, please refer to Austin et al. (2017) or the NICE Guidelines (2015).

Psychological approaches

In this section, we review cognitive-behavioral therapy, compassion focused therapy, mindfulness, and supportive counseling. When reported, we provide details of the sample, the materials and interventions used, and the type of anxiety assessed and conclude with some recommendations.

COGNITIVE BEHAVIORAL THERAPY

Several studies have examined cognitive behavior therapy as an intervention for perinatal anxiety. Green et al. (2020) conducted an intervention among 86 pregnant (36% of the sample) and postpartum (up to 6 months) women aged 22–41 years (M_{age} = 31.91, SD = 3.61) with a diagnosed DSM-V anxiety disorder. Five women were assigned to a cognitive behavior therapy group and they participated in 6 weekly 2-hour group sessions (six per group). This intervention used techniques such as psychoeducation and cognitive restructuring and the content included research on why anxiety may increase during this period and identifying problematic behaviors such as excessive reassurance-seeking. A significant and greater reduction in non-specific anxiety (State-Trait Inventory for Cognitive and Somatic Anxiety), worry (Penn State Worry Questionnaire – PSWQ), stress (Perceived Stress Scale – PSS), and depression (Edinburgh Postnatal Depression Scale – EPDS) was noted, pre-to post-intervention, for the cognitive behavior therapy group (N = 44) in comparison to controls.

In an earlier study, Green et al. (2015) examined ten women (20% pregnant, 80% up to 12 months postpartum, M_{age} = 31.20, SD = 4.50) with a diagnosed DSM-IV anxiety disorder. The women attended 6 weekly 2-hour cognitive behavior therapy group interventions (similar to the study mentioned earlier). These researchers concluded that cognitive-behavioral therapy significantly reduced non-specific anxiety, depression, worry, and stress assessed using the measures detailed earlier. These treatment outcomes were also independent of medication use and whether the woman was pregnant or postpartum. The gains in symptom reduction were maintained at 3-months follow-up but given that only two women in this sample were pregnant, it is unclear the gains were directly relevant to them.

The aforementioned results are consistent with other randomized control trials (RCTs) that assessed cognitive behavior therapy in pregnancy. These include Lowndes et al. (2019) who examined 60 pregnant women in their third trimester (N = 60, M_{age} = 32.41, SD = 3.63) who were randomly allocated to a treatment or control (i.e., a wait-list) group. The treatment comprised of a 4-week, guided self-help program with a booklet and a brief weekly phone call from a therapist. The treatment was not pregnancy-specific but rather "a summarized version of self-help CBT for perfectionism" (p. 109). There were reductions in perfectionism, non-specific anxiety (EPDS anxiety subscale), and depression (EPDS depression subscale) for the treatment group. Correspondingly, a recent systematic review (18 studies) of perinatal anxiety management concluded that given the available scientific evidence, cognitive behavior therapy should be the first-line recommended treatment for perinatal anxiety (Marchesi et al., 2016). While there is limited research on the efficacy of this therapy for pregnancy-related anxiety, it is conceivable, given the studies reviewed earlier, that tailored interventions could be effective.

COMPASSION-FOCUSED THERAPY

Compassion-focused therapy aims to strengthen the capacity for experiencing inner warmth, safeness, soothing, and kindness directed to oneself and others (Gilbert, 2015). Applied to pregnant women, the goal of this therapy is to develop self-compassion and compassion for her infant and relationship (Cree, 2010). To date, perinatal research exploring compassion-focused therapy has focused on depression, few studies have examined anxieties in pregnancy. The one study located that examined anxiety (Kelman et al., 2018) did so with 123 women (aged 18–54 years) predominantly from the United States (79%) or India (21%) who were pregnant (48%), intending to fall pregnant (39%) or given birth in the last 12 months (13%). Women were randomly assigned to one of two internet-based interventions: compassionate mind training (N = 61) or cognitive behavior therapy (N = 62), both administered over 2 weeks. The compassionate mind training included four meditation sessions and was based on standard cognitive behavior therapy concepts with some pregnancy-specific content (e.g., affect regulation and pregnancy). The cognitive behavior therapy consisted of four brief exercises focused on thoughts, activities, assertiveness, and sleep. The Patient Health Questionnaire 4 (PHQ-4) assessed depression (2-items) and the GAD-2 (2-items) assessed anxiety. Overall, near equivalence in reductions in anxiety for both interventions was found with both deemed useful as brief symptom reduction tools. While this study provides some evidence for compassionate mind training as an intervention for perinatal women, it is worth highlighting that this evidence is only preliminary given that it was not reported whether any of the women had clinical levels of anxiety and depression. More importantly, nearly 40% of the sample included women who were not pregnant, and the data analyses did not examine the outcomes specific to the three groups of women.

MINDFULNESS

Mindfulness is an awareness that comes from "paying attention on purpose, in the present moment, and non-judgmentally to the unfolding of experience moment-to-moment." (Kabat-Zinn, 2003, p. 145). Therapy approaches based on this philosophy aim to increase mindfulness, improve tolerance and regulation of negative affect, and increase psychological flexibility. Symptom reduction and mood improvement are not the primary goals but are common outcomes (Kabat-Zinn).

Single treatment group studies on mindfulness-based interventions in pregnancy have found reductions in outcomes such as anxiety, stress, and depression and increases in maternal-fetal attachment (e.g., Dunn et al., 2012; Muzik et al., 2012; Vieten et al., 2018). Duncan and Bardacke (2010) examined 27 pregnant women (M_{age} = 34.61, SD = 4.22, 93% nulliparous) in mid to late pregnancy who were well educated (nearly 80% had a bachelor's degree or higher). These women completed the *Mindfulness-based Childbirth and Parenting Program* which consisted of 9 weekly 3-hour sessions, a 7-hour silent retreat, and postpartum reunion. This program integrated mindfulness with pregnancy-specific content, such as a guided reflection around hopes/fears of pregnancy, childbirth, and parenting (see Duncan & Bardacke for detailed information). In this study, they used a pregnancy-related anxiety scale that included concerns about childbirth and the baby (e.g., I have a lot of fear regarding the health of my baby). They also assessed stress (PSS), depression (Center for Epidemiological Studies-Depression [CES-D]), and positive and negative affect. There were significant decreases for depression and some measures of positive and negative affect pre-and posttreatment. Pregnancy-related anxiety, comparatively, had the largest decrease with the largest effect size (Cohens d = 0.81).

Goodman et al. (2014) examined a mindfulness-based cognitive behavior therapy intervention for pregnant women with anxiety called *Coping with Anxiety through Living Mindfully* (CALM). This program consisted of 8 weekly 2-hour sessions, which include psychosocial education, group exercises aimed at cognitive skill development, and leader-facilitated group discussion. The content was tailored to anxieties around childbirth, the baby's well-being, and motherhood. In this study, they assessed 24 pregnant women (18 nulliparous) with a diagnosed anxiety disorder or prominent anxiety symptoms assessed by a trained therapist, recruited from a large hospital (M_{age} = 33.50, SD = 4.40; $M_{gestation}$ = 15.54, SD = 5.83). The women participated in group sessions of 6–12 women. The results indicated statistically significant improvements (p < 0.01) on a range of measures, including non-specific anxiety (Beck Anxiety Inventory – BAI), worry (PSWQ), depression (Beck Depression Inventory – BDI), self-compassion (Self-Compassion Scale – SCS), all with strong effect sizes ranging from 0.36 for anxiety to 0.58 for self-compassion (eta-squared). Of note is that of the 16 women who completed CALM and had previously met the diagnostic criteria for Generalized Anxiety Disorder at baseline, only one woman still met these criteria, post-intervention.

While single group studies support the effectiveness of mindfulness, RCTs are needed to draw causal inferences. Of the five RCTs reported in the literature, three have reported significant reductions in anxiety during the antenatal period (reviewed later) and two have reported significant reductions in stress (e.g., Lönnberg et al., 2020; Pan et al., 2019). Vieten and Astin (2008, p. 69) recruited pregnant women (M_{age} = 33.90, SD = 3.80, $M_{gestation}$ = 25.00, SD = 4.00) with a self-reported history of a mood disorder and allocated 13 to mindfulness therapy and 18 to a wait-list control group. The therapy, called the *Mindful Mother Program* included 8 weekly 2-hour sessions that were pregnancy-specific (e.g., awareness of the developing fetus and belly, an intervention manual is available from Vieten and Astin). Those who received the mindfulness therapy had significant reductions in non-specific anxiety (State Trait Anxiety Inventory – STAI), stress (PSS), and depression (CES-D) after the program, compared to controls.

Woolhouse et al. (2014) assessed the *MindBabyBody* program, a 6-week, 2-hour group program for pregnant women within a large Australian maternity hospital. The program comprised of pregnancy-specific formal and informal mindfulness practices. For example, one session includes mindfulness of physical and emotional pain, and how this relates to labor (see Woolhouse et al. for more detailed information). Women were randomly allocated to the intervention (N = 17, M_{age} = 30.81, SD = 0.75, 94% nulliparous), or a care as usual control group (N = 15, M_{age} = 34.08, SD = 0.90, 73% nulliparous). Only anxiety (Depression Anxiety Stress Scale – DASS) significantly reduced pre- to post-intervention for the mindfulness group (pre-test M = 8.62, SD = 7.72; post-test M = 4.62, SD = 3.95, p = 0.02). For all other measures (i.e., depression [CES-D, DASS], non-specific anxiety [STAI], stress [PSS, DASS]), there were no significant within- or between-group differences. It should be noted however that the DASS' anxiety items have a greater focus on somatic symptoms (e.g., feeling shaky, perspiring) than the STAI, and mindfulness may be more conducive to alleviating these symptoms (Kabat-Zinn, 2003).

To the best of our knowledge, only one study has examined pregnancy-related anxiety and mindfulness. Guardino et al. (2014) conducted an RCT with 40 pregnant women (M_{age} = 33.13, SD = 4.79; $M_{gestation}$ = 17.78, SD = 5.10), equally assigned to either a 6 weekly 2-hour mindfulness group or the control group who received a healthy pregnancy book that they read/referred to over the same period. The mindfulness training included sitting and walking meditations and managing difficult thoughts and feelings but was not pregnancy-specific. On average the women attended 4.75 (SD = 1.07) of the six classes and all but one of the participants in the control group read/referred to the book. Participants were assessed for prenatal stress and anxiety using two measures of pregnancy-related anxiety: pregnancy-specific anxiety and pregnancy-related thoughts.[2] Non-specific anxiety (STAI) and stress (PSS) were also assessed. The intervention resulted in a reduction of the pregnancy-specific anxiety/stress measures for both groups with a greater decrease for the mindfulness group post-intervention. However, this change was not sustained when assessed 6 weeks later. For the remaining measures (i.e., PSS, STAI), there were decreases, but they were not statistically significant. The findings suggest that the interventions may be effective for pregnancy-related anxiety, but further examination is needed. Moreover, the lack of pregnancy-specific content, in this intervention, compared to the more pregnancy-specific control measure, is problematic when drawing strong conclusions on the efficacy of this program for pregnancy-related anxiety.

Finally, two systematic reviews examined mindfulness-based interventions and their efficacy in reducing pregnancy anxiety. Dhillon et al. (2017), based on statistical pooling, concluded that there were no differences between the outcomes for mindfulness interventions and control groups. However, this conclusion was based on the three studies reviewed earlier and given they used heterogeneous measures of anxiety (i.e., Guardino et al. assessed pregnancy-related anxiety, whereas the others assessed non-specific anxiety), it is difficult to draw this conclusion. Conversely, when Dhillon et al. pooled the results of six non-RCTs that assessed non-specific anxiety as an outcome measure, they found a significant benefit for the mindfulness group. Given there were more studies included in this second analysis and the outcome measures were more homogeneous (i.e., all used the STAI or DASS), this result is more likely indicative of the efficacy of this therapy for pregnancy anxiety.

As described, mindfulness therapies currently have greater evidence concerning their efficacy for both non-specific pregnancy anxiety and pregnancy-related anxiety. Specific RCTs that have examined pregnancy anxiety using known measures and interventions, when tailored to pregnancy-related anxiety, were effective. Therefore, the use of psychoeducation *and* techniques that calm the mind and body may be useful in providing effective short-term symptom relief and longer-term benefits.

SUPPORTIVE COUNSELING

Both Australian (Austin et al., 2017) and United Kingdom (NICE, 2015) national perinatal mental health guidelines endorse supportive counseling (i.e., therapy with a client-centered approach) for postnatal anxiety but acknowledge there is less evidence for its efficacy for antenatal anxiety. In an Iranian RCT (Esfandiari et al., 2020), 80 pregnant women between 6 and 32 weeks gestation were assigned to either a supportive counseling group or routine care. The counseling group comprised of 6 weekly 2-hour sessions and addressed areas of pregnancy-related worries (e.g., parenting, baby's health, childbirth), all fears consistent with pregnancy-related anxiety (Bayrampour et al., 2016). In this trial, supportive counseling reduced non-specific anxiety (STAI) and pregnancy-specific distress (Revised Prenatal Distress Scale, includes medical/financial problems, health, parenting, childbirth). The routine care group, who received no intervention, showed no reduction in anxiety or distress. However, it is worth noting that these reductions in anxiety levels were not supported by changes in cortisol levels, a biomarker of anxiety, from pre-to post-intervention.

Ong et al. (2019) found that a trusting therapeutic relationship, empathic support, and engaging partners in the treatment process were important to Singaporean perinatal women in a cross-sectional study of 66 women pregnant women with anxiety or depression. The client-centered approach that characterizes supportive therapy provides women with a priority toward building the therapeutic relationship, empathic listening, and can include problem-solving, goal setting, and psychoeducation (Winston et al., 2004). These aspects of this therapy are all conducive to addressing problematic cognitions, which are an attribute of pregnancy-related anxiety.

CONCLUSION AND RECOMMENDATIONS

Psychoeducation, a feature of all the aforementioned therapies and the ability to target therapies to pregnancy concerns and fears, we believe is a necessary component of any intervention. Increasing a woman's capacity to tolerate uncertainty and reduce suffering, the hallmarks of supportive counseling are also critical features in dealing with the feeling of helplessness in the face of future worries (e.g., childbirth, baby concerns, motherhood). Qualities such as "allowing" and "sitting with" rather than avoidance of pregnancy-related cognitions may help address cognitive avoidance, which interferes with engaging in developmental processes. Additionally, the art of mindfulness is a precursor to accessing a reflective mind about the self and baby (called *early maternal mind-mindedness*) and identified as predictive of mother-infant attachment security (Meins et al., 2002). Therefore, based on the available evidence, these therapies hold potential for pregnancy-related anxiety interventions, but all require further investigation before stronger conclusions can be drawn.

Psychosocial approaches

In this section, we review current psychosocial approaches for pregnancy anxiety. These include massage therapy, physical activity, psychoeducation, relaxation training, and social support and we conclude with recommendations.

MASSAGE THERAPY

Field and colleagues have explored the role of massage in pregnancy as an anxiety reduction intervention. Field et al. (1999) assigned 26 pregnant women (M_{age} = 29.50, SD = 2.70; $M_{gestation}$ = 23.50, SD = 4.60) to either a 20-minute massage or relaxation therapy twice weekly over 5 weeks. They assessed the women pre-and post-therapy for non-specific anxiety (STAI) and pregnancy-related anxiety using the Perinatal Anxieties and Attitudes scale that assesses pregnancy and childbirth attitudes/anxieties (e.g., were you frightened when you reached the hospital). They also assessed depressed mood (CES-D, Profile of Mood Symptoms [POMS]), maternal-fetal attachment using a measure that includes perceived social support (Maternal-Fetal Attachment scale, e.g., I talk to my unborn baby), and other outcome measures such as mood, sleep, and obstetrics (e.g., delivery complications). For pregnancy anxiety, the massage therapy group reported a more optimal pregnancy experience and less pregnancy-specific worries, whereas the relaxation group reported *more* worries. Of note is that neither therapy made a significant difference in maternal-fetal attachment apart from the massage therapy group indicating improved perceived social support, whereas the relaxation therapy reported *less* perceived support. For anxiety, both groups showed initial decreases; however, the massage group showed a longer-term decrease compared to the relaxation group.

Thomas (2019) reported similar results in anxiety reduction for pregnant women (N = 12, M_{age} = 32.00, SD = 3.86, 67% nulliparous) whose partners provided them with a chair massage twice weekly. They compared group differences for pre- and post-measures of mood (EPDS) and non-specific anxiety (STAI). Significant improvements were noted for both groups with anxiety having a larger effect size (d = 0.87 and d = 1.03, respectively). However, there were several limitations in this pilot study that included the small sample size, lack of a control group, and a reliance on self-report measures, which are more susceptible to social desirability effects and sympathy/compassion for investigator effects. These limitations are likely to have influenced the results toward inflating the responses in favor of massage.

One study examined pregnancy-related anxiety using the Pregnancy Related Anxiety Questionnaire-Revised (Khojasteh et al., 2016). In this RCT, 50 nulliparous pregnant women from Iran were randomly allocated to a massage group (M_{age} = 22.76, SD = 3.85; $M_{gestation}$ = 22.12, SD = 0.93), who received 6 weekly 20-minute massages or a group who received guided imagery techniques over the same duration/frequency (M_{age} = 23.76, SD = 3.74; $M_{gestation}$ = 22.2, SD = 0.87). The control group received routine pregnancy care (M_{age} = 23.92, SD = 4.41, $M_{gestation}$ = 22.12, SD = 0.93). Both interventions showed decreases in pregnancy-related anxiety, whereas the control group did not. These findings suggest that both massage therapy and guided imagery are efficacious for pregnancy-related anxiety. However, it should be noted that the researchers indicated that education may have confounded results. The education level of those in the guided imagery group meant they were more persistent and committed to continuing the exercises, but education had no effect in the massage therapy group.

PHYSICAL ACTIVITY

Physical activity is recommended for depression in pregnancy (Austin et al., 2017; NICE, 2015), yet few studies have examined the efficacy of physical activity on antenatal anxiety (Dipietro et al., 2019). A recent systematic review and meta-analyses of 52 studies concluded from pooled results of RCTs that exercise (e.g., 150 minutes of moderate-intensity exercise) reduced antenatal depressive symptoms, but the same decrease was not evident for prenatal or postnatal non-specific anxiety symptoms (predominantly assessed as state/trait anxiety, Davenport et al., 2018). However, in this review, they regarded the evidence from the eight RCTs reviewed as potentially biased, thus the efficacy of antenatal exercise as a treatment for non-specific pregnancy anxiety symptoms is unclear.

Field et al. (2013b) examined the efficacy of yoga for pregnant women with anxiety. Yoga is considered advantageous as a physical activity for pregnant women as it is cost-effective and convenient (i.e., can be done in multiple locations) and once learned can be practiced at home. In this study, they examined 92 pregnant women (22 weeks gestation) with a clinical diagnosis of antenatal depression (structured clinical interview) who were mainly Hispanic or African American with high school education and were from low-income areas. Women were allocated to social support or yoga groups and both received 12 weekly 20-minute group interventions. The social support group ($N = 46$, $M_{age} = 24.50$, SD = 5.02) consisted of a leaderless discussion with free-flowing interactions, the staff member present remained silent. The yoga group ($N = 46$, $M_{age} = 24.40$, SD = 4.70) participated in a yoga class that was designed for women in late pregnancy and conducted by a trained instructor. Pre-to post-intervention comparisons confirmed that the yoga group had greater decreases in depression (EPDS), non-specific anxiety (STAI), and anger (State Anger Inventory, STAIX) compared to the support group who showed no significant changes. However, when the longer-term effect was assessed, that is pre-intervention to 1–3 weeks post-birth, both groups showed decreased depression (CES-D, POMS) and non-specific anxiety (STAI) suggesting both interventions may provide longer-term benefits.

PSYCHOEDUCATION

Psychoeducation has well-established effectiveness in reducing the severity of anxiety symptoms in non-perinatal adults (Rodrigues et al., 2018 provides a review). Applied to pregnant women, there is strong evidence for the use of structured psychoeducation for the treatment of mild to moderate depression (Austin et al., 2017) but less evidence for psychologically informed psychoeducation providing clinically significant benefits for anxiety symptom reduction in pregnancy (NICE, 2015).

In an RCT with pregnant Australian women in their second trimester (Toohill et al., 2014), psychoeducation was provided via midwife-led telephone counseling. This was part of the *Birth Emotions and Looking to Improve Expectant Fear* (BELIEF) program. BELIEF was adapted from the midwifery counseling framework, which aims to reduce women's fear during pregnancy and includes listening to and responding to women's feelings and providing consistent and accurate information. Women who scored high for fear of childbirth (Wijma Delivery Expectancy/Experience Questionnaire) were randomly allocated to groups.

Fear of childbirth is common in both nulliparous and multiparous women and associated with concerns about pain, obstetric experiences, birth capabilities, and baby concerns, all fears consistent with key dimension of pregnancy-related anxiety (Bayrampour et al., 2016; Saisto & Halmesmäki, 2003). The intervention group received pregnancy-specific psychoeducation via telephone at 24- and 34-week gestation. The control group received standard care. The treatment group ($N = 101$, $M_{age} = 29.00$, SD = 5.90, 57% nulliparous, $M_{gestation} = 18.20$, SD = 3.17) compared to the control group ($N = 97$, $M_{age} = 29.20$, SD = 4.98, 60% nulliparous, $M_{gestation} = 17.90$, SD = 2.80) had significant differences in post-intervention scores on the fear of childbirth measure (medium effect size). That is, women who received the intervention reported less childbirth fear than controls. Fenwick et al. (2015) reported findings from a secondary analysis from this RCT with 91 women in the intervention group and 93 controls on various outcomes such as depression (EPDS), parenting confidence, distressing childbirth flashbacks, and other obstetric outcomes (e.g., cesarean section). They reported that the intervention was efficacious in reducing flashbacks, but no other statistical differences were found between the intervention and control groups. Of note was that fewer women in the intervention group had emergency cesarean sections (18% vs. 25%), but this was not statistically significant.

RELAXATION TRAINING

Despite relaxation training being a staple anxiety management strategy, surprisingly little research has focused on the use of relaxation as a stand-alone treatment for pregnancy anxiety. In the few available studies reviewed here, anxiety symptom reduction has been evidenced in pregnant women.

Bastani et al. (2005) randomly assigned 110 nulliparous pregnant women ($M_{age} = 23.80$, SD = 3.10, $M_{gestation} = 17.80$, SD = 1.80) recruited from prenatal clinics in Iran to equal groups. The experimental group received 7 weekly 90-minute group education sessions on applied relaxation training, and they were asked to practice these techniques at home. The relaxation intervention contained some pregnancy-specific information such as a discussion about stress-related pregnancy issues. The control group received standard care. A significant reduction in non-specific anxiety (STAI) and stress (PSS) for the experimental group was noted but no significant reduction for the control group. The control group did show increased stress scores pre-to post-intervention.

More convincing evidence supporting relaxation training comes from Teixeira et al. (2005) who randomly assigned 58 pregnant women (28–32 weeks gestation) recruited from an antenatal clinic to either a passive (e.g., sitting quietly reading) and active relaxation to induce feelings of comfort. The narrative was based on hypnotherapeutic methods and developed by the stress management expert who directed the relaxation technique (see Teixeira et al. for further details). Both interventions were given once for 45 minutes and were effective in reducing maternal heart rate and self-rated non-specific pregnancy anxiety (STAI). The active relaxation however significantly lowered anxiety scores more than passive relaxation. Blood samples showed that the passive relaxation reduced cortisol and noradrenaline, whereas there was no significant change for either group for adrenaline or uterine blood flow. The authors concluded that given the interventions did not have a significant effect on the biological indices of anxiety, different interventions may be necessary to reduce both the psychological and biological effects of anxiety.

Toosi et al. (2017) examined stress and anxiety in 80 nulliparous women who conceived using IVF. Women were randomly allocated to the relaxation group or a control group that received standard care. The relaxation group consisted of 4 weekly 90-minute classes that were pregnancy-specific. For example, one session included information on signs of risk in pregnancy and coping, maternal-fetal attachment, and fetal growth. When compared pre-and post-intervention, non-specific anxiety (STAI) reduced for the intervention group but *increased* for the control group. In regard to maternal-fetal attachment, this also increased for the intervention group with no difference for the control group. These findings indicate that relaxation therapy, with a pregnancy-specific focus, could be a viable treatment for reducing non-specific anxiety during pregnancy, but given that not all studies include biological indices of anxiety, the extent to which it is effective is unknown.

SOCIAL SUPPORT

The absence of social support is a known risk factor for non-specific pregnancy anxiety (assessed with the Hospital Anxiety and Depression Scales [HADS] and BAI; Lee et al., 2007; Leigh & Milgrom, 2008). McLeish and Redshaw (2017) conducted a qualitative study with 47 pregnant women (aged 19–40+, 57% nulliparous) who received organized peer support (e.g., emotional, informational, and practical support). These women identified this support as positively impacting their emotional well-being during pregnancy (e.g., reduced low mood and anxiety). The women also said that peer-support helped them to contain their emotional distress as they could self-disclose in a safe space, and their anxieties were reduced through enhanced self-esteem and reduced isolation. The women also reported that they felt more comfortable confiding in their peers than health professionals such as midwives and doctors.

Field and colleagues (2013a) compared two interventions with pregnant women recruited from prenatal clinics. These women were primarily low-income, Hispanic or African American with high school education and diagnosed with antenatal depression using structured clinical interviews. One intervention consisted of 24 women randomly allocated to one of three groups who received weekly peer support for 12 weeks. The peer-support groups informally discussed different topics with all members actively participating. A staff member, who was not a trained therapist, attended but did not participate. The second intervention also consisted of 24 women randomly allocated into three equal groups who attended 12 weekly 1-hour interpersonal therapy group sessions. The therapy focused on pregnancy experiences and relationship problems and was based on published principles of interpersonal psychotherapy, which included the active participation of the trained therapist and the use of techniques such as encouragement of affect, communication analysis, and behavior change (see Weismann et al., 1977). Both groups experienced significant decreases in non-specific anxiety (STAI), depression (EPDS), and anger (STAIX) and salivary cortisol levels, but the decreases were greater for the peer-support group.

CONCLUSION AND RECOMMENDATIONS

Massage therapy, physical activity, and relaxation training all showed some efficacy in reducing anxiety in pregnancy. However, while they may provide an intervention that reduces anxiety symptomology, they do not target the antecedents of pregnancy-related anxiety, that is, the fears and worries that characterize it. For specific anxiety such as pregnancy-related anxiety, targeting these antecedents would seem a necessary inclusion. Therefore, as a primary intervention, the efficacy of these therapies may be limited and may serve better as complementary to psychological therapies. The evidence for peer support indicates that it may offer a cost- and time-effective intervention for anxiety in pregnancy. While social support has therapeutic benefits for well-being in pregnancy (Lebel et al., 2020), the limitation of this method, when conducted in an informal setting, is the lack of opportunity to correct misbeliefs or inaccurate perceptions that may contribute to a woman's anxieties. Indeed uncorrected, these misperceptions may be exacerbated (Smith et al., 2020).

Psychoeducation has the benefit of correcting misperceptions and is brief and can be incorporated into routine care. Psychoeducation is a feature of all the psychological therapies reviewed, yet the evidence for it providing clinically significant benefits for anxiety in pregnancy as a stand-alone intervention is limited (NICE, 2015). Notwithstanding this, based on the available evidence concerning its efficacy with fear of childbirth, it is conceivable that psychoeducation could be effective as an intervention for pregnancy-related anxiety. Therefore, future research with a broader focus that includes other dimensions of pregnancy-related anxiety (e.g., baby concerns, body image, and future motherhood) is needed. Additionally, psychoeducation concerning the psychological processes of pregnancy focusing on normative developmental and relational changes is also an area worthy of future research.

Overall conclusion

Pregnancy can bring a state of uncertainty for both the present (e.g., the developing baby) and the future (e.g., childbirth). Fears and worries from this uncertainty may manifest as pregnancy-related anxiety, which can interrupt a woman's developmental trajectory and circumvent her reflective capacity. These are both necessary activities important in developing the motherhood mindset. The development of a motherhood mindset requires a capacity for sustained reflective thought across a range of domains (e.g., self as mother, baby as a person), which a woman who is anxious about her baby's health, childbirth, or body image may find difficult. This chapter has presented current interventions for pregnancy anxiety and while some interventions have been examined for pregnancy-related anxiety and shown promise as an intervention, an urgent need exists for more research. Treatment interventions that integrate symptom management in a frame of developmental and relational change within pregnancy are likely to meet the needs of women more comprehensively during this significant life phase.

Notes

1 Previous chapters have defined pregnancy-related anxiety, see Part I of this book.
2 Both scales are reviewed in Chapter 8 of this book.

References

Austin, M.-P., Highet, N., & the Expert Working Group. (2017). *Mental health care in the perinatal period: Australian clinical practice guideline.* Centre of Perinatal Excellence.

Bastani, F., Hidarnia, A., Kazemnejad, A., Vafaei, M., & Kashanian, M. (2005). A randomized controlled trial of the effects of applied relaxation training on reducing anxiety and perceived stress in pregnant women. *Journal of Midwifery & Women's Health, 50,* 36–40. https://doi.org/10.1016/j.jmwh.2004.11.008

Bayrampour, H., Ali, E., McNeil, D. A., Benzies, K., MacQueen, G., & Tough, S. (2016). Pregnancy-related anxiety: A concept analysis. *International Journal of Nursing Studies, 55,* 115–130. https://doi.org/10.1016/j.ijnurstu.2015.10.023

Cree, M. (2010). Compassion focused therapy with perinatal and mother-infant distress. *International Journal of Cognitive Therapy, 3*(2), 159–171. https://doi.org/10.1521/ijct.2010.3.2.159

Davenport, M. H., McCurdy, A. P., Mottola, M. F. Skow, R. J., Meah, V. L., Poitras, V. J., Garcia, A. J., Gray, C. E., Barrowman, N., Riske, L., Sobierajski, F., James, M., Nagpal, T., Marchand, A., Nuspl, M., Slater, L. G., Barakat, R., Adamo, K. B., Davies, G. A., & Ruchat, M. (2018). Impact of prenatal exercise on both prenatal and postnatal anxiety and depressive symptoms: A systematic review and meta-analysis. *British Journal of Sports Medicine, 52*(21), 1376–1385. http://doi.org/10.1136/bjsports-2018-099697

Dhillon, A., Sparkes, E., & Duarte, R. V. (2017). Mindfulness-based interventions during pregnancy: A systematic review and meta-analysis. *Mindfulness, 8,* 1421–1437. https://doi.org/10.1007/s12671-017-0726-x

Dipietro, L., Evenson, K. R., Bloodgood, B., Sprow, K., Troiano, R. P., Piercy, K. L., Vaux-Bjerke, A., Powell, K. E., & 2018 Physical Activity Guidelines Advisory Committee. (2019). Benefits of physical activity during pregnancy and postpartum: An umbrella review. *Medicine and Science in Sports and Exercise, 51*(6), 1292–1302. https://doi.org/10.1249/MSS.0000000000001941

Duncan, L. G., & Bardacke, N. (2010). Mindfulness-based childbirth and parenting education: Promoting family mindfulness during the perinatal period. *Journal of Child and Family Studies, 19,* 190–202. https://doi.org/10.1007/s10826-009-9313-7

Dunn, C., Hanieh, E., & Roberts, R. (2012). Mindful pregnancy and childbirth: Effects of a mindfulness-based intervention on women's psychological distress and well-being in the perinatal period. *Archives of Women's Mental Health, 15,* 139–143. https://doi.org/10.1007/s00737-012-0264-4

Esfandiari, M., Faramarzi, M., Nasiri-Amiri, F., Parsian, H., Chehrazi, M., Pasha, H., Omidvar, S., & Gholinia, H. (2020). Effect of supportive counseling on pregnancy-specific stress, general stress, and prenatal health behaviors: A multi-center randomized controlled trial. *Patient Education and Counseling, 103*(11), 2297–2304. https://doi.org/10.1016/j.pec.2020.04.024

Fenwick, J., Toohill, J., Gamble, J., Creedy, D. K., Buist, A., Turkstra, E., Sneddon, A., Scuffman, P. A., & Ryding, E. L. (2015). Effects of a midwife psycho-education intervention to reduce childbirth fear on women's birth outcomes and postpartum psychological wellbeing. *BMC Pregnancy & Childbirth, 15,* 284. https://doi.org/10.1186/s12884-015-0721-y

Field, T., Diego, M., Delgado, J., & Medina, L. B. S. (2013a). Peer support and interpersonal psychotherapy groups experienced decreased prenatal depression, anxiety and cortisol. *Early Human Development, 89*(9), 621–624. http://dx.doi.org/10.1016/j.earlhumdev.2013.04.006

Field, T., Diego, M., Delgado, J., & Medina, L. B. S. (2013b). Yoga and social support reduce prenatal depression, anxiety and cortisol. *Journal of Bodywork & Movement Therapies, 17*(4), 397–403. http://dx.doi.org/10.1016/j.jbmt.2013.03.010

Field, T., Hemandez-Reif, M., Hart, S., Theakston, H., Schanberg, S., & Kuhn, C. (1999). Pregnant women benefit from massage therapy. *Journal of Psychosomatic Obstetrics & Gynecology, 20*(1), 31–38. https://doi.org/10.3109/01674829909075574

Gilbert, P. (2015). Affiliative and prosocial motives and emotions in mental health. *Dialogues in Clinical Neuroscience, 17*(4), 381–389.

Goodman, J. H., Guarino, A., Chenausky, K., Klein, L., Prager, J., Petersen, R., Forget, A., & Freeman, M. (2014). CALM pregnancy: Results of a pilot study of mindfulness-based cognitive therapy for perinatal anxiety. *Archives of Women's Mental Health, 17*(5), 373–387. https://doi.org/10.1007/s00737-013-0402-7

Green, S. M., Donegan, E., McCabe, R. E., Streiner, D. L., Agako, A., & Frey, B. N. (2020). Cognitive behavioral therapy for perinatal anxiety: A randomized controlled trial. *Australian & New Zealand Journal of Psychiatry, 54*(4), 423–432. https://doi.org/10.1177%2F0004867419898528

Green, S. M., Haber, E., & Frey, B. N. (2015). Cognitive-behavioral group treatment for perinatal anxiety: A pilot study. *Archives of Women's Mental Health, 18,* 631–638. https://doi.org/10.1007/s00737-015-0498-z

Guardino, C. M., Dunkel Schetter, C., Bower, J. E., Lu, M. C., & Smalley, S. L. (2014). Randomised controlled pilot trial of mindfulness training for stress reduction during pregnancy. *Psychology and Health, 29,* 334–349. https://doi.org/10.1080/08870446.2013.852670

Harpel, T. S. (2008). Fear of the unknown: Ultrasound and anxiety about fetal health. *Health, 12*(3), 295–312. https://doi.org/10.1177/1363459308090050

Hart, R., & McMahon, C. A. (2006). Mood state and psychological adjustment to pregnancy. *Archives of Women's Mental Health, 9*(6), 329–337. https://doi.org/10.1007/s00737-006-0141-0

Kabat-Zinn, J. (2003). Mindfulness-based interventions in context: Past, present, and future. *Clinical Psychology: Science and Practice, 10*(2), 144–156. https://doi.org/10.1093/clipsy/bpg016

Kelman, A. R., Evare, B. S., Barrera, A. Z., Muñoz, R. F., & Gilbert, P. (2018). A proof-of-concept pilot randomized comparative trial of brief internet-based compassionate mind training and cognitive-behavioral therapy for perinatal and intending to become pregnant women. *Clinical Psychology and Psychotherapy*, 25(4), 608–619. https://doi.org/10.1002/cpp.2185

Khojasteh, F., Rezaee, N., Safarzadeh, A., Sahlabadi, R., & Shahrakipoor, M. (2016). Comparison of the effects of massage therapy and guided imagery on anxiety of nulliparous women during pregnancy. *Der Pharmacia Lettre*, 8(19), 1–7. www.scholarsresearchlibrary.com/archive.html

Leach, L. S., Poyser, C., & Fairweather-Schmidt, K. (2017). Maternal perinatal anxiety: A review of prevalence and correlates. *Clinical Psychologist*, 21(1), 4–19. https://doi.org/10.1111/cp.12058

Lebel, C., MacKinnon, A., Bagshawe, M., Tomfohr-Madsen, L., & Giesbrecht, G. (2020). Elevated depression and anxiety symptoms among pregnant individuals during the COVID-19 pandemic. *Journal of Affective Disorders*, 277, 5–13. https://doi.org/10.1016/j.jad.2020.07.126.

Lederman, R. P., & Weiss, K. (2009). *Psychosocial adaptation to pregnancy* (3rd ed.). Springer Publishing Company.

Lee, A. M., Lam, S. K., Sze Mun Lau, S. M., Chong, C. S., Chui, H. W., & Fong, D. Y. (2007). Prevalence, course, and risk factors for antenatal anxiety and depression. *Obstetrics & Gynecology*, 110(5), 1102–1112. https://doi.org/10.1111/appy.12036

Leigh, B., & Milgrom, J. (2008). Risk factors for antenatal depression, postnatal depression and parenting stress. *BMC Psychiatry*, 8(24). https://doi.org/10.1186/1471-244X-8-24

Lönnberg, G., Jonas, W., Unternaehrer, E., Bränström, R., Nissen, E., & Niemi, M. (2020). Effects of a mindfulness based childbirth and parenting program on pregnant women's perceived stress and risk of perinatal depression – results from a randomized controlled trial. *Journal of Affective Disorders*, 262, 133–142. https://doi.org/10.1016/j.jad.2019.10.048

Loughnan, S. A., Wallace, M., Joubert, A. E., Haskelberg, H., Andrews, G., & Newby, J. M. (2018). A systematic review of psychological treatments for clinical anxiety during the perinatal period. *Archives of Women's Mental Health*, 21, 481–490. https://doi.org/10.1007/s00737-018-0812-7

Lowndes, T. A., Egan, S. J., & McEvoy, P. M. (2019). Efficacy of brief guided self-help cognitive behavioral treatment for perfectionism in reducing perinatal depression and anxiety: A randomized controlled trial. *Cognitive Behaviour Therapy*, 48(2), 106–120. https://doi.org/10.1080/16506073.2018.1490810

Marchesi, C., Ossola, P., Amerio, A., Daniel, B. D., Tonna, M., & De Panfilis, C. (2016). Clinical management of perinatal anxiety disorders: A systematic review. *Journal of Affective Disorders*, 190, 543–550. https://doi.org/10.1016/j.jad.2015.11.004

Matthey, S., & Souter, K. (2019). Is pregnancy-specific anxiety more enduring than general anxiety using self-report measures? A short-term longitudinal study. *Journal of Reproductive and Infant Psychology*, 37(4), 384–396. https://doi.org/10.1080/02646838.2019.1578869

McLeish, J., & Redshaw, M. (2017). Mothers' accounts of the impact on emotional wellbeing of organised peer support in pregnancy and early parenthood: A qualitative study. *BMC Pregnancy & Childbirth*, 17(28). https://doi.org/10.1186/s12884-017-1220-0

Meins, E., Fernyhough, C., Wainwright, R., Das Gupta, M., Fradley, E., & Tuckey, M. (2002). Maternal mind-mindedness and attachment security as predictors of theory of mind understanding. *Child Development, 73*(6), 1715–1726. https://doi.org/10.1111/1467-8624.00501

Muzik, M., Hamilton, S., Rosenblum, K. L., Waxler, E., & Hadi, Z. (2012). Mindfulness yoga during pregnancy for psychiatrically at-risk women: Preliminary results from a pilot feasibility study. *Complementary Therapies in Clinical Practice, 18*, 235–240. http://dx.doi.org/10.1016/j.ctcp.2012.06.006

NICE. (2015). *Antenatal and postnatal mental health. The NICE guideline on clinical management and service guidance.* National Institute for Health and Care Excellence.

Nillni, Y. I., Mehralizade, A., Mayer, L., & Milanovic, S. (2018). Treatment of depression, anxiety, and trauma-related disorders during the perinatal period: A systematic review. *Clinical Psychology Review, 66*, 136–148. https://doi.org/10.1016/j.cpr.2018.06.004

Ong, L. L., Ch'ng, Y. C., Chua, T. E., & Chen, H. Y. (2019). A cross-sectional survey of what patients find most therapeutic in perinatal mental healthcare in Singapore. *Asian Journal of Psychiatry, 43*, 57–59. https://doi.org/10.1016/j.ajp.2019.05.007

Pan, W.-L., Chang, C.-W., Chen, S.-M., & Gau, M.-L. (2019). Assessing the effectiveness of mindfulness-based programs on mental health during pregnancy and early motherhood – A randomized control trial. *BMC Pregnancy & Childbirth, 19*(1), 346–348. https://doi.org/10.1186/s12884-019-2503-4

Rodrigues, F., Bártolo, A., Pacheco, E., Pereira, A., Silva, C. F., & Oliveira, C. (2018). Psycho-education for anxiety disorders in adults: A systematic review of its effectiveness. *Journal of Forensic Psychology, 3*(1). https://doi.org/10.4172/2475-319X.1000142

Saisto, T., & Halmesmäki, E. (2003). Fear of childbirth: A neglected dilemma. *Acta Obstetricia et Gynecologica Scandinavica, 82*(3), 201–208. https://doi.org/10.1034/j.1600-0412.2003.00114.x

Sinesi, A., Maxwell, M., O'Carroll, R., & Cheyne, H. (2019). Anxiety scales used in pregnancy: A systematic review. *BJPsych Open, 5*(1), 1–13. https://doi.org/10.1192/bjo.2018.75

Smith, M., Mitchell, A. S., Townsend, M. L., & Herbert, J. S. (2020). The relationship between digital media use during pregnancy, maternal psychological well-being, and maternal-fetal attachment. *PLos One, 15*(12), e0243898. https://doi.org/10.1371/journal.pone.0243898

Stern, D. N., & Bruschweiler-Stern, N. (1998). *The birth of a mother: How the motherhood experience changes you forever.* Basic Books.

Teixeira, J., Martin, D., Prendiville, O., & Glover, V. (2005). The effects of acute relaxation on indices of anxiety during pregnancy. *Journal of Psychosomatic Obstetrics & Gynecology, 26*(4), 271–276. https://doi.org/10.1080/01674820500139922

Thomas, L. (2019). A pilot study of partner chair massage effects on perinatal mood, anxiety, and pain. *International Journal of Therapeutic Massage & Bodywork, 12*(2), 3–11. https://pubmed.ncbi.nlm.nih.gov/31191783/

Toohill, J., Fenwick, J., Gamble, J., Creedy, D., Buist, A., Turkstra, E., & Ryding, E.-L. (2014). A randomized controlled trial of a psycho-education intervention by midwives in reducing childbirth fear in pregnant women. *Birth, 41*(4), 384–394.

Toosi, M., Akbarzadeh, M., & Ghaemi, Z. (2017). The effect of relaxation on mother's anxiety and maternal-fetal attachment in primiparous IVF mothers. *Journal of the National Medical Association, 109*(3), 164–171. https://doi.org/10.1016/j.jnma.2017.03.002

Vieten, C., & Astin, J. (2008). Effects of a mindfulness-based intervention during pregnancy on prenatal stress and mood: Results of a pilot study. *Archives of Women's Mental Health*, *11*(1), 67–74. https://doi.org/10.1007/s00737-008-0214-3

Vieten, C., Laraia, B. A., Kristeller, J., Adler, N., Coleman-Phox, K., Bush, N. R., Wahbeh, H., Duncan, L. G., & Epel, E. (2018). The mindful moms training: Development of a mindfulness-based intervention to reduce stress and overeating during pregnancy. *BMC Pregnancy & Childbirth*, *18*(1), 201–214. https://doi.org/10.1186/s12884-018-1757-6

Weismann, M. M., Sholomskas, D., Pottenger, M., Prusoff, B. B., & Locke, B. Z. (1977). Assessing depressive symptoms in five psychiatric populations: A validation study. *American Journal of Epidemiology*, *106*, 203–214. https://doi.org/10.1093/oxfordjournals.aje.a112455

Winston, A., Rosenthal, R. N., & Pinsker, H. (2004). *Core competencies in psychotherapy. Introduction to supportive psychotherapy.* American Psychiatric Publishing, Inc.

Woolhouse, H., Mercuri, K., Judd, F., & Brown, S. J. (2014). Antenatal mindfulness intervention to reduce depression, anxiety and stress: A pilot randomised controlled trial of the MindBabyBody program in an Australian tertiary maternity hospital. *BMC Pregnancy & Childbirth*, *14*(369). www.biomedcentral.com/1471-2393/14/369

Part III
Future directions

10 Cross-cultural perspectives of pregnancy-related anxiety

Katherine S. Bright and Shahirose Sadrudin Premji

Cross-cultural perspectives of pregnancy-related anxiety

Pregnancy-related anxiety is a specific anxiety defined by pregnancy-specific fears and worries (Huizink et al., 2004). Pregnancy may give rise to many concerns because of anticipated uncertainties around pregnancy, labor, birth-related problems, the health of the infant, and parenting (Madhavanprabhakaran et al., 2015). Pregnancy-related anxiety can affect pregnant women's health and impact labor outcomes, including preterm delivery, prolonged labor, cesarean birth, and low birth weight (Hernández-Martínez et al., 2011; Rose et al., 2016).

Globally, the prevalence of pregnancy-related anxiety is high and varied ranging from 14% to 60% (Faisal-Cury & Menezes, 2007; Heron et al., 2004; Madhavanprabhakaran et al., 2015; Nasreen et al., 2011). The prevalence is generally higher in low-and middle-income countries (e.g., Brazil is reported to be up to 60%, Bangladesh is reported to be 29%; Faisal-Cury & Menezes, 2007; Nasreen et al., 2011) than high income countries (UK prevalence rates are reported to be up to 27%; Heron et al., 2004).

The timing of the assessment of pregnancy-related anxiety may partially explain these differences in prevalence. Pregnancy-related anxiety can fluctuate at different trimesters of pregnancy with higher levels noted in the first and third trimesters (Teixeira et al., 2009). Higher levels of pregnancy-related anxiety in early pregnancy is attributed to feelings about being pregnant (unwanted pregnancy) or concerns for the baby, while later in pregnancy the approaching birth and fear of birth may increase concerns (Sandman et al., 2012; Wadhwa et al., 2011), which is increasingly common in nulliparous pregnant women (Grant et al., 2008, 2009). Pregnancy-related anxiety is also influenced by cultural factors, which may explain the varied rates globally and across trimesters (Nasreen et al., 2011). Anxiety disorders occur across societies with cross-cultural variations in the presentation, symptomology, etiology, and how individuals seek care for their mental health concerns. These cultural variations are a product of the implicit values, social structure, and shared beliefs within systems (Akhtar, 1988). Several studies exploring perinatal psychological disorders have examined the role that social functioning has on women's adjustment, including attitudes and feelings to pregnancy and the postpartum period (Dunkel-Schetter et al., 2016; Gurung

DOI: 10.4324/9781003014003-14

et al., 2005; Shapiro et al., 2017). These cultural factors include differences in social norms/social issues such as emotional expression, shame, power distance, collectivism, spirituality, and religion (Gopalkrishnan, 2018).

Examples of culturally specific anxiety disorders

High-income countries

Research on pregnancy-related anxiety has predominantly been situated in high-income countries. In the recent concept analysis by Bayrampour et al. (2016), they reviewed 38 studies that identified nine dimensions of pregnancy-related anxiety. These dimensions included anxiety about fetal health, fetal loss, childbirth, parenting and caring for the child, mother's well-being, body image, health-care-related issues, financial issues, and family and social support. Additionally, they identified three critical attributes (affective responses [emotions], cognitions, and somatic complaints), three antecedents (a real or anticipated threat to pregnancy or its outcome, low perceived control, and cognitive activity and excessive thinking), and four consequences of pregnancy-related anxiety (negative attitudes and difficulty concentrating, excessive reassurance-seeking behaviors, and avoiding behaviors) (Bayrampour et al., 2016). The overall benefit of this concept analysis is that there is a precise theoretical and operational definition of pregnancy-related anxiety for high-income countries.

Low- to middle-income countries

Studies examining pregnancy-related anxiety or anxiety during pregnancy in low-to middle-income countries are sparse with most studies published in the last 15 years. These include studies of pregnant women from Vietnam, Bangladesh, Brazil, Ethiopia, Nigeria, Tanzania, Turkey, and Pakistan that focus on the prevalence of anxiety during pregnancy. Only the studies from Tanzania and Turkey looked at pregnancy-related anxiety, suggesting that pregnancy-related anxiety is an understudied concept. Qualitative studies have examined the cultural context of anxiety as it relates to local customs and beliefs that influence maternal thoughts and feelings about pregnancy and prenatal care. Overall, there have been difficulties in establishing pregnancy-related anxiety as a clear concept independent of anxiety during pregnancy. Often the literature uses pregnancy-related anxiety and anxiety during pregnancy interchangeably, resulting in a lack of understanding about pregnancy-related anxiety.

In a recent descriptive phenomenological study designed to explore and understand the experiences of pregnancy-related anxiety, Rosario et al. (2017) interviewed ten pregnant and postpartum women from Mwanza, Tanzania, who had obtained high scores on a pregnancy-related anxiety scale (i.e., the PRT, Rini et al. (1999) as reviewed in Chapter 8). While some of the themes in the women's experiences reflected the five domains addressed in the PRT (i.e., labor, delivery, baby's and mother's health, care of the baby), additional themes such as lack of knowledge, partner relationship, interactions with the health care system, spirituality, and fear of HIV/AIDS were domains identified for women in this region.

Within the domain of lack of knowledge and understanding, women reported being worried because they did not know what was "normal" in pregnancy and motherhood. Women in Mwanza also reported that their pregnancy-related anxiety stemmed from worries because their partners were absent and they felt unsupported. Additionally, these women reported that they experienced anxiety as a result of their interactions with the health care system, including access to care and quality of the care they received. One woman reported that her health care provider did not communicate information clearly, provided contradictory information, and poor advice. In this case, the woman reported that the health care provider added to her worries and her pregnancy-related anxiety.

These strained relationships with health care providers, the inability to access additional services, and lost time at work were underlying issues for many women. Additionally, these women reported that their spirituality and religion often reduced their worries and was a positive coping strategy. Women from Mwanza also reported feeling consumed with fears of HIV/AIDS, worrying about the possible impact on the developing fetus, or who would care for their baby if they (or their partners) died. These new domains of worry depict the sociocultural context of pregnancy-related anxiety and need consideration for accurate assessment of pregnancy-related anxiety in this low- and middle-income country.

In a recent best-fit framework synthesis of nine studies situated in South Asia (i.e., Pakistan, Bangladesh, Eastern India, and Nepal), Bright et al. (2018) found that pregnancy-related anxiety for South Asian women mapped onto 9 of the 11 cognitive dimensions of pregnancy-related anxiety identified by Bayrampour et al. (2016). In particular, the eight domains were fetal health, loss of fetus, childbirth, mother's well-being, parenting and care for child, health care related, financial, and family and social support. The one cognitive dimension not relevant for South Asian women was body image. Four additional pregnancy-related anxiety domains were identified for these women, which included general pregnancy concerns (i.e., worries about feeling unwell during pregnancy, that the pregnancy may interfere with household duties, and anxiety as a result of an unplanned or unwanted pregnancy), confidence and control, gender inequality (i.e., a general preference for sons, women not having decision-making control over daily household expenditures or their health-seeking behaviors, and women not permitted to work outside the home), and domestic violence (i.e., sexual, physical, and verbal abuse by any family member; sexual, physical, and verbal abuse within 6 months of their current pregnancy; verbal abuse from their husband; and generalized harassment). These additional pregnancy-related anxiety domains are important to consider in this culture to capture this specific sociocultural aspect of pregnancy-related anxiety.

Cultural factors influencing pregnancy-related anxiety

Culture is a complex concept and the context in which all human emotions, experiences, and actions are understood. Cultural factors contributing to pregnancy-related anxiety are associated with ethnopsychology and ethnophysi-ology, and/or contextual factors (Howard, 1993). Ethnopsychology is how individuals from different cultures conceptualize themselves, their emotions, per-sonality, interpretation of experiences, and human nature (Kohrt & Hruschka, 2010; White, 1992). For example, Puerto Rican women describe anxiety as feelings of nervousness, agitation, and restlessness. The experience of anxiety in this culture is often accompanied by physical complaints such as disrupted sleep, headaches, fatigue, weakness, and chest pains (Koss-Chioino, 1989). For these women, the symptoms of anxiety can also include hostility, crying episodes, and hallucinations. These characteristics of anxiety are not commonly reported in Western psychiatric literature and support the notion that culture contributes to the nature of anxiety disorders.

Ethnophysiology is the culturally guided mental process by which an indi-vidual makes sense of an idea or concept by assimilating it into the body of ideas or concepts they already hold, of the mind/body (i.e., apperception; Hinton & Hinton, 2002). Ethnophysiology may profoundly influence the understanding, experience, and treatment seeking of pregnancy-related anxiety. For example, in Puerto Rico, anxiety can present as trembling attributed to "atague de nerv-ios," a culture-bound syndrome thought to result in a loss of control, acting-out behaviors, and possibly insanity (Hinton & Pollack, 2009). Complex cultural ethnopsychological and ethnophysiological factors could possibly contribute to pregnancy-related anxiety being embodied differently cross-culturally (Csordas, 2002). These factors are not independent, rather they exist in a complex interac-tive relationship in different cultures and could uniquely influence this anxiety.

Contextual factors are associated with societal social norms and rules (Hofstede, 1984), and collectively may play a role in the development of pregnancy-related anxiety. Contextual factors of pregnancy-related anxiety include environmental (e.g., lack of support and resources, health care, low socioeconomic status) and psychological vulnerabilities (e.g., low self-esteem, helplessness; Johnson et al., 2012; Onah et al., 2017). Cultural groups express pregnancy-related anxiety according to their own understanding and beliefs about the human body's func-tioning (Hofmann & Hinton, 2014).

The autonomic arousal symptoms associated with pregnancy-related anxiety might be consistent cross-culturally, but apperception may vary (Hinton & Hin-ton, 2002). Due to a complex interaction of arousal, attention, and expecta-tion, a person becomes acutely aware of and focuses on certain bodily sensations, called an attentional amplification of physiological shifts (Hinton & Hinton, 2002). While these sensations and symptoms result from the activation of the sympathetic nervous system and thus have a biological basis, certain cultures are more prone to certain sensations during stress and anxiety. Thus, there are inherent problems in measuring pregnancy-related anxiety when using self-report measures designed without cultural considerations to assess anxiety symptoms. The complex ethnophysiologies and local epistemologies of cultures serve as a form of embodiment and a manner of naturalizing dominant social order and both aesthetic and gender ideas (Good & Good, 1982). For example, in South Asia, domestic violence is viewed as normative behavior when conflict exists in the home (Bright et al., 2018). Thus, it is reasonable to assume that biological responses to pregnancy-related anxiety may vary in cultures where domestic violence is not condoned.

Given that a society may have specific beliefs and metaphoric associations regarding symptoms and sensations of pregnancy-related anxiety, no neat boundaries exist among these realms. Therefore, a presupposed dichotomous mind-body approach to psychological and somatic manifestations of pregnancy-related anxiety must be considered. The most commonly reported physiological presentations of pregnancy-related anxiety may include sleep problems, fatigue, trembling, heart palpitations, breathlessness, hyperventilation, and tremors (Bayrampour et al., 2016). For example, in higher-income countries (e.g., the United States, Australia, and Canada), individuals with pregnancy-related anxiety tend to present within their health systems with more cognitive-based symptoms and in the acute stages of mental distress (Gopalkrishnan, 2018; Nguyen & Bornheimer, 2014). In low- and middle-income countries, such as Asia and Southeast Asia, individuals are more likely to present with somatic symptoms, yet access the health care systems less frequently due to shame-related reasons (Bright et al., 2018; Gopalkrishnan, 2018). Relatively little research around the development of pregnancy-related anxiety screening tools has focused on capturing the experience of low- and middle-income countries. Rather, these screening tools have been developed in high-income Western cultures and there is debate about whether these constructs have transferability, validity, and acceptability in different cultural settings (Bright et al., 2018; Wall et al., 2018). Women may also assign different meaning and emphasis on the various dimensions of pregnancy-related anxiety based on their cultural context (Bayrampour et al., 2016; Wall et al., 2018).

Cross-cultural cognitive dimensions of pregnancy-related anxiety

Given the recent best-fit framework (Bright et al., 2018), concept analysis (Bayrampour et al., 2016), and the research included in this chapter, we propose 14 cross-cultural cognitive dimensions of pregnancy-related anxiety (Table 10.1). These include the most frequently reported dimensions of pregnancy-related anxiety (e.g., fetal, childbirth, and parenting concerns) and issues around health care and pregnancy, finances, family, support, and decision-making and confidence. Within higher-income countries, an additional dimension is body image. More prevalent in low- and middle-income countries are gender inequality, community, and domestic violence. Understanding the dimensions of pregnancy-related anxiety can inform the development of culturally sensitive screening tools and interventions to reduce pregnancy-related anxiety. Current screening tools measure various dimensions of pregnancy-related anxiety, but none of these scales cover all the domains relevant in accurately assessing pregnancy-related anxiety cross-culturally.

Table 10.1 Cross-cultural cognitive dimensions of pregnancy-related anxiety

Dimension	Description	Dimension	Description
Fetal health Childbirth	Health and well-being of the fetus. Previous method of delivery and adverse outcomes of pregnancies	Loss of fetus Body image	Previous losses, stillbirth, neonatal and childhood death One's appearance, gaining weight and shame about pregnant appearance
Mother's well-being	Health problems in pregnancy, delivery, and postpartum (somatic symptoms). Increased maternal age, stressful life events, more perceived stress and previous mental health concerns	Parenting and newborn/child/children care	Higher parity. Looking after the children and concerns about children's illness
Health care related	Antenatal care received, access to quality reproductive health services with integrated mental health services. Quality of care provided by health care professionals and untrained health care aids	Family and social support	Insufficient partner and/or immediate family/in-law support during the perinatal period. Loss of freedom and concerns around the acceptance of the gender of the baby
Financial Community	Concerns about financial security, housing security, employment security, and food security. Resident status: lack of social support. Immigrant status: length of time in host residence, refugee or asylum-seeker status, proficiency in host country's spoken language, marriage as a reason for migration	Gender inequality Domestic violence	Gender preference (for sons). Maternal decision-making control over daily household expenditures and health-seeking behaviors for herself. Low household decision-making power and female employment outside the home Sexual, physical, and verbal abuse by any family member and/or within 6 months of the current pregnancy
Decision-making control and confidence	Concerns about control and not having the freedom to make decisions. Husband and in-laws making decisions around reproductive health and/or around daily household expenditures. Feelings of helplessness. Having nothing to be proud of	General pregnancy concerns	Willingness of pregnancy, unplanned pregnancy. Concerns about feeling unwell in pregnancy and/or not being able to meet work/caretaking/housework demands

Health care

Socioeconomic disadvantages generate hardship and stress leaving women of low- and middle-income countries susceptible to mental health conditions and deteriorating health overall (Baker et al., 2010). Additionally, the values of clinicians and service systems of low- and middle-income countries influences the nature of broader perinatal health services (Bright et al., 2018; Wall et al., 2018). The foremost barriers of access to health services include cost, societal stigma, and fragmented organization of services (Brown et al., 2007).

Access to antenatal services

Antenatal care is an important component of maternal health care in order to optimize both neonatal and maternal outcomes (Sharma, 2018). However, antenatal care in low- and middle-income countries may be less comprehensive, and the quality of care may be poor (Mbuagbaw et al., 2015). Moreover, women from relatively lower socioeconomic status are less likely to access antenatal services, let alone mental health care, even if provided (Simkhada et al., 2008). Quite often, women consider that available services are inadequate, and that the benefits of antenatal care (including mental health services) do not outweigh the potential harms (e.g., loss of family resources or physical dangers associated with travel to services) (Finlayson & Downe, 2013).

Health literacy

Health literacy refers to a set of skills that people need to function effectively in the health care environment. We propose the examination of health literacy from the health care provider perspective. Health literacy refers to the capacities of providers to understand the context of pregnancy-related anxiety, what factors are influencing it, and knowing how to address these factors (Budhathoki et al., 2019; Kwan et al., 2006; Sørensen et al., 2012). When health literacy levels are inadequate, it impacts assessment and communication with women (Coelho, 2018). This hinders a woman's own health literacy and the ability to take responsibility for their individual health in addition to their family's health and the greater community health (Lambert et al., 2014; McQueen et al., 2007). Lower levels of health literacy among health care providers can negatively impact women's health, while low health literacy among pregnant women contributes to low quality of life; both are associated with poorer health outcomes and poorer use of health care services (Berkman et al., 2011; Coelho, 2018).

Health literacy is highly influenced by personal factors (e.g., social support), cultural factors (e.g., religion and spiritual beliefs), and societal and environmental determinants (e.g., demographic situation) (Lambert et al., 2014; Sørensen et al., 2012; Zarcadoolas et al., 2003). Research into health literacy has largely been conducted in high-income countries with participants who have the ability to identify their mental health disorders (Jorm et al., 2006). Identifying pregnancy-related anxiety in low- and middle-income countries is highly influenced by culture and likely includes culture-specific dimensions such as gender inequality, as discussed earlier. Lack of recognition of these influences may be barriers to health literacy (Rowther et al., 2020). For health professionals with low health literacy, this can create a power dynamic in the prenatal relationship, which may take the voice away from pregnant women, altering the preparation they choose to undertake in health care (Rowther et al., 2020). As a result, this dynamic alters elements of problem-solving and informed choice from a shared collaboration to a more authoritarian approach to care on the part of the health care provider (Sanders & Crozier, 2018). Advancing the level of health literacy cross-culturally in relation to pregnancy-related anxiety among health care professionals requires education and improved understanding of pregnancy-related anxiety within the cultural context in which they work. Increased health literacy means more effective communication with pregnant women that in turn will improve their readability of the health system (Zarcadoolas et al., 2003) and access mental health services.

Mental health stigma

Some individuals may not seek professional help or access treatment because they feel stigmatized. Mental health stigma has the potential to impact the prevention, early detection, and treatment of pregnancy-related anxiety (Papadopoulos et al., 2013). Moore et al. (2016) identified three subthemes of stigma: internal, external, and treatment stigma.

Internal stigma refers to stigmatizing attitudes women have toward themselves such as feelings of maternal inadequacy. Internal stigma also occurs when individuals endorse external stigma (e.g., being perceived by others as a bad mother), and apply a negative evaluation to themselves (Moore & Ayers, 2017). Internal stigma may contribute to concealment of symptoms and not seeking help (Hatzenbuehler, 2016). For example, in Western-centric cultures, approximately 50% of women with perinatal mental health report stigma as the barrier to disclosing and seeking help (Moore et al., 2016). High levels of internal stigma are associated with lowered self-esteem and being perceived as an unfit mother and concerns about the forced removal of children (Moore & Ayers, 2017).

External stigma comes from stigmatizing attitudes from health care providers such as fearing that professionals would view them as an inadequate mother if they disclose anxiety symptoms. In collective cultures where conformity to norms is highly valued, it is unsurprising that mental health disorders are perceived as outside the norm and as a result are rejected and stigmatized (Hall, 1989; Heller et al., 1980). Therefore, external stigma is considered a major barrier to mental health treatment seeking (Corrigan, 2004; Keating et al., 2002).

Internal and external stigma can cause individuals to feel shame, hide their feelings, and not seek treatment (Gopalkrishnan, 2018; Hechanova & Waelde, 2017). An individual's concern about seeking and adhering to professional treatment can lead to underutilization of mental health services (Wu et al., 2017). In addition, structural issues (e.g., knowledge and availability of resources, ease of accessing services, service costs; Bright et al., 2020), are highly influenced by demographic and socioeconomic factors across countries and cultures (Gopalkrishnan, 2018). Structural stigma is an underrecognized process that produces pregnancy-related mental health inequalities (Hatzenbuehler, 2016). Individuals with pregnancy-related anxiety living in countries with higher levels of structural stigma related to mental illness will have higher rates of self-stigma and of perceived discrimination than those women in countries with lower levels of structural stigma (Thornicroft et al., 2016).

A range of complex and interactive cultural factors and systems such as norms, values, and the dimensions of individualism-collectivism can mediate the likelihood of mental health stigma occurring within a culture (Brewer & Chen, 2007; Wu et al., 2017). While there is cultural external stigma, internal stigma may also exist with pregnancy-related anxiety (Moore & Ayers, 2017).

Summary and discussion

Pregnancy is a time where there are changes in physiology, hormones, and decreased social support, potentially increasing women's risk of pregnancy-related anxiety (Huizink et al., 2004; Mulder et al., 2002). There are considerable differences in the way that pregnancy-related anxiety presents, which results in variety in the detection, reporting, and prevalence rates across cultures (Faisal-Cury & Menezes, 2007; Heron et al., 2004; Madhavanprabhakaran et al., 2015; Nasreen et al., 2011). Cultural differences encompass social norms and societal issues such as the way in which emotions are expressed as well as concepts such as shame, power, collectivism, spirituality, and religious beliefs (Gopalkrishnan, 2018). Fourteen cognitive dimensions of pregnancy-related anxiety have been proposed in this chapter that include dimensions common to most cultures (fetal and childbirth concerns, mother's well-being and body image, parenting and health care concerns, finances and family, social support; general pregnancy concerns; decision-making and confidence) and culture-specific dimensions (gender inequality; community; domestic violence).

Cultural differences in the experience and expression of pregnancy-related anxiety are largely related to ethnopsychology and ethnophysiology, that is, a pregnant woman's view of herself, which may differ from her culture (Kohrt & Hruschka, 2010). The assimilation of complex ethnopsychology and ethnophysiologies plays a significant role in the ways that pregnancy-related anxiety is personified and provides insight into the direction required to manage this anxiety (Csordas, 2002).

In this chapter we proposed the examination of health literacy from the health care provider perspective. Examining health literacy from this perspective considers the factors that contribute to pregnant women's health literacy, while stigma explains the relationship between health literacy and health outcomes (Squiers et al., 2012). Culture exerts an influence across both these areas and "affect the extent and development of health literacy skills, but they also influence how they are applied in health care systems and interactions with health care providers" (Squiers et al., 2012, p. 45).

Conclusion

Pregnancy-related anxiety is a common mental health concern among women, present across all pregnancy trimesters (Teixeira et al., 2009). Culturally, there are significant differences in the way that human emotions, experiences, and actions are expressed leading to multiple dimensions in the way pregnancy-related anxiety is understood. Health care provider's knowledge of the culture and expressed dimensions of pregnancy-related anxiety can influence communication, assessment, and health literacy of pregnant women. Stigma and health/help-seeking attitudes, beliefs, and behaviors can influence pregnant women's ability to use health literacy skills to improve quality of life and health outcomes. The perspectives presented in this chapter are intended to advance our knowledge and provide direction for future research to operationalize the complex construct of pregnancy-related anxiety. Furthermore, they should challenge us to consider the role of health literacy in both health care providers and women when considering health outcomes.

References

Akhtar, S. (1988). Four culture-bound psychiatric syndromes in India. *The International Journal of Social Psychiatry, 34*(1), 70–74. https://doi.org/10.1177% 2F002076408803400109

Baker, T. A., Buchanan, N. T., & Spencer, T. R. (2010). Disparities and social inequities: Is the health of African American women still in peril? *Ethnicity & Disease, 20*(3), 304–309. https://europepmc.org/article/med/20828107

Bayrampour, H., Ali, E., McNeil, D. A., Benzies, K., MacQueen, G., & Tough, S. (2016). Pregnancy-related anxiety: A concept analysis. *International Journal of Nursing Studies, 55*, 115–130. https://doi.org/10.1016/j.ijnurstu.2015.10.023

Berkman, N. D., Sheridan, S. L., Donahue, K. E., Halpern, D. J., & Crotty, K. (2011). Low health literacy and health outcomes: An updated systematic review. *Annals of Internal Medicine, 155*(2), 97–107. https://doi.org/10.7326/0003-4819-155-2-201107190-00005

Brewer, M. B., & Chen, Y-R. (2007). Where (who) are collectives in collectivism? Toward conceptual clarification of individualism and collectivism. *Psychological Review, 114*(1), 133–151. https://doi.org/10.1037/0033-295X.114.1.133

Bright, K. S., Charrois, E. M., Mughal, M. K., Wajid, A., McNeil, D., Stuart, S., Hayden, K. A., & Kingston, D. (2020). Interpersonal psychotherapy to reduce psychological distress in perinatal women: A systematic review. *International Journal of Environmental Research and Public Health, 17*(22), 8421. https://doi.org/10.3390/ijerph17228421

Bright, K. S., Norris, J. M., Letourneau, N. L., King Rosario, M., & Premji, S. S. (2018). Prenatal maternal anxiety in South Asia: A rapid best-fit framework synthesis. *Frontiers in Psychiatry, 9*, 467. https://doi.org/10.3389/fpsyt.2018.00467

Brown, J. S., Meadows, S. O., & Elder, G. H., Jr. (2007). Race-ethnic inequality and psychological distress: Depressive symptoms from adolescence to young adulthood. *Developmental Psychology*, *43*(6), 1295–1311. https://doi.org/10.1037/0012-1649.43.6.1295

Budhathoki, S. S., Pokharel, P. K., Jha, N., Moselen, E., Dixon, R., Bhattachan, M., & Osborne, R. H. (2019). Health literacy of future healthcare professionals: A cross-sectional study among health sciences students in Nepal. *International Health*, *11*(1), 15–23. https://doi.org/10.1093/inthealth/ihy090

Coelho, R. (2018). Perceptions and knowledge of health literacy among healthcare providers in a community based cancer centre. *Journal of Medical Imaging and Radiation Sciences*, *49*(1), S11–S12. https://doi.org/10.1016/j.jmir.2018.02.033

Corrigan, P. (2004). How stigma interferes with mental health care. *American Psychologist*, *59*(7), 614–625. https://doi.org/ 10.1037/0003-066X.59.7.614

Csordas, T. J. (2002). Embodiment as a paradigm for anthropology. In *Body/meaning/healing* (pp. 58–87). Springer Publishing Company.

Dunkel-Schetter, C., Niles, A. N., Guardino, C. M., Khaled, M., & Kramer, M. S. (2016). Demographic, medical, and psychosocial predictors of pregnancy anxiety. *Paediatric and Perinatal Epidemiology*, *30*(5), 421–429. https://doi.org/10.1111/ppe.12300

Faisal-Cury, A., & Menezes, P. R. (2007). Prevalence of anxiety and depression during pregnancy in a private setting sample. *Archives of Women's Mental Health*, *10*(1), 25–32. https://doi.org/ 10.1007/s00737-006-0164-6

Finlayson, K., & Downe, S. (2013). Why do women not use antenatal services in low-and middle-income countries? A meta-synthesis of qualitative studies. *PLoS Medicine*, *10*(1). https://doi.org/10.1371/journal.pmed.1001373

Good, B. J., & Good, M.-J. D. (1982). Toward a meaning-centered analysis of popular illness categories: "fright illness" and "heart distress" in Iran. In A. J. Marsella & G. M. White (Eds.). *Cultural conceptions of mental health and therapy. Culture, illness, and healing (studies in comparative cross-cultural research)* (Vol. 4, pp. 141–166). Springer Publishing Company.

Gopalkrishnan, N. (2018). Cultural diversity and mental health: Considerations for policy and practice. *Frontiers in Public Health*, *6*, 179. https://doi.org/10.3389%2Ffpubh.2018.00179

Grant, K. A., McMahon, C., & Austin, M. P. (2008). Maternal anxiety during the transition to parenthood: A prospective study. *Journal of Affective Disorders*, *108*(1–2), 101–111. https://doi.org/ 10.1016/j.jad.2007.10.002

Grant, K. A., McMahon, C., Austin, M. P., Reilly, N., Leader, L., & Ali, S. (2009). Maternal prenatal anxiety, postnatal caregiving and infants' cortisol responses to the still-face procedure. *Developmental Psychobiology*, *51*(8), 625–637. https://doi.org/10.1002/dev.20397.

Gurung, R. A., Dunkel-Schetter, C., Collins, N., Rini, C., & Hobel, C. J. (2005). Psychosocial predictors of prenatal anxiety. *Journal of Social and Clinical Psychology*, *24*(4), 497–519. https://doi.org/10.1136/bmjopen-2017-020056

Hall, E. T. (1989). *Beyond culture*. Anchor Books Doubleday.

Hatzenbuehler, M. L. (2016). Structural stigma: Research evidence and implications for psychological science. *American Psychologist*, *71*(8), 742–751. https://doi.org/ 10.1037/amp0000068

Hechanova, R., & Waelde, L. (2017). The influence of culture on disaster mental health and psychosocial support interventions in Southeast Asia. *Mental Health,*

Religion & Culture, *20*(1), 31–44. https://doi.org/10.1080/13674676.2017.1 322048

Heller, P. L., Chalfant, H. P., Worley, M. D. C. R., Quesada, G. M., & Bradfield, C. D. (1980). Socio-economic class, classification of 'abnormal' behaviour and perceptions of mental health care: A cross-cultural comparison. *British Journal of Medical Psychology*, *53*(4), 343–348. https://doi.org/10.1111/j.2044-8341.1980.tb02561.x

Hernández-Martínez, C., Val, V. A., Murphy, M., Busquets, P. C., & Sans, J. C. (2011). Relation between positive and negative maternal emotional states and obstetrical outcomes. *Women & Health*, *51*(2), 124–135. http://doi.org/10.1080/036 30242.2010.550991

Heron, J., O'Connor, T. G., Evans, J., Golding, J., & Glover, V. (2004). The course of anxiety and depression through pregnancy and the postpartum in a community sample. *Journal of Affective Disorders*, *80*(1), 65–73. https://doi.org/10.1016/j. jad.2003.08.004

Hinton, D., & Hinton, S. (2002). Panic disorder, somatization, and the new cross-cultural psychiatry: The seven bodies of a medical anthropology of panic. *Culture, Medicine and Psychiatry*, *26*(2), 155–178. https://doi.org/10.1023/ A:1016374801153

Hinton, D. E., & Pollack, M. H. (2009). Introduction to the special issue: Anxiety disorders in cross-cultural perspective. *CNS Neuroscience & Therapeutics*, *15*, 207–209. https://doi.org/10.1111/j.1755-5949.2009.00097.x

Hofmann, S. G., & Hinton, D. E. (2014). Cross-cultural aspects of anxiety disorders. *Current Psychiatry Reports*, *16*(6), 450. https://doi.org/10.1007%2Fs 11920-014-0450-3

Hofstede, G. (1984). The cultural relativity of the quality of life concept. *Academy of Management Review*, *9*(3), 389–398. https://doi.org/10.2307/258280

Howard, R. (1993). Transcultural issues in puerperal mental illness. *International Review of Psychiatry*, *5*(2–3), 253–260. https://doi.org/10.3109/09540269309028315

Huizink, A. C., Mulder, E. J. H., de Medina, P. G. R., Visser, G. H. A., & Buitelaar, J. K. (2004). Is pregnancy anxiety a distinctive syndrome? *Early Human Development*, *79*(2), 81–91. https://doi.org/10.1016/j.earlhumdev.2004.04.014

Johnson, M., Schmeid, V., Lupton, S. J., Austin, M. P., Matthey, S. M., Kemp, L., . . . Yeo, A. E. (2012). Measuring perinatal mental health risk. *Archives of Women's Mental Health*, *15*(5), 375–386.

Jorm, A. F., Barney, L. J., Christensen, H., Highet, N. J., Kelly, C. M., & Kitchener, B. A. (2006). Research on mental health literacy: What we know and what we still need to know. *Australian and New Zealand Journal of Psychiatry*, *40*(1), 3–5. https://doi.org/10.1111/j.1440-1614.2006.01734.x

Keating, F., Robertson, D., McCulloch, A., & Francis, E. (2002). *Breaking the circles of fear: A review of the relationship between mental health services and African and Caribbean communities.* The Sainsbury Centre for Mental Health. www.centrefor mentalhealth.org.uk/sites/default/files/breaking_the_circles_of_fear.pdf

Kohrt, B. A., & Hruschka, D. J. (2010). Nepali concepts of psychological trauma: The role of idioms of distress, ethnopsychology and ethnophysiology in alleviating suffering and preventing stigma. *Culture, Medicine, and Psychiatry*, *34*(2), 322–352. https://doi.org/10.1007/s11013-010-9170-2.

Koss-Chioino, J. D. (1989). Experience of nervousness and anxiety disorders in Puerto Rican women: Psychiatric and ethnopsychological perspectives. *Health Care for Women International*, *10*(2–3), 245–272. https://doi.org/10.1080/ 07399338909515852

Kwan, B., Frankish, J., Rootman, I., Zumbo, B., Kelly, K., Begoray, D., Kazanijan, A., Mullet, J., & Hayes, M. (2006). *The development and validation of measures of "health literacy" in different populations.* UBC Institute of Health Promotion Research and University of Victoria Community Health Promotion Research. http://blogs.ubc.ca/frankish/files/2010/12/HLit-final-report-2006-11-24.pdf

Lambert, M., Luke, J., Downey, B., Crengle, S., Kelaher, M., Reid, S., & Smylie, J. (2014). Health literacy: Health professionals' understandings and their perceptions of barriers that Indigenous patients encounter. *BMC Health Services Research*, *14*(1), 614. https://doi.org/10.1186/s12913-014-0614-1

Madhavanprabhakaran, G. K., D'Souza, M. S., & Nairy, K. S. (2015). Prevalence of pregnancy anxiety and associated factors. *International Journal of Africa Nursing Sciences*, *3*, 1–7. https://doi.org/10.1016/j.ijans.2015.06.002

Mbuagbaw, L., Medley, N., Darzi, A. J., Richardson, M., Garga, K. H., & Ongolo-Zogo, P. (2015). Health system and community level interventions for improving antenatal care coverage and health outcomes. *Cochrane Database of Systematic Reviews*, *1*(12). https://doi.org/10.1002/14651858.cd010994.pub2

McQueen, D., McQueen, D. V., Kickbusch, I., Potvin, L., Balbo, L., Abel, T., & Pelikan, J. M. (2007). *Health and modernity: The role of theory in health promotion.* Springer Science & Business Media.

Moore, D., & Ayers, S. (2017). Virtual voices: Social support and stigma in postnatal mental illness Internet forums. *Psychology, Health & Medicine*, *22*(5), 546–551. https://doi.org/10.1080/13548506.2016.1189580

Moore, D., Ayers, S., & Drey, N. (2016). A thematic analysis of stigma and disclosure for perinatal depression on an online forum. *JMIR Mental Health*, *3*(2), e18. https://doi.org/10.2196/mental.5611

Mulder, E. J., De Medina, P. R., Huizink, A. C., Van den Bergh, B. R., Buitelaar, J. K., & Visser, G. H. (2002). Prenatal maternal stress: Effects on pregnancy and the (unborn) child. *Early Human Development*, *70*(1–2), 3–14.

Nasreen, H. E., Kabir, Z. N., Forsell, Y., & Edhborg, M. (2011). Prevalence and associated factors of depressive and anxiety symptoms during pregnancy: A population based study in rural Bangladesh. *BMC Women's Health*, *11*(1), 22. https://doi.org/10.1186/1472-6874-11-22

Nguyen, D., & Bornheimer, L. A. (2014). Mental health service use types among Asian Americans with a psychiatric disorder: Considerations of culture and need. *The Journal of Behavioral Health Services & Research*, *41*(4), 520–528. https://doi.org/10.1007/s11414-013-9383-6

Onah, M. N., Field, S., Bantjes, J., & Honikman, S. (2017). Perinatal suicidal ideation and behaviour: Psychiatry and adversity. *Archives of Women's Mental Health*, *20*(2), 321–331. https://doi.org/10.1007/s00737-016-0706-5

Papadopoulos, C., Foster, J., & Caldwell, K. (2013). 'Individualism-collectivism' as an explanatory device for mental illness stigma. *Community Mental Health Journal*, *49*(3), 270–280. https://doi.org/10.1007/s10597-012-9534-x

Rini, C. K., Dunkel-Schetter, C., Wadhwa, P. D., & Sandman, C. A. (1999). Psychological adaptation and birth outcomes: The role of personal resources, stress, and sociocultural context in pregnancy. *Health Psychology*, *18*(4), 333–345. https://doi.org/10.1037/0278-6133.18.4.333

Rosario, M. K., Premji, S. S., Nyanza, E. C., Bouchal, S. R., & Este, D. (2017). A qualitative study of pregnancy-related anxiety among women in Tanzania. *BMJ Open*, *7*(8), e016072. https://doi.org/10.1136/bmjopen-2017-016072

Rose, M. S., Pana, G., & Premji, S. (2016). Prenatal maternal anxiety as a risk factor for preterm birth and the effects of heterogeneity on this relationship: A systematic review and meta-analysis. *BioMed Research International, 2016,* 8312158. https://doi.org/10.1155%2F2016%2F8312158

Rowther, A. A., Kazi, A. K., Nazir, H., Atiq, M., Atif, N., Rauf, N., Malik, A., & Surkan, P. J. (2020). "A woman is a puppet." women's disempowerment and prenatal anxiety in Pakistan: A qualitative study of sources, mitigators, and coping strategies for anxiety in pregnancy. *International Journal of Environmental Research and Public Health, 17*(14), 4926. https://doi.org/10.3390/ijerph17144926

Sanders, R. A., & Crozier, K. (2018). How do informal information sources influence women's decision-making for birth? A meta-synthesis of qualitative studies. *BMC Pregnancy Childbirth, 18*(1), 21. https://doi.org/10.1186/s12884-017-1648-2

Sandman, C., Davis, E., Glynn, L., & Morrison, J. (2012). Psychobiological stress and preterm birth. In J. Morrison (Ed.), *Preterm birth: Mother and child.* IntechOpen. https://doi.org/10.5772/1284

Shapiro, G. D., Séguin, J. R., Muckle, G., Monnier, P., & Fraser, W. D. (2017). Previous pregnancy outcomes and subsequent pregnancy anxiety in a Quebec prospective cohort. *Journal of Psychosomatic Obstetrics & Gynecology, 38*(2), 121–132. https://doi.org/10.1080/0167482x.2016.1271979

Sharma, J., O'Connor, M., & Jolivet, R. R. (2018). Group antenatal care models in low-and middle-income countries: A systematic evidence synthesis. *Reproductive Health, 15*(1), 38. https://doi.org/10.1186/s12978-018-0476-9

Simkhada, B., Teijlingen, E. R., Porter, M., & Simkhada, P. (2008). Factors affecting the utilization of antenatal care in developing countries: Systematic review of the literature. *Journal of Advanced Nursing, 61*(3), 244–260. https://doi.org/10.1111/j.1365-2648.2007.04532.x.

Sørensen, K., Van den Broucke, S., Fullam, J., Doyle, G., Pelikan, J., Slonska, Z., & Brand, H. (2012). Health literacy and public health: A systematic review and integration of definitions and models. *BMC Public Health, 12*(1), 80. https://doi.org/10.1186/1471-2458-12-80

Squiers, L., Peinado, S., Berkman, N., Boudewyns, V., & McCormack, L. (2012). The health literacy skills framework. *Journal of Health Communication, 17*(sup3), 30–54. https://doi.org/10.1080/10810730.2012.713442

Teixeira, C., Figueiredo, B., Conde, A., Pacheco, A., & Costa, R. (2009). Anxiety and depression during pregnancy in women and men. *Journal of Affective Disorders, 119*(1–3), 142–148. https://doi.org/10.1016/j.jad.2009.03.005

Thornicroft, G., Mehta, N., Clement, S., Evans-Lacko, S., Doherty, M., Rose, D., Koschorke, M., Shidhaye, R., O'Reilly, C., & Henderson, C. (2016). Evidence for effective interventions to reduce mental-health-related stigma and discrimination. *The Lancet, 387*(10023), 1123–1132. https://doi.org/10.1016/S0140-6736(15)00298-6

Wadhwa, P. D., Entringer, S., Buss, C., & Lu, M. C. (2011). The contribution of maternal stress to preterm birth: Issues and considerations. *Clinics in Perinatology, 38*(3), 351–384. https://doi.org/10.1016%2Fj.clp.2011.06.007

Wall, V., Premji, S. S., Letourneau, N., McCaffrey, G., & Nyanza, E. C. (2018). Factors associated with pregnancy-related anxiety in Tanzanian women: A cross sectional study. *BMJ Open, 8*(6), e020056. http://doi.org/10.1136/bmjopen-2017-020056

White, G. M. (1992). Ethnopsychology. In T. Schwartz, G. M. White, & C. A. Lutz (Eds.), *New directions in psychological anthropology.* Cambridge University Press.

Wu, I. H., Bathje, G. J., Kalibatseva, Z., Sung, D., Leong, F. T., & Collins-Eaglin, J. (2017). Stigma, mental health, and counseling service use: A person-centered approach to mental health stigma profiles. *Psychological Services, 14*(4), 490. https://doi.org/10.1037/ser0000165

Zarcadoolas, C., Pleasant, A., & Greer, D. S. (2003). Elaborating a definition of health literacy: A commentary. *Journal of Health Communication, 8*(S1), 119–120. https://doi.org/10.1080/713851982

11 Acculturation and antenatal anxiety in migrant women

Anna Sharapova and Betty Goguikian Ratcliff

Acculturation and antenatal anxiety in migrant women

Motherhood is a major transition in a woman's life at individual and interpersonal levels. It is a physical and psychological experience that includes major changes on biological and hormonal levels but also in the woman's identity. The latter include redefining of self, changes in personal commitments, reconsidering relationships with others, and review of professional goals (Stern, 1998). These identity transformations occur during the whole perinatal period, that is during pregnancy and postpartum. New mothers are particularly vulnerable during this time, as they need to adapt to their new role, leaving behind their usual lifestyle, accepting new responsibilities, and modifying their everyday behaviors and thoughts to adjust to the new life with the baby (Stern, 1998). The perinatal period is often characterized by disruptions and sacrifices, physical and emotional exhaustion, and loss of control over one's life (Nelson, 2003; Sardas, 2016). Given this, it is not surprising that the transition to motherhood is often accompanied by many conflicting emotions, such as intense love, joy, excitement, pride, but also fear, frustration, ambivalence, stress, anxiety, uncertainty, confusion, guilt, and loss of self-esteem (Nanzer, 2009; Sardas, 2016).

Most research about psychological distress during pregnancy focuses on depression, while anxiety has been less studied (Faisal-Cury & Rossi Menezes, 2007; Matthey et al., 2003). Scarce work in this area may be due to methodological issues, such as absence of clear definitions of antenatal anxiety, few validated instruments for the assessment of anxiety during pregnancy, or the use of measures that include physical symptoms, as well as comorbidity with depression (Heron et al., 2004; Johnson & Slade, 2003). These methodological issues are discussed in more detail in other chapters of this book and will therefore not be examined in this chapter.

Many pregnant women experience clinically significant anxiety symptoms and pregnancy-related worries. Therefore, the construct of pregnancy-related anxiety as a distinct syndrome has been proposed (Huizink et al., 2004). However, most studies on antenatal and postnatal anxiety focus on general anxiety and/ or specific anxiety disorders (Ross & McLean, 2006), with few studies that have specifically examined pregnancy-related anxiety. Consequently, in this chapter,

DOI: 10.4324/9781003014003-15

we will use the term of antenatal anxiety and refer to research related to general antenatal anxiety, including pregnancy-related anxiety, leaving aside specific anxiety disorders.

Antenatal anxiety

Anxiety during pregnancy may occur as an independent disorder or represent a significant feature of antenatal depression (Heron et al., 2004; Lee et al., 2007; Ross & McLean, 2006) Anxiety and depression disorders are highly comorbid during pregnancy (Austin et al., 2007; Field et al., 2003; Heron et al., 2004; Lee et al., 2007). However, the importance of separate assessment of antenatal anxiety and depression needs to be stressed. Clinically significant antenatal anxiety has major negative consequences: it not only represents an independent risk factor for the occurrence of postpartum depression (Austin et al., 2007; Heron et al., 2004), but it has also been associated with adverse obstetric and neonatal outcomes, such as small gestational age, low birth weight, slow fetal growth and development (Dole et al., 2003; Orr et al., 2007), preterm birth (Sandman et al., 1994), and behavior/emotional problems in the child (Foss et al., 2004; O'Connor et al., 2002).

Anxiety during pregnancy is common and often temporary, reflecting a normal psychological adjustment to a complex process of transition to motherhood (Ross & McLean, 2006). Different studies have evaluated the prevalence of general antenatal anxiety and have reported it to be as high as 21%–50% (Faisal-Cury & Rossi Menezes, 2007; Heron et al., 2004; Lee et al., 2007). Its prevalence increases during the first and the last trimesters of pregnancy (Rubertsson et al., 2014), and decreases after the birth (Heron et al., 2004; Sharapova & Goguikian Ratcliff, 2018).

Research on pregnancy-specific worries has shown that during the first trimester of pregnancy, women report experiencing anxiety as they become aware of the upcoming life transition and may also experience uncomfortable physical symptoms (Rubertsson et al., 2014). At the end of pregnancy, women usually report worries about coping with delivery, pain of childbirth, bodily changes, a safe outcome for the infant, and parenting (Faisal-Cury & Rossi Menezes, 2007; Koleva et al., 2011). Furthermore, pregnant women tend to worry about potential financial issues, work, and reconciling professional and family lives (Koleva et al., 2011). Antenatal anxiety may persist for several months, even after delivery. Mothers' worries during the postpartum period mostly concern baby's health, breastfeeding, lack of sleep, changes in the relationship with partner, financial problems, home reorganization, and returning back to work (Lugina et al., 2004; Sharapova et al., 2021). In fact, for many women who live in Western societies, decision-making concerning matters related to returning to work is a major cause of ambivalence and anxiety (Nelson, 2003).

Many internal and external factors may add to the stress inherent in the maternal transition, putting women at increased risk for antenatal anxiety. Women who have been exposed to lifetime traumatic events (Breslau et al., 1995; Heron et al.,

2004), or who have a history of anxiety disorders (Rubertsson et al., 2014), present particularly high levels of antenatal and postnatal anxiety. Those who live in precarious or disadvantaged conditions must cope with socioenvironmental stressors such as lack of personal, financial, social, or legal resources (Foss et al., 2004; Goguikian Ratcliff et al., 2015b; Razurel & Kaiser, 2015). As proposed by the cumulative stress model (Rutter, 1995), the accumulation and interaction of adversity and stressful events or daily hassles have a greater negative impact on mental health than a single major stressful event. In the following, we will discuss the impact of migration and cultural adjustment as specific risk factors for antenatal anxiety in migrant women.

Antenatal anxiety in migrant women

In this chapter, we refer to migrant women as foreign-born women who migrated as adults and went through pregnancy in the host country. Migrant mothers have been identified as being two to three times at higher risk for antenatal depression than non-migrant women, with prevalence estimates varying between 25% and 42% (Goguikian Ratcliff et al., 2015b; Lara et al., 2009; Zelkowitz et al., 2004, 2008). Migrant women appear to also be at a higher risk for antenatal anxiety. However, research that has directly examined this issue is lacking.

Several psychological, psychosocial, and sociocultural factors specific to migration explain the increased vulnerability of migrant women to antenatal distress. We will first consider sociocultural factors as they have received less attention in the literature than psychosocial or environmental factors.

In our view, culture is a set of practices executed in a tangible and observable way by a social group, as well as internal patterns and belief systems, each level mutually reinforcing the other (Licata & Heine, 2012). Human development is thus embedded in social networks, interpersonal relations, and the local cultural environment. Therefore, culture plays an important role in shaping our identity and personality within a specific historical and cultural context (Guerraoui & Troadec, 2000). At the same time, important interindividual differences may exist within the same cultural community (Moro, 1994). Culture is not a static and concrete reality, as members of a social group continually adapt to ever-changing environments and modify cultural norms (Jahoda, 2012).

Migration involves moving from one political, socioeconomic, and cultural system to another. Therefore, pregnant migrant women, especially primiparas, are experiencing overlapping life transitions: a sociocultural transition calling for an acculturation process and a developmental transition to motherhood (Foss et al., 2004; Goguikian Ratcliff et al., 2015a). For migrant women, the disruption that characterizes the transition to motherhood as a major life event is magnified as they are far from their familiar cultural environment and lack support from family and community.

Childbirth and child-rearing are culturally loaded human activities. Culture determines how the future mother will perceive her pregnancy and prepare her for motherhood. Pregnancy and childbirth are not only biological events, they are also associated with culturally based rituals, and each culture has its own beliefs and practices related to the perinatal period. The latter mainly refer to how to protect the mother and the child during this time of vulnerability and how to recognize and welcome a new member of the group (Bina, 2008; Team et al., 2009). This cultural frame links the woman to her social group, strengthening her sense of belonging, embodying the intergenerational continuity, actualizing the family ties, and increasing the sense of support and security (Goguikian Ratcliff et al., 2015a; Mestre, 2016).

Pregnancy and delivery in a different cultural environment often force migrant women to get to know the local society with its requirements, traditions, practices, and institutional functioning. They need to go through the confrontation of two cultural frameworks, which may represent a source of contradiction, incongruity, and, as stated by certain authors, anxiety (Baubet & Moro, 2013). Migrant mothers may face contradictory recommendations and therefore report elevated pregnancy-related anxiety concerning the choice of appropriate practices, the baby's health, and doubts related to their maternal competence (Fortin & Le Gall, 2007). The stress is magnified when the cultural distance between the two cultural frameworks is significant (Hanlon et al., 2008), as it may be the case when women from collectivistic traditional societies (e.g., Western Africa rural areas) where biomedicine and medical technology is poorly developed move to more individualistic and modern societies (e.g., urban Western countries).

Acculturation and pregnancy

Migrants who move from one cultural context to another must go through the process of acculturation to achieve cultural adjustment. Acculturation is defined as a dynamic and ongoing process of cultural modification of an individual or a group by adapting to or borrowing traits from the new culture they enter in contact with (host culture). Modification occurs in terms of values, behavior, character, and language skills (Berry, 1970, 1980; Ryder et al., 2000). However, acculturation is more than a cultural learning. For instance, the psychological integration of new views requires flexibility and complexifies the previous self-identity (Berry, 1997).

In the age of globalization, one's identity may be a result of multiple cultural affiliations (Berry, 1997; Chanson, 2011). Thus, in recent studies, acculturation is defined and measured as a bi- or multidimensional process in which different belongings may coexist: individuals may maintain their heritage culture and at the same time choose to adopt new practices (Berry, 1997; Gibson, 2001; Ryder et al., 2000; Tadmor et al., 2009). Therefore, migrant parents do not simply replicate the original or local practices but find themselves in an intercultural frame and may consciously create mixed parenting practices (Goguikian Ratcliff & Diaz-Marchand, 2019; Guerraoui & Troadec, 2000).

For pregnant migrant women, acculturation occurs through the process of conciliation of culturally different pregnancy-related knowledge and practices. For example, in many non-Western societies, especially rural and traditional ones, pregnancy is seen as a natural phenomenon that does not call for medical intervention (Team et al., 2009). In collectivistic traditional societies, pregnancy and postpartum is a period when family and community support of the elder women of the families is crucial for the future mother, while marital support is more peripheral. Elder women provide guidance, knowledge, and know-how (Choudhry, 1997; Simkhada et al., 2007). These women also ensure emotional support that can reduce pregnancy-related and general antenatal anxiety (Capponi & Horbacz, 2007). Traditional practices and rituals are brought into play to protect the mother and the baby from spirits and other dangers and negative outcomes (Team et al., 2009). These practices may include special diet, songs, gifts, religious ceremonies, sleep routines, activities, and a set of prohibitions. These practices are transmitted from generation to generation and are underpinned by a coherent set of cultural representations (Team et al., 2009; Von Overbeck Ottino, 2011).

In comparison, in individualistic Western societies, medical assistance is perceived as an essential component of pregnancy and childbirth. Expectant mothers benefit from a medical follow-up from the first weeks of pregnancy and may partake in birth preparation classes provided by a midwife, often with their partner. Western pregnant women tend to focus on professional assistance and their nuclear family rather than on extended family or community support (Moro & Drain, 2009). Furthermore, the social context related to pregnancy and birth has changed in the past few decades. Several authors have introduced the concept of "modern motherhood" (van Doorne-Huiskes & Doorten, 2010), which reflects motherhood as a woman's personal accomplishment and entails conciliation of professional and family life. In these societies, kin networks and the role and importance of kinship during the perinatal period are in decline. With the use of contraception, maternity has become for many women a conscious choice and a personal responsibility, so that transition to parenthood is perceived as an individual or marital matter (van Doorne-Huiskes & Doorten, 2010). Therefore, the quality of the marital relationship and marital support are central factors in Western women's perinatal mental health (Fortin & Le Gall, 2007; Zelkowitz et al., 2004).

Acculturation and its impact on antenatal anxiety

Migrant mothers face a complex situation in which they need to strike a balance between preserving the intergenerational and family bonds and adopting a number of new practices that are relevant in the new cultural context. The challenge consists therefore in transformation and creation of mixed or hybrid practices (Goguikian Ratcliff & Diaz-Marchand, 2019). As a result of continuous contact with the host culture, acculturating migrants may start to adapt representations and practices of their culture of origin to those of the local culture (Fortin & Le Gall, 2007; Rabain-Jamin & Wornham, 1990). As highlighted earlier, culture is not static, and human behavior interacts with the cultural context within which it occurs (Berry, 1997). Most migrant women follow practices of both cultural references simultaneously (e.g., taking medication and traditional herbal drink); some women choose between the two recommendations (e.g., for a cold, she will see a doctor, and for nausea, she will refer to traditional practices). Only few women choose to follow exclusively practices of their home country (Baubet & Moro, 2013; Rabain-Jamin & Wornham, 1990; Sharapova et al., 2021). The latter strategy may represent the lack of mental flexibility associated with adaptation capacities.

Little is known about the impact of the acculturation process on antenatal or postnatal anxiety in first-generation migrant women (Beck, 2006; Bornstein & Cote, 2006; Fung & Dennis, 2010). Most studies have focused on postpartum depression in second-generation migrant women (Heilemann et al., 2004; Martinez-Schallmoser et al., 2003). Given the scarcity of research specific to pregnancy-related anxiety and acculturation, in comparison to the research available on depression, we present some results concerning depression. Considering the high comorbidity between antenatal and postnatal anxiety and depression, it may be hypothesized that similar findings could be found for antenatal anxiety.

Research on acculturation and antenatal and/or postnatal depression has shown inconsistent results. These inconsistencies may relate to the definition of migrant women or the definition and operationalization of the concept of acculturation. First, a key methodological issue is related to the population of the studies. Most studies include or exclusively focus on second-generation migrant women. This raises important questions as acculturating people have been initially defined as migrants who enter in contact with a new culture and who are going through the process of adaptation to that culture (Berry, 1970, 1980). Second-generation migrant women were born and brought up in the dominant culture and therefore were not exposed to the migration experience, nor to the process of acculturation. Thus, measuring acculturation in second-generation women, who belong to ethnic minority groups, essentializes their cultural difference, and might rather represent a measure of perceived discrimination and marginalization.

Second, acculturation has been often defined as a unidimensional construct, that is, the degree of cultural learning or assimilation of the host culture's practices or features. Acculturation is often measured with unidimensional scales or through proxies such as country of birth or language preference. Studies using the unidimensional model of acculturation have resulted in contradictory results. Some of them have reported that women who assimilated with the local culture are less likely to suffer from postpartum depression (Foss, 2001; Zelkowitz & Milet, 1995). While other studies have stressed that a high level of acculturation to the host culture represented a risk factor for antenatal and postnatal depression (Acevado, 2000; Heilemann et al., 2004; Martinez-Schallmoser et al., 2003), as acculturated women were more prone to adopt health risk behaviors (e.g., smoking, bad eating habits) and have poorer perinatal outcomes (e.g., premature birth, low birth weight) than their less acculturated counterparts.

Few studies have measured acculturation as a bidimensional process of psychological integration leading to a bicultural identity, that is, maintaining traditions of heritage culture and simultaneous adoption of local practices related to child-rearing views. The study of Abbott and Williams (2006) using structured interviews showed that first- and second-generation migrant women from Pacific Islands in New Zealand were at risk of postpartum depression if they rejected the values of both their heritage and host cultures. This strategy is described in Berry's model (1997) as marginalization. Conversely, women who maintained their heritage culture and at the same time adopted the host culture reported less depression. These authors suggested that women who strongly identified with the Pacific culture also belonged to a strong religious and cultural community and therefore benefitted from strong social support. Further, the association of marginalization and postpartum depression might be explained as a lack of anchoring in either cultural frame, especially in a time where transgenerational family ties are essential. The study of Sharapova and Goguikian Ratcliff (2018) examining the role of acculturation process, using a bidimensional acculturation questionnaire (the Vancouver Index of Acculturation) and family and social support in antenatal anxiety (measured with the State Trait Anxiety Inventory – STAI) and depression (measured with the Edinburgh Postnatal Depression Scale – EPDS), showed the complexity of the mechanisms involved. Unexpectedly, results indicated that a strong attachment to the heritage culture in migrant women represented a risk factor for antenatal depression but not anxiety. On the other hand, migrant women who had family members living in the same city reported significantly less anxiety symptoms than women who did not. These results might reflect the migrant women's longing for the familiar cultural environment and family ties and stress the importance of social support during the perinatal period.

The discrepancies in findings concerning the impact of acculturation on antenatal and postnatal depression may also be explained by interindividual differences in the importance given by women to the conservation of their heritage culture and to the establishment of social contacts with the host culture. For some foreign-born individuals, who adhere to individualistic principles, cultural tradition does not represent a significant part of their identity, while career does (Hunt et al., 2004). Furthermore, cultural elements and traditions to maintain may also differ from one woman to another. In her ethnographic literature review on the impact of cultural factors on postpartum depression, Bina (2008) underlines that the maintenance of cultural traditions, beliefs, and rituals has an alleviating impact on depression only if these rituals are relevant to women's expectations and educational level. Otherwise, their maintenance may be perceived as a constraint and lead to psychological distress. For instance, a mother who gives particular importance to mother-child bonding and feels the need to spend time alone with her newborn will not always appreciate the presence and increased support from the extended family.

Even though existing studies on the role of acculturation in perinatal mental health show contradictory results, the findings suggest that for many migrant mothers it is important to maintain their cultural heritage and at the same time to adapt to the local cultural norms. Cognitive flexibility, openness to the host culture, but also preservation of some meaningful cultural practices in the migratory context might represent protective factors against perinatal anxiety and depression

(Bina, 2008; Kim & Omizo, 2006; Moro & Drain, 2009). However, more qualitative or mixed methods research using bidimensional measures of acculturation is needed to better understand how first-generation migrant mothers manage to construct a bicultural identity and how it acts as a risk or a protective factor for perinatal anxiety and depression (Beck, 2006; Fung & Dennis, 2010).

Finally, in quantitative research with women coming from traditional non-Western backgrounds, it is essential to address specific methodological issues and to be careful when interpreting scores and establishing cutoffs. Instruments used to measure antenatal or postnatal anxiety in migrant women (e.g., STAI; Beck Anxiety Inventory) have been conceptualized in Western countries and therefore may lack cultural sensitivity or validity. The translation of a scale designed to assess psychological constructs such as depression and anxiety in one social context does not guarantee its cultural validity in another social context (Van de Vijver & Tanzer, 1997). Even the validation of a scale and the adaptation of items may not suppress certain culture-related bias, such as familiarity with the screening process. Moreover, valid intercultural comparison supposes that global scores of a scale should have the same psychological meaning through cultures and refer to the same concept or perceived illness state (Van de Vijver & Leung, 2000).

Psychosocial risk factors and antenatal anxiety in migrant women

Several psychological and psychosocial risk factors increase the vulnerability of migrant women to antenatal anxiety. *Psychological risk factors* include pre-migratory traumatic or stressful events (e.g., war, political instability, sexual violence, natural disasters, living in refugee camps, hunger, poverty, and torture), domestic violence, and unwanted pregnancy (Wolff et al., 2008). Post-migratory *psychosocial risk factors* include precarious legal status, socioeconomic difficulties, inappropriate housing, social isolation, separation with family, lack of marital support, cultural difference, barriers to care, and communication difficulties with health care professionals (Bollini et al., 2009; Da Silva et al., 1998; Gagnon et al., 2010; Zelkowitz et al., 2004). Migrant women with precarious legal status (e.g., undocumented, asylum seekers, temporary residence permit) face multiple psychosocial difficulties, and the accumulation of adverse circumstances exacerbates their stress level during pregnancy (Foss et al., 2004; Goguikian Ratcliff et al., 2015a).

Undocumented, refugees, and asylum seekers are particularly exposed to psychological and psychosocial risk factors. Most women who experienced forced migration are likely to have also been exposed to pre-migratory traumatic events (as listed earlier) and might develop chronic post-traumatic stress disorder (PTSD), depression, or generalized anxiety symptoms (Kennedy & Murphy-Lawless, 2003). Early separation from children is also considered a highly traumatic experience (McLeish, 2005). History of abuse and traumatic experiences represent risk factors for pregnancy-related anxiety (Brunton et al., 2020; Coles & Jones, 2009). Abuse survivors often express anxiety about obstetric care itself. They report heightened fear of childbirth compared to women without abuse histories (Heimstad et al., 2006). Obstetric follow-up procedures may be perceived by migrant women of rural background as invasive and may trigger negative emotions such as fear, shame, anger, or irritability (Moro & Drain, 2009), or invoke extreme distress in women with active trauma symptoms (Ackerson, 2012; Coles & Jones, 2009). The study of Punamäki et al. (2017) in Palestine showed that war trauma and associated PTSD represented a risk factor for poor mother-fetus attachment.

Post-migratory risk factors for increased antenatal or postnatal anxiety include different psychosocial difficulties and life circumstances associated with migration experience and sociocultural transition (Goguikian Ratcliff et al., 2015a; Sharapova et al., 2021). In recent years, the impact of legal status on the perinatal distress of migrant women has been studied as a major post-migratory stressor. Asylum seekers arrive to the host country and find themselves more socially isolated than other migrants, as they are often separated from their families and live in isolated districts of the town (Pumariega et al., 2005). The stress associated with the legal processes around asylum-seeking, the fear of an unsuccessful claim and subsequent deportation, insecure feelings about collective housing in refugees' camps, and lack of social support may be overwhelming and beyond their coping capacities. Becoming pregnant soon after arrival (Goguikian Ratcliff et al., 2011) with uncertainty about their future can further increase woman's vulnerability to mental health problems. In several Western countries, pregnant asylum-seeking women often report feelings of confusion, uncertainty, and difficulties to project into the future (McLeish, 2005; Mestre, 2016). Under these circumstances, these women are likely to present with anxiety, depression, or PTSD symptoms that persist over time or reemerge during pregnancy (Collins et al., 2011).

The study of Sharapova et al. (2021) compared undocumented economic migrants (precarious migrant women) and highly skilled economic migrants (non-precarious migrant women) to native Swiss (non-migrant) women for perinatal depression (measured with the EPDS) and anxiety (measured with the STAI). Results indicate that non-precarious migrant women, who were professionally active and reported a solid social network, did not suffer from greater anxiety and depression symptoms than native Swiss women during pregnancy and after birth. Conversely, precarious migrant women facing cumulative stressors (financial and housing difficulties, lack of social and marital support) were three to four times at higher risk for depression and anxiety during the perinatal period. For most of these women, pregnancy represented as an additional stressor. The burden of non-pregnancy-related psychosocial stressors made it difficult for them to project into the future as mothers. Furthermore, these women reported little pregnancy-related anxiety, but mostly general anxiety related to precarious living conditions.

Conclusion

Pregnancy and childbirth represent a major life transition in a woman's life. Multiple changes occurring in the mother's identity and daily routines pose significant adjustment problems to many women. In that sense, anxiety during pregnancy is a normal phenomenon, but several negative life circumstances may add to the anxiety inherent to the transition to motherhood and lead to greater psychological distress. Migrant women often report greater anxiety during the perinatal period, as they face the double transition of motherhood and migration. Furthermore, migrant women may be exposed to cumulative environmental stressors related to migration. Therefore, even though a history of migration does not constitute a risk factor for antenatal anxiety, it represents a major life event involving many losses (e.g., loss of social network, family resources, and cultural context), exposure to post-migratory environmental stressors, but also a need for acculturation and cultural identity self-redefinition. Thus, the conditions of the migration experience and the available psychological, economic, and cultural resources must be assessed. It seems crucial that perinatal health care providers assess migrant women's legal status, which is often closely related to their socio-economic status, living conditions, and available social support. All these factors may represent protective or risk factor for perinatal anxiety and depression. Undocumented migrant women are particularly vulnerable because they often lack health insurance and early pregnancy follow-up. They face multiple stressors, may feel overwhelmed by daily hassles, and at the same time be unable to seek help due to low acculturation, access to health care, or social services due to their "invisible" condition (Davoudian, 2012; Mestre, 2016).

Routine screening of anxiety and depression symptoms in migrant women should take place during pregnancy, as women are regularly seen by different health care professionals. Moreover, it is crucial to stress the importance of increased tolerance to diverse cultural views and expectations by perinatal health care professionals when working with this population. Further, perinatal health professionals should be open to question the universality of Western models of assessment and intervention and be flexible to understand and use other models of health care and traditional practices. Finally, when working with migrant women, it seems important to know the existing network of medical, social, and psychological assistance for migrants, in order to set up multidimensional and integrated interventions (Baubet & Moro, 2013; Mestre, 2016; Moro, 2016).

Prevention and intervention programs need to meet precarious or disadvantaged migrant women's specific needs. Precarious women often face cumulative stressors, which make it difficult for them to endorse their new role as a mother. Early interventions for migrant women who report psychosocial difficulties or psychological distress include programs aiming to improve access to health care services, with home visits by midwives, nurses, or social workers (Hollowell et al., 2012). Further, parenting-guidance groups represent a specific kind of prevention for isolated and low-income migrant women. Such groups offer them a place for sharing their representations, experiences, and know-how related to motherhood in an empathetic and non-judgmental atmosphere, but also a social network of migrant women sharing a similar perinatal experience (Adohane, 2007).

168 *Anna Sharapova and Betty Goguikian Ratcliff*

References

Abbott, M. W., & Williams, M. M. (2006). Postnatal depressive symptoms among Pacific mothers in Auckland: Prevalence and risk factors. *Australian and New Zealand Journal of Psychiatry, 40*, 230–238. https://doi.org/10.1080/j.1440-1614. 2006.01779.x

Acevado, M. C. (2000). The role of acculturation in explaining ethnic differences in the prenatal health-risk behaviors, mental health, and parenting beliefs of Mexican American and European American at-risk women. *Child Abuse & Neglect, 24*(1), 111-127. https://doi.org/10.1016/s0145-2134(99)00121-0

Ackerson, K. (2012). A history of interpersonal trauma and the gynecological exam. *Qualitative Health Research, 22*, 679–688. https://doi.org/10.1177/1049732311424730

Adohane, T. (2007). Parentalité d'exil: naissance à venir d'un enfant "porte-parent" et "fondateur de lignée". *La clinique lacanienne, 12*, 75–86. https://doi.org/10.3917/cla.012.0075

Austin, M.-P., Tully, L., & Parker, G. (2007). Examining the relationship between antenatal anxiety and postpartum depression. *Journal of Affective Disorders, 101*, 1–3. https://doi.org/10.1016/j.jad.2006.11.015

Baubet, T., & Moro, M. R. (2013). *Psychopathologie transculturelle.* Elsevier-Masson.

Beck, C. T. (2006). Acculturation: Implications for perinatal research. *The American Journal of Maternal and Child Nursing, 31*(2), 114–120. https://doi.org/10.1097/00005721-200603000-00011

Berry, J. W. (1970). Marginality, stress and ethnic identification in an acculturated aboriginal community. *Journal of Cross-Cultural Psychology, 1*, 239–252. https://doi.org/10.1177%2F135910457000100303

Berry, J. W. (1980). Acculturation as varieties of adaptation. In A. M. Padilla (Ed.), *Acculturation: Theory, models and some new findings* (pp. 9–25). Westview Press.

Berry, J. W. (1997). Immigration, acculturation and adaption. *Applied Psychology, 46*, 5–34. https://doi.org/ 10.1111/j.1464-0597.1997.tb01087.x

Berry, J. W., & Sam, D. L. (1997). Acculturation and adaptation. In J. W. Berry, M. H. Segall, & C. Kagitcibasi (Eds.), *Handbook of cross-cultural psychology, vol. 3: Social behaviour and applications* (pp. 291–326). Allyn & Bacon.

Bina, R. (2008). The impact of cultural factors upon postpartum depression: A literature review. *Health Care for Women International, 29*, 568–592. https://doi.org/10.1080/07399330802089149

Bollini, P., Pampallona, S., Wanner, P., & Kupelnick, B. (2009). Pregnancy outcome of migrant women and integration policy: A review of the international literature. *Social Science and Medicine, 68*, 452–461. https://doi.org /10.1016/j.socscimed.2008.10.018

Bornstein, M. H., & Cote, L. R. (2006). Parenting cognitions and practices in the acculturative process. In M. H. Bornstein & L. R. Cote (Eds.), *Acculturation and parent-child relationships* (pp. 135–173). Lawrence Erlbaum Associates.

Breslau, N., Schultz, L., & Peterson, E. (1995). Sex differences in depression: A role of preexisting anxiety. *Psychiatry Research, 58*(1), 1–12. https://doi.org/10.1016/0165-1781(95)02765-O

Brunton, R., Wood, T., & Dryer, R. (2020). Childhood abuse, pregnancy- related anxiety and the mediating role of resilience and social support. *Journal of Health Psychology*, 1-11. https://doi.org/10.1177/1359105320968140

Capponi, I., & Horbacz, C. (2007). Femmes en transition vers la maternité: sur qui comptent-elles? *Dialogue, 175*(1), 115–127. https://doi.org/10.3917/dia. 175.0115.

Chanson, P. (2011). *Variations métisses. Dix métaphores pour penser le métissage.* Bruylant-Academia.

Choudhry, U. K. (1997). Traditional practices of women from India: Pregnancy, childbirth, and newborn care. *Journal of Obstetric, Gynecologic and Neonatal Nursing, 26*, 533-539. https://doi.org/10.1111/j.1552-6909.1997.tb02156.x

Coles, J., & Jones, K. (2009). Universal precautions: Perinatal touch and examination after childhood sexual abuse. *Birth, 36*, 230–236. https://doi.org/10.1111/j.1523-536X.2009.00327.x

Collins, C. H., Zimmerman, C., & Howard, L. M. (2011). Refugee, asylum seeker, immigrant women and postnatal depression: Rates and risk factors. *Archives of Women's Mental Health, 14*, 3-11. https://doi.org/10.1007/s00737-010-0198-7

Da Silva, V. A., Moares-Santos, A. R., Carvalho, M. S., Martins, M. L. P., & Teixeira, N. A. (1998). Prenatal and postnatal depression among low income Brazilian women. *Brazilian Journal of Medical and Biological Research, 31*, 799–804. https://doi.org/10.1590/s0100-879x1998000600012

Davoudian, C. (2012). *Mères et bébés sans papiers. Une nouvelle clinique à l'épreuve de l'errance et de l'invisibilité?* Erès.

Dole, N., Savitz, D. A., Hertz-Picciotto, I., Siega-Riz, A. M., McMahon, M. J., & Buekens, P. (2003). Maternal stress and preterm birth. *American Journal of Epidemiology, 157*, 14–24. https://doi.org/10.1093/aje/kwf176

Faisal-Cury, A., & Rossi Menezes, P. (2007). Prevalence of anxiety and depression during pregnancy in a private setting sample. *Archives of Women's Mental Health, 10*, 25–32. https://doi.org/10.1007/s00737-006-0164-6

Field, T., Diego, M., Hernandez-Reif, M., Schanberg, S., Kuhn, C., Yando, R., & Bendell, D. (2003). Pregnancy anxiety and comorbid depression and anger: Effects on the fetus and neonate. *Depression and Anxiety, 17*, 140–151. https://doi.org/10.1002/da.10071

Fortin, S., & Le Gall, J. (2007). Néonatalité et constitution des savoirs en contexte migratoire: familles et services de santé. Enjeux théoriques, perspectives anthropologiques. *Enfances, Familles, Générations, 6*, 16–37. https://doi.org/10.7202/016481ar

Foss, G. F. (2001). Maternal sensitivity, posttraumatic stress and acculturation in Vietnamese and Hmong mothers. *The American Journal of Maternal/Child Nursing, 26*(5), 257–263. https://doi.org/10.1097/00005721-200109000-00009

Foss, G. F., Andjukenda, W. C., & Hendrickson, S. (2004). Maternal depression and anxiety and infant development: A comparison of foreign-born and native mothers. *Public Health Nursing, 21*, 237–246. https://doi.org/10.1111/j.0737-1209.2004.21306.x

Fung, K., & Dennis, C. L. (2010). Postpartum depression among immigrant women. *Current Opinion in Psychiatry, 23*, 342–348. https://doi.org/10.1097/YCO.0b013e32833ad721

Gagnon, A. J., Zimbeck, M., & Zeitlin, J. (2010). Migration and perinatal health surveillance: An international survey. *European Journal of Obstetrics, Gynecology and Reproductive Biology, 149*, 37–43. https://doi.org/10.1016/j.ejogrb.2009.12.002

Gibson, M. A. (2001). Immigrant adaptation and patterns of acculturation. *Human Development, 44*, 19–23. https://doi.org/10.1159/000057037

Goguikian Ratcliff, B., Borel, F., Suardi, F., & Sharapova, A. (2011). Devenir mère en terre étrangère. *Cahiers de la puéricultrice, 252,* 26–29.

Goguikian Ratcliff, B., & Diaz-Marchand, N. (2019). Élever son enfant loin des siens: petits gestes, grands enjeux. In C. Barras & A. Manço (Eds.), *L'accompagnement des familles: entre réparation et créativité* (pp. 67–81). L'Harmattan.

Goguikian Ratcliff, B., Sharapova, A., Pereira Kraft, C., Grimard, N., & Borel Radeff, F. (2015a). Dépression périnatale et complications obstétricales chez des migrantes primo-arrivantes à Genève [Perinatal depression and obstetrical complications in newcomers in Geneva]. *Devenir, 2*(27), 77–99. https://doi.org/10.3917/dev. 152.0077

Goguikian Ratcliff, B., Sharapova, A., Suardi, F., & Borel, F. (2015b). Factors associated with antenatal depression and obstetric complications in immigrant women in Geneva. *Midwifery, 31*(9), 871–878. https://doi.org/10.1016/j.midw. 2015.04.010

Guerraoui, Z., & Troadec, B. (2000). *Psychologie interculturelle.* Armand Colin.

Hanlon, C., Medhin, G., Alem, A., Araya, M., Abdulahi, A., Hughes, M., Tesfaye, M., Wondimagegn, D., Patel, V., & Prince, M. (2008). Detecting perinatal common mental disorders in Ethiopia: Validation of the self-reporting questionnaire and Edinburgh Postnatal Depression Scale. *Journal of Affective Disorders, 108*(3), 251–262. https://doi.org/10.1016/j.jad.2007.10.023.

Heilemann, M. S., Frutos, L., Lee, K., & Kury, F. S. (2004). Protective strength factors, resources, and risks in relation to depressive symptoms among childbearing women of Mexican descent. *Health Care for Women International, 25*(1), 88–106. https://doi.org/10.1080/07399330490253265

Heimstad, R., Dahloe, R., Laache, I., Skogvoll, E., & Schei, B. (2006). Fear of childbirth and history of abuse: Implications for pregnancy and delivery. *Acta Obstetrica et Gynecologica Scandinavica, 85*(4), 435–440. https://doi.org/10.1080/ 00016340500432507

Heron, J., O'Connor, T. G., Evans, J., Golding, J., & Glover, V. (2004). The course of anxiety and depression through pregnancy and the postpartum in a community sample. *Journal of Affective Disorders, 80,* 65–73. https://doi.org/10.1016/j. jad.2003.08.004

Hollowell, J., Oakey, L., Vigus, C., Barnett-Page, E., Kavanagh, J., & Oliver, S. (2012). *Increasing the early initiation of antenatal care by black and minority ethnic women in the United Kingdom: A systematic review and mixed methods synthesis of women's views and the literature of intervention effectiveness.* Final report for National Perinatal Epidemiology Unit, University of Oxford.

Huizink, A. C., Mulder, E. J. H., Robles de Medina, P. G., Visser, G. H. A., & Buitelaar, J. K. (2004). *Is pregnancy anxiety a distinctive syndrome? Early Human Development, 79*(2), 81–91. https://doi.org/10.1016/j.earlhumdev.2004.04.014

Hunt, L. M., Schneider, S., & Comer, B. (2004). Should "acculturation" be a variable in health research? A critical review of research on US Hispanics. *Social Science & Medicine, 59*(5), 973–986. doi:10.1016/j.socscimed.2003.12.009

Jahoda, G. (2012). Critical reflexions on some recent definitions of "culture". *Culture and Psychology, 18*(3), 289–303. https://doi.org/10.1177/1354067X12446229

Johnson, R. C., & Slade, P. (2003). Obstetric complications and anxiety during pregnancy: Is there a relationship? *Journal of Psychosomatic Obstetrics & Gynecology, 24*(1), 1-14, https://doi.org/10.3109/01674820309042796

Kennedy, P., & Murphy-Lawless, J. (2003). The maternity care needs of refugee and asylum-seeking women in Ireland. *Feminist Review*, *73*(1), 39–53. https://doi.org/10.1057/palgrave.fr.9400073

Kim, B. S., & Omizo, M. M. (2006). Behavioural acculturation and enculturation and psychological functioning among Asian American college students. *Cultural Diversity and Ethnic Minority Psychology*, *12*(2), 245–258. https://doi.org/10.1037/1099-9809.12.2.245

Koleva, H., Stuart, S., O'Hara, M. W., & Bowman-Reif, J. (2011). Risk factors for depressive symptoms during pregnancy. *Archives of Women's Mental Health*, *14*, 99-105. https://doi.org/10.1007/s00737-010-0184-0

Lara, M. A., Le, H.-N., Letechipia, G., & Hochhausen, L. (2009). Prenatal depression in Latinas in the U.S. and Mexico. *Maternal and Child Health Journal*, *13*(4), 567–576. https://doi.org/10.1007/s10995-008-0379-4

Lee, A. M., Keung Lam, S., Sze Mun Lau, S. M., Shiu Yin Chong, C., Wai Chui, H., & Yee Tak Fong, D. (2007). Prevalence, course, and risk factors for antenatal anxiety and depression. *Obstetrics and Gynecology*, *110*, 1102–1112. https://doi.org/10.1097/01.AOG.0000287065.59491.70

Licata, L., & Heine, A. (2012). *Introduction à la psychologie clinique interculturelle*. De Boeck.

Lugina, H. I., Nyström, L., Christensson, K., & Lindmark, G. (2004). Assessing mothers' concerns in the postpartum period: Methodological issues. *Journal of Advanced Nursing*, *48*(3), 279–290. https://doi.org/10.1111/j.1365-2648.2004.03197.x

Martinez-Schallmoser, L., Telleen, S., & Macmullen, N. J. (2003). The effect of social support and acculturation on postpartum depression in Mexican American women. *Journal of Transcultural Nursing*, *14*(4), 329–338. https://doi.org/10.1177/1043659603257162.

Matthey, S., Barnett, B., Howie, P., & Kavanagh, D. J. (2003). Diagnosing postpartum depression in mothers and fathers: Whatever happened to anxiety? *Journal of Affective Disorders*, *74*(2), 139–147. https://doi.org/10.1016/S0165-0327(02)00012-5

McLeish, J. (2005). Maternity experiences of asylum seekers in England. *British Journal of Midwifery*, *13*(12), 782–785. https://doi.org/10.12968/bjom.2005.13.12.20125

Mestre, C. (2016). *Bébés d'ici, mères d'exil*. Erès.

Moro, M. R. (1994). *Parents en exil: psychopathologie et migrations*. Presses Universitaires de France.

Moro, M.-R. (2016). Préface. Être et faire: être femme, être mère en situation transculturelle. In C. Mestre (dir.), *Bébés d'ici, mères d'exil* (pp. 9–25). Erès.

Moro, M. R., & Drain, E. (2009). Parentalité en exil. *Soins Pédiatrie*, *30*, 16–19. https://doi.org/SPP-10-2009-30-250-1259-4792-101019-200906265

Nanzer, N. (2009). *La dépression postnatale, sortir du silence*. Editions Favre.

Nelson, A. M. (2003). Transition to motherhood. *Journal of Obstetric, Gynecologic and Neonatal Nursing*, *32*, 465–477. https://doi.org/10.1177/0884217503255199

O'Connor, T. G., Heron, J., Glover, V., & the ALSPAC Study Team. (2002). Antenatal anxiety predicts child behavioral/emotional problems independent of postnatal depression. *Journal of American Academy of Child and Adolescent Psychiatry*, *41*, 1470–1477. https://doi.org/10.1097/00004583-200212000-00019

Orr, S., Reiter, J., Blazer, D., & James, S. (2007). Maternal prenatal pregnancy-related anxiety and spontaneous preterm birth in Baltimore, Maryland. *Psychosomatic Medicine, 38,* 10–16. https://doi.org/10.1097/PSY.0b013e3180cac25d

Pumariega, A., Rothe, E., & Pumariega, J. (2005). Mental health of immigrants and refugees. *Community Mental Health Journal, 41*(5), 581–597. https://doi.org/10.1007/s10597-005-6363-1

Punamäki, R.-L., Isosävi, S., Qouta, S. R., Kuittinen, S., & Diab, S. Y. (2017). War trauma and maternal – fetal attachment predicting maternal mental health, infant development, and dyadic interaction in Palestinian families. *Attachment & Human Development, 19*(5), 463–486. https://doi.org/10.1080/14616734.2017.1330833

Rabain-Jamin, J., & Wornham, W. L. (1990). Transformation des conduites de maternage et des pratiques de soin chez les migrantes originaires d'Afrique de l'Ouest. *Psychiatrie de l'enfant, 33*(1), 287–319.

Razurel, C., & Kaiser, B. (2015). The role of satisfaction with social support on the psychological health of primiparous mothers in the perinatal period. *Women & Health, 55*(2), 167–186. https://doi.org/10.1080/03630242.2014.979969

Ross, L. E., & McLean, L. M. (2006). Anxiety disorders during pregnancy and the postpartum period. A systematic review. *Journal of Clinical Psychiatry, 67*(8), 1285-1298. https://doi.org/10.4088/JCP.v67n0818

Rubertsson, C., Hellström, J., Cross, M., & Sydsjö, G. (2014). Anxiety in early pregnancy: Prevalence and contributing factors. *Archives of Women's Mental Health, 17,* 221–228. https://doi.org/10.1007/s00737-013-0409-0

Rutter, M. (1995). Psychosocial adversity: Risk, resilience and recovery. *Southern African Journal of Child and Adolescent Mental Health, 7*(2), 75–88. https://doi.org/10.1080/16826108.1995.9632442

Ryder, A. G., Lynn, E. A., & Delroy, L. E. (2000). Is acculturation unidimensional or bidimensional? A head-to-head comparison in the prediction of personality, self-identity, and adjustment. *Journal of Personality and Social Psychology, 79*(1), 49-65. doi: 10.1037//0022-3514.79.1.49

Sandman, C. A., Wadhwa, P. D., Dunkel-Schetter, C., Chicz-Demet, A., Belman, J., Porto, M., Murata, Y., Garite, T. J., & Crinella, F. M. (1994). Psychobiological influences of stress and HPA regulation on the human fetus and infant birth outcomes. *Annals of the New York Academy of Sciences, 739,* 198–210. https://doi.org/10.1111/j.1749-6632.1994.tb19822.x

Sardas, F. (2016). *Maman blues. Du bonheur et de la difficulté de devenir mère.* Eyrolles.

Sharapova, A., & Goguikian Ratcliff, B. (2018). Anxiété et dépression périnatales chez des femmes migrantes à Genève: une étude longitudinale. *Devenir, 30*(4), 309–330. https://doi.org/10.3917/dev.184.0309

Sharapova, A., Torche, B., Epiney, M., & Goguikian Ratcliff, B. (2021). Dépression périnatale chez les femmes migrantes: le rôle du statut légal sur les difficultés éprouvées. *L'Autre, 22*(1), 22–37.

Simkhada, B., Van Teijlingen, E. R., Porter, M., & Simkhada, P. (2007). Factors affecting the utilization of antenatal care in developing countries: Systematic review of the literature. *Journal of Advanced Nursing, 61*(3), 244–260. https://doi.org/10.1111/j.1365-2648.2007.04532.x

Stern, D. N. (1998). *La naissance d'une mère.* Editions Odile Jacob.

Tadmor, C. T., Tetlock, P. E., & Peng, K. (2009). Acculturation strategies and integrative complexity the cognitive implications of biculturalism. *Journal of Cross Cultural Psychology, 40,* 105-139. https://doi.org/10.1177/0022022108326279

Team, V., Vasey, K., & Manderson, L. (2009). *Cultural dimensions of pregnancy, birth and post-natal care.* www.health.qld.gov.au/multicultural/support_tools/14MCSR-pregnancy.pdf.

Van de Vijver, F. J. R., & Leung, K. (2000). Methodological issues in psychological research on culture. *Journal of Cross-Cultural Psychology, 31*(1), 33–51. https://doi.org//10.1177/0022022100031001004

Van de Vijver, F. J. R., & Tanzer, N. K. (1997). Bias and equivalence in cross-cultural assessment: An overview. *European Review of Applied Psychology, 54*(2), 119–135. https://doi.org/10.1016/j.erap.2003.12.004

Van Doorne-Huiskes, A., & Doorten, I. (2010). The complexity of parenthood in modern societies. In G. Beets, J. Schippers, & E. R. de Velde (Eds.), *The future of motherhood in western societies* (pp. 107–124). Springer Publishing Company.

Von Overbeck Ottino, S. (2011). Tous parents, tous différents. Parentalités dans un monde en mouvement. *L'Autre, 3*(12), 304–315. https://doi.org/10.3917/lautr.036.0304

Wolff, H., Epiney, M., Lourenco, A. P., Costanza, M. C., Delieutraz-Marchand, J., Andreoli, N., Dubuisson, J.-B., Gaspoz, J.-M., & Irion, O. (2008). Undocumented migrants lack access to pregnancy care and prevention. *BMC Public Health, 8*, 93. https://doi.org/10.1186/1471-2458-8-93

Zelkowitz, P., & Milet, T. H. (1995). Screening for post-partum depression in a community sample. *The Canadian Journal of Psychiatry, 40*(2), 80–86. https://doi.org/10.1177/070674379504000205

Zelkowitz, P., Saucier, J. F., Wang, T., Katofsky, L., Valenzuela, M., & Westreich, R. (2008). Stability and change in depressive symptoms from pregnancy to two months postpartum in childbearing immigrant women. *Archives of Women's Mental Health, 11*, 1–11. https://doi.org/10.1007/s00737-008-0219-y

Zelkowitz, P., Schinazy, J., Katofsky, L., Saucier, J.-F., Valenzuels, M., Westereich, R., & Dayan, J. (2004). Factors associated with depression in pregnant immigrant women. *Transcultural Psychiatry, 41*, 445–464. https://doi.org/10.1177/1363461504047929

12 Psychosocial functioning and childhood sexual abuse

Robyn Brunton

Psychosocial functioning and childhood sexual abuse

This chapter examines the implications of a history of child sexual abuse on pregnancy and childbirth. While the focus of this chapter is on child sexual abuse, it is acknowledged that physical and emotional abuse experienced in childhood are also pervasive with long-term effects and may potentially co-occur. Also, while this book has a focus on pregnancy-related anxiety, the research into child sexual abuse and pregnancy-related anxiety is limited. While we highlight research on this topic of pregnancy-related anxiety and child sexual abuse, we also identify the similarity in outcomes between these two so-called experiences that suggest a causal relationship. In doing so, we draw on theory and research. The intent of this chapter is to encourage further research into an area that has important implications for the health and well-being of women and their progeny.

In this chapter, child sexual abuse is first defined and its prevalence examined. Following this, there is a detailed list of possible sequelae of this abuse, both generally and in pregnancy particularly. The commonalities between child sexual abuse and pregnancy-related anxiety are then explored with an additive effect proposed. The chapter concludes with a discussion of the implications of antenatal care for sexual abuse survivors and recommendations for future directions such as antenatal screening.

Defining child sexual abuse

Violence against women and girls occurs in all societies and countries in varying degrees and is indiscriminate of socioeconomic status and culture (WHO, 2015, p. 139). Child sexual abuse, one type of sexual violence, is defined as sexual acts that involve a child who is developmentally unprepared or does not fully comprehend the acts, cannot give consent, and the acts violate societal laws or are considered social taboos (WHO, 2017). The perpetrator of this abuse is usually in a position of responsibility, trust, or power over the victim and the act is intended to gratify the perpetrators' needs (WHO, 2017, p. vii). While definitions of child sexual abuse may vary due to differing age limits (can vary from 14 to 18 years) and the inclusion of different behaviors (ranging from contact to non-contact), it is generally agreed that definitions require two elements, that the sexual activities involve a

DOI: 10.4324/9781003014003-16

child and an abusive condition (see Finkelhor, 1994 for a discussion on definitional controversies).

Globally, estimates of girls subjected to child sexual abuse range from 2% to 64% (Iran and Japan, respectively; Mohammadi et al., 2014; Tanaka et al., 2017). One review estimated that around 20% of women in North America and Australia have experienced this abuse (Moody et al., 2018). However, accurate approximations of child sexual abuse are challenging due to issues around reporting (e.g., inconsistencies in definitions; see Hulme, 2004 for a detailed discussion) and disclosure, with many women choosing never to disclose (McElvaney, 2015). Culture is an additional influence with some cultures having greater ease in talking about abuse than others (Pereda et al., 2009). Taken together, child sexual abuse is pervasive and prevalent; however, inconsistencies in defining and reporting this abuse may mean that many survivors are undetected by systems or by their own intention.

Child sexual abuse and pregnancy

Despite the issues in determining an accurate occurrence of child sexual abuse, a significant proportion of pregnant women will likely have this history. This is probable as approximately 85% of women will experience pregnancy more than once in their lifetime (Livingston, 2015). In one Australian study, (N = 638), 28% of pregnant women reported the occurrence of child sexual abuse (Brunton et al., 2020). Other systematic reviews noted prevalence ranging from 12% to 37% (Brunton & Dryer, 2021; Leeners et al., 2006b, respectively) with variabilities in estimates likely reflecting, varying approaches, measurement, and methodologies.

These prevalence rates indicate that approximately one third of pregnant women will likely have a history of abuse. Therefore, the well-documented sequelae of child sexual abuse that includes a range of adverse adult outcomes is concerning. As shown in Figure 12.1, these outcomes can be broadly classified as *psychiatric*,

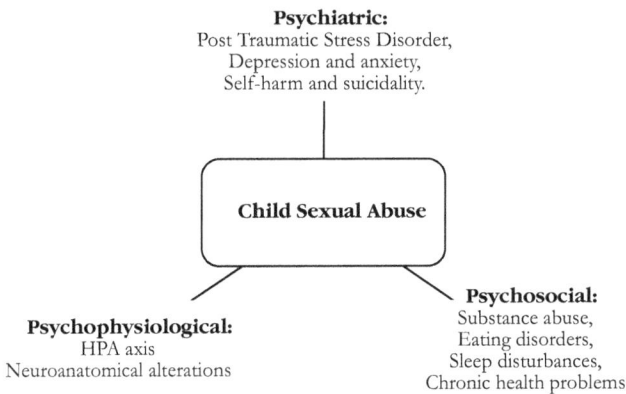

Note. HPA axis = hypothalamic pituitary axis which is the central stress response system.

Figure 12.1 Adverse outcomes associated with child sexual abuse

psychosocial, and *psychophysiological,* (Maniglio, 2009; Putnam, 2003; Wilson, 2010).

Furthermore, during pregnancy, these deleterious outcomes may be more likely to occur, or existing pathologies exacerbated possibly due to the nature of prenatal care and childbirth which involves intimate procedures and sometimes positions of powerlessness, which may amplify a sexual abuse survivor's trauma (Yampolsky et al., 2010). Many of the psychosocial outcomes of sexual abuse, such as sleeplessness, substance use/abuse, and physical symptoms (e.g., asthma, migraines, pelvic pain), occur more frequently and are experienced more intensely for pregnant women who are child sexual abuse survivors than other expectant mothers (Brunton & Dryer, 2021; Hulme, 2000; Leeners et al., 2006b, 2014). This increased and intensified symptomology may explain why some pregnant women with this history have more primary care visits than other women (Leeners et al., 2006b).

Psychiatric

Childhood sexual abuse is linked to anxiety, depression, and suicide ideation and identified as a "clear risk factor" and strong predictor of antenatal anxiety (Biaggi et al., 2016, p. 66; Plant et al., 2013). Robertson-Blackmore et al. (2013) noted that women with a history of child abuse were nearly 2.5 times more likely to have antenatal anxiety compared to other women. Martini et al. (2015) identified sexual trauma as associated with anxiety during pregnancy, theorizing it may be due to anxieties about the upcoming birth and birth-related fears. Increased depressive symptomology and suicide ideation are also seen in child sexual abuse survivors during pregnancy (Leeners et al., 2006b). In one study of pregnant women who experienced sexual abuse in their childhood, around 25% self-reported depression compared to less than 2% of women with no abuse history (Leeners et al., 2014). The increased risk of suicidality in pregnant women with a history of childhood sexual abuse is evidenced by these women nearly four times more likely to attempt suicide than other women with an exponential risk if multiple incidences of abuse were experienced (Lara et al., 2015).

Post-traumatic stress disorder (PTSD) is common among child sexual abuse survivors. In pregnancy, it is estimated that around 16% of women who present with this history will have PTSD, and around 39% if they suffered both childhood and adult sexual abuse (Wosu et al., 2015). For women with a child sexual abuse history, they may experience higher levels of all PTSD symptomologies (e.g., flashbacks, arousal, disassociation, avoidance) compared to other women (Lev-Wiesel et al., 2009). Pregnancy and childbirth may be particularly triggering with some women reporting memories of the abuse returning at this time and for some, it could be the first time memories have resurfaced since childhood (Leeners et al., 2007, 2013, 2016). Arousal (increased hypervigilance) in some cases may be counterproductive with hypervigilant women more aware of every sensation in their body and thus more prone to seeking care. Conversely, disassociation or detachment during childbirth may prevent some women from the awareness of knowing something is wrong and avoidance may mean some women do not seek care when needed (Leeners et al., 2006b; Lev-Wiesel et al., 2009; Zambaldi et al., 2011). This sequela of PTSD could compromise optimal prenatal and obstetrical care.

Psychosocial

Eating disorders and weight gain during pregnancy are also common for survivors of child sexual abuse. Women with this history are frequently more obese and often have eating disorder symptomologies such as anorexia and bulimia and self-induced vomiting and laxative use (Brunton & Dryer, 2021; Leeners et al., 2006b). These disorders/behaviors may be due to anxiety underlying these issues with pregnancy a triggering "event" (Leeners et al., 2006b).

Child sexual abuse is also linked to increased common complaints with pregnant women who are abuse survivors experiencing more discomfort and health complaints such as nausea and vomiting, tiredness, and headache than other women (Lukasse et al., 2009). Moreover, these women have been identified as having more medical conditions associated with a high-risk pregnancy such as hypertension, deep vein thrombosis, diabetes mellitus, or chronic nephropathy (Leeners et al., 2010). These outcomes may be the result of health risk behaviors linked to child sexual abuse (e.g., poor self-care, substance abuse) and serve to increase the number of unscheduled health care visits (Leeners et al., 2006b).

SUBSTANCE USE/ABUSE

Substance use/abuse (i.e., alcohol, smoking, and illicit drugs) is an area of critical concern, with these behaviors introducing harmful teratogens into the prenatal environment. Alcohol is known to cause congenital disabilities and malformation with *fetal alcohol syndrome* having a long-term sequela for the child (Keegan et al., 2010). Around 12%–15% of women with a child sexual abuse history continue to smoke in pregnancy (Keegan et al., 2010) with a dose-response relationship between tobacco use and adverse maternal and fetal outcomes (e.g., spontaneous abortion, low birth weight, and birth before 37 weeks gestation [preterm birth]; Keegan et al., 2010). The prevalence of antenatal drug use for child sexual abuse survivors ranges from 1% to 21% depending on the drug, with opioids related to a sixfold increase in maternal obstetric complications such as puerperal morbidity and stillbirth. Cocaine is linked to spontaneous abortion and amphetamine use associated with congenital abnormalities such as heart defects and cleft lip and palate. All drugs are associated with maternal and fetal withdrawal (Keegan et al., 2010).

Despite the harmful effects of these behaviors, few studies have examined child sexual abuse and substance use/abuse during pregnancy (see Brunton & Dryer, 2021 for a review). Of those who have examined this issue, there are inconsistent findings that are likely due to methodological issues. Nonetheless, it would seem that, generally, pregnant women who were sexually abused in childhood are more likely to have increased substance use in pregnancy than other women (Brunton & Dryer, 2021; Leeners et al., 2006b). Given the findings in the general population (e.g., see Wilson, 2010), the potential for increased substance use/abuse is likely high.

Psychophysiological

Child sexual abuse survivors may suffer psychophysiological outcomes, including effects on the hypothalamic-pituitary-adrenal (HPA) axis, the sympathetic nervous system, and potentially the immune system (Putnam, 2003). Some studies have noted several neuroanatomical alterations in survivor's brains such as reduced hippocampal volume, an area involved in the regulation of the HPA axis. Decreases in the corpus callosum whose primary function is transferring information between the brain hemispheres have also been noted. Decreases in this volume are associated with PTSD and dissociative symptoms with all psychophysiological outcomes similar to those noted in combat-related PTSD (Putnam, 2003).

Other areas of concern

In addition to the areas detailed in Figure 12.1, in the context of pregnancy, additional areas of concern for women with a child sexual abuse history have been identified. These include preterm birth and baby concerns, childbirth, medical staff, and intimate partner violence. For many of these areas, they are consistent with key areas of concern that characterize pregnancy-related anxiety (e.g., childbirth, baby concerns, and concerns toward medical staff). Moreover, for some of these adverse outcomes such as preterm birth, they are associated with pregnancy-related anxiety and this is discussed further later.

PRETERM BIRTH AND BABY CONCERNS

Child sexual abuse is a risk factor for preterm birth, which is a significant global health issue (Romero et al., 2014). Leeners' (2014) study matched expectant mothers who experienced sexual abuse in childhood to women with no such history. Of the 255 children born overall, women who experienced child sexual abuse had more preterm births than women who had not experienced abuse (18.8% *cf.* 8.2%, $p = 0.02$). Others have found that women with a child sexual abuse history are more likely (in some cases nearly three times more likely) to have a preterm birth (than other women) with heightened maternal cortisol significantly related to their preterm status (Noll et al., 2007). While other researchers have not found any significant association between preterm birth and sexual abuse (e.g., Benedict et al., 1999; Grimstad & Schei, 1999; Jacobs, 1992), these studies were limited by their sample size and measurement choice (see Brunton & Dryer, 2021 for a detailed review).

While the etiology of preterm birth is complex and subject to ongoing investigation, one proposition is that the early life stress caused by the trauma of child sexual abuse may disrupt neuroendocrine pathways in the stress response system, as indicated earlier (Horan et al., 2000). During pregnancy, this disruption is further exacerbated by the natural elevation of maternal cortisol concentrations, which exponentially rise during pregnancy to nearly three times more than normal levels (Liapi et al., 1996). The increased cortisol from the trauma and that which occurs naturally in pregnancy may contribute to a chronic overproduction of cortisol, enhancing the sense of fear associated with the early sexual abuse and contributing to the earlier onset of labor (Horan et al., 2000).

In addition to preterm birth, expectant mothers with a child sexual abuse history may also have profound fears for their unborn child (Leeners et al., 2006b). These fears may stem from concerns for the vulnerability of the child and doubts about the mother's ability to protect the child or be "good enough" to parent them. While studies into this specific area are scarce, qualitative research has shown that survivors of sexual abuse have an innate need to protect their offspring (LoGiudice, 2016).

CHILDBIRTH

For many women who experienced child sexual abuse, childbirth is a negative experience characterized by intense fear and difficulties in birthing (i.e., longer duration, increased pain; Leeners et al., 2016). For some women, repressed memories of abuse may surface, and these have been linked to more pain, an inability to cooperate with clinicians, and the cessation of contractions. Disassociation may occur as a means to cope with pain and other overwhelming aspects of childbirth, such as perceived powerlessness and intimate procedures (Leeners et al., 2016). Indeed, for some women who were sexually abused in childhood, childbirth is seen as a repetition of the abuse and more emotionally painful (Leeners et al., 2006b).

MEDICAL STAFF

Expectant mothers with a child sexual abuse history may have difficulties trusting caregivers (e.g., medical staff) and may avoid prenatal care or have difficulty in communicating their needs (Brunton & Dryer, 2021; Leeners et al., 2006b). The implication of this is in their clinical care and is discussed in more detail in the next section on clinical considerations.

INTIMATE PARTNER VIOLENCE

Another area linked to child sexual abuse survivors is experiencing violence in pregnancy (Brunton & Dryer, 2021; Leeners et al., 2006b, 2016). Intimate partner violence is physical, sexual, emotional violence, or coercive control by an intimate partner (WHO, 2011, p. 1). One disturbing aspect of intimate partner violence is the intention to harm the pregnancy or unborn child by targeting the violence toward the woman's abdomen (WHO, 2003). Global estimates of intimate partner violence range from 15% to 40% depending on age. The highest occurrence for this violence is between 20–44 years, aligning with the peak childbearing years of 15–44 (Australian Institute of Health & Welfare, 2015). Regional estimates can vary with the occurrence of intimate partner violence greater in low-middle-income regions (e.g., Africa, Americas, and Europe, up to 38%). Around half of the countries report a lifetime prevalence of 30% (WHO, 2015).

Concerningly, among women subjected to child sexual abuse, at least 60%–80% may also suffer intimate partner violence with an exponential risk for multiple abuse types (Classen et al., 2005). Indeed, child sexual abuse represents a particular vulnerability for this violence (Cloitre et al., 1996; Mezey et al., 2005) consistent with theoretical explanations for revictimization, including *experiential avoidance*, the proposition that dissociation and PTSD symptoms influence revictimization, and the *vulnerability hypothesis* that proposes that early sexual experiences present a particular vulnerability for later victimization (Bell & Higgins, 2015; Koss & Dinero, 1989).

Sexual abuse and pregnancy-related anxiety

Given the previously mentioned links between child sexual abuse and adverse outcomes in later life and the compelling evidence that anxiety, in particular, is common, it is conceivable that child sexual abuse is a risk factor for pregnancy-related anxiety. As depicted in Figure 12.2, commonalities between the deleterious

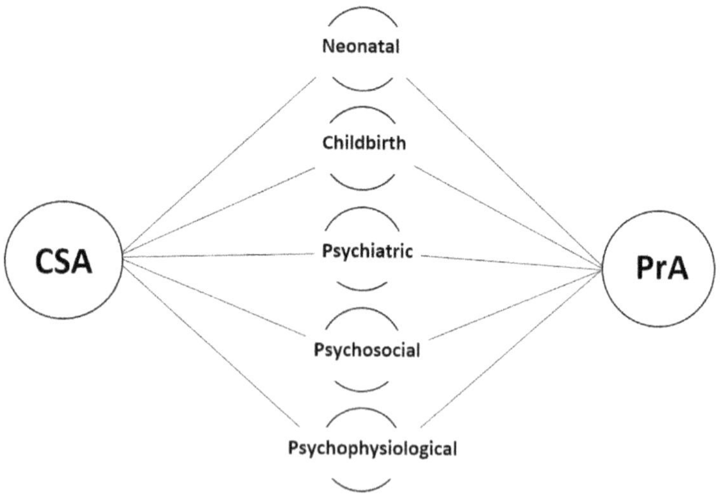

Note. CSA = child sexual abuse, PrA = pregnancy-related anxiety

Figure 12.2 Commonalities between child sexual abuse and pregnancy-related anxiety

outcomes for pregnant women with a history of sexual abuse in their childhood and identified dimensions of pregnancy-related anxiety include fear of childbirth, concerns for the unborn baby, attitudes to medical staff, and avoidance. This proposition is consistent with *developmental cascade theories* (also known as chain reactions, snowball, or progressive effects), which explain the cumulative consequences of trauma and abuse that alter the course of human development. Cascade effects (the processes that influence development) explain why some child sexual abuse survivors have more difficulties and adverse outcomes in adulthood than others who have less to no difficulties (Masten & Cicchetti, 2010).

There is limited research in this area, with a search of the psychological databases Psychinfo, ProQuest, and EBSCO since 2000 returning only one result. In this study, physical, sexual, and psychological abuse were examined as risk factors for pregnancy-related anxiety in a community sample ($N = 638$). Women with at least one instance of any abuse (physical. sexual, or emotional) had significantly higher pregnancy-related anxiety (measured by the *Pregnancy-related Anxiety Scale* – PrAS), $M_{abused} = 64.40$ cf. $M_{nonabused} = 55.36$ than other women. In this study three models were examined, one for each abuse type. For each model, pregnancy-related anxiety was the outcome variable and resilience and social support were examined as mediators of the relationship between the abuse type and this anxiety. All three abuse types independently predicted pregnancy-related anxiety with resilience and social support fully mediating the child sexual abuse model and partially mediating the other two models (Brunton et al., 2020).

FEAR OF CHILDBIRTH AND BABY CONCERNS

Other studies have focused on certain dimensions of pregnancy-related anxiety such as fear of childbirth and fears for the unborn child. Heimstad et al. (2006) in a large community study of 4,695 pregnant women found that of the women exposed to child sexual abuse, 8.2% had a greater fear of childbirth compared to other women. Also, of the abused women, nearly half (46.0%) had a complicated vaginal delivery compared to 25.0% of women with no abuse history.

Eide and colleagues (2010, p. 1) examined baby worry as part of a large pregnancy cohort study ($N = 58,139$) noting that women with an experience of sexual abuse in childhood were more likely to have strong worries about the unborn baby (OR = 4.8) than other women (OR = 3.5). Indeed, experiencing both physical and sexual abuse increased the odds ratio to 8.2. The authors acknowledged that baby worry explained some variance in pregnancy-related anxiety, and concluded that together with a fear of childbirth, baby worry might be part of "a more complex context of anxiety in pregnancy" (p. 8).

Studies have also documented links between child sexual abuse, intimate partner violence, and fear of childbirth. Oliveira et al. (2017) explored pathways from child sexual abuse to postpartum PTSD in 456 women with high-risk pregnancies. In this sample, 11.4% of women experienced child sexual abuse at least once (upper age limit: 14 years), with 71.8% and 21.2% of women reporting psychological and physical intimate partner violence, respectively. While there was a link from both types of intimate partner violence to PTSD, only psychological violence had a direct pathway from child sexual abuse to fear of childbirth and PTSD. The authors concluded that for some child sexual abuse survivors, pregnancy might be "marked by disagreements and violence with her partner, marred by fears and anxieties" (p. 303).

Other commonalities exist, with pregnancy-related anxiety and child sexual abuse both risk factors for preterm birth (e.g., Roesch et al., 2004; Wadhwa et al., 1993). Hoyer et al. (2020) noted that for women with pregnancy-related anxiety, they were nearly 1.5 times more likely to have a preterm birth and this relationship was potentially mediated by other variables such as age, maternal health, socioeconomic status, and social support. Wadhwa et al. (1993) noted that for every one-unit increase in pregnancy-related anxiety, there was an associated three-day decrease in gestational age at birth (β = –0.31, p < 0.01), a result independent of other biomedical risk factors such as hypertension and diabetes. Reasons for the association between pregnancy-related anxiety and preterm birth are similar to those proposed earlier for child sexual abuse and preterm birth. That is, the associated increase in stress hormones from pregnancy-related anxiety together with elevated cortisol as part of pregnancy lead to *hypercortisolism* (Mastorakos & Ilias, 2003). Given this, the potential for an additive effect is likely with women with child sexual abuse *and* pregnancy-related anxiety at greater risk of preterm birth than those with either "condition" alone. Initial findings in an ongoing study are indicative of this additive effect; however, as yet, this is a relatively unexamined area in the literature (Brunton & Dryer, 2020 *unpublished manuscript*).

The aforementioned studies show that research is emerging concerning child sexual abuse and pregnancy-related anxiety. The commonalities in regard to the deleterious outcomes associated with both child sexual abuse and pregnancy-related anxiety and the evidence to date indicate that child sexual abuse contributes to and is a risk factor for pregnancy-related anxiety.

Implications and clinical considerations

Given the potential for the adverse sequelae in pregnancy for women with a child abuse history, the need for identifying such women and providing them with more sensitive antenatal care is evident. However, concerningly, child sexual abuse has been described as an underestimated factor in perinatal care (Leeners et al., 2006a), suggesting that such consideration may be uncommon. However, the need for additional consideration in clinical care is underscored by child sexual abuse being identified as a potential risk factor for high-risk pregnancy (Yampolsky et al., 2010).

Considerations in care

A history of child sexual abuse can have differing effects on women in terms of antenatal care with some seeking more care, whereas other women may avoid any interactions with medical staff (Leeners et al., 2006b). For those who have higher prenatal care visits, it may be due to child sexual abuse linked to a greater number of physical conditions known to affect their pregnancy. In one study, pregnant women with more physical ailments were subjected to more interactions with clinicians and had more non-routine invasive examinations than other women. These intimate medical procedures, focused on areas of a woman's body typically associated with sexual abuse, are possibly retraumatizing (Leeners et al., 2016), with some women refusing to participate and others being unable to communicate their needs (Leeners et al., 2013). Moreover, pregnancy and childbirth and their related intimate procedures may be triggering by reminding survivors of the prior abuse and associated powerlessness (Kitzinger, 1992).

While childbirth is not recognized as a traumatic event per se, childbirth and its related procedures may include traumatic elements for abuse survivors. Indeed, the likelihood of birth-related PTSD is higher for women with a child sexual abuse history than other women (Lev-Wiesel et al., 2009). Thus, the likelihood of unintentionally exacerbating psychological distress for pregnant women with a child sexual abuse history is exceptionally high, particularly when the obstetric provider is unaware of the abuse history or unaware of the implications of such a history for their prenatal care.

Identifying sexual abuse survivors

There are consistent calls for antenatal screening or changes in clinical practice to allow for greater consideration of a history of child sexual abuse when treating pregnant women (Collin-Vézina et al., 2015; Lukasse et al., 2009; Plant et al., 2013; Robertson-Blackmore et al., 2013). While most developed countries advocate that child sexual abuse history be specifically screened, it is not a widespread practice. In 2013, it was estimated that only 10% of obstetricians routinely assess a history of child sexual abuse (Leeners et al., 2006a) with low awareness among clinicians of the potential impact on perinatal care of a child sexual abuse history. In one study, despite all participants reporting at least one incidence of child abuse at intake, only 22% of obstetricians detected this information (Stevens et al., 2017).

The American College of Obstetricians and Gynecologists (2011) specifically recommends screening for child sexual abuse, whereas in Australia and the United Kingdom recommendations include a conversation about "sensitive issues" as part of a psychosocial assessment (Austin, 2014; NICE, 2008). Despite child sexual abuse not specifically named, these conversations may be a step toward identifying women at risk; however, considerations of the specific training in the particularities of such a conversation are needed (Rollans et al., 2013).

With the increased use of midwife-led continuity of care models in many countries (Sandall et al., 2016), these conversations may come in the form of the trusted relationships developed through these models. These relationships may foster environments conducive to disclosure for women who experienced child sexual abuse as they may feel safe to share their concerns and anxieties. For those who choose not to disclose, they also offer opportunities for the trained professional to recognize that all is not well without the abuse explicitly verbalized (Montgomery et al., 2015). Of interest in one study, nearly 20% of women with a child sexual abuse history felt dissatisfied with their prenatal care due to not having an opportunity to discuss their child sexual abuse (Leeners et al., 2013). Given that close to 30% of women may never disclose (McElvaney, 2015) due to (but not limited to) barriers such as internalized blame and protective mechanisms such as minimization and repression or an awareness of the impact of telling (Collin-Vézina et al., 2015), the importance of these conversations cannot be underestimated. With increased calls for the need to screen for pregnancy-related anxiety, opportunities may arise for specific insights into a woman's history using more comprehensive screening tools such as the PrAS (see Brunton et al., 2015 for further details).

Conclusion

This chapter has detailed the possible deleterious outcomes associated with child sexual abuse, a highly prevalent occurrence. Pregnancy presents a time that may exacerbate existing pathologies or create new ones given its contextualized nature and focus on areas of the women's body associated with sexual acts. Commonalities between child sexual abuse and pregnancy-related anxiety were detailed with the proposition of an additive effect for those women who have both a history of this abuse and the distinct pregnancy-related anxiety. While screening for child sexual abuse is not specifically advocated in most countries, the possibilities of screening and identifying those at risk may come through continuity of care models with the trusted relationships formed through these models may offer opportunities for disclosure or identification and more comprehensive screening tools.

References

Austin, M.-P. (2014). Marcé international society position statement on psychosocial assessment and depression screening in perinatal women. Best practice & research *Clinical Obstetrics & Gynaecology, 28*(1), 179–187. https://doi.org/10.1016/j.bpobgyn.2013.08.016

Australian Institute of Health & Welfare. (2015). *Australia's mothers and babies 2013 – in brief.* Perinatal Statistics Series No. 31.

Bell, K. M., & Higgins, L. (2015). The impact of childhood emotional abuse and experiential avoidance on maladaptive problem solving and intimate partner violence. *Behavioral Sciences, 5*(2), 154–175. https://doi.org/10.3390/bs5020154

Benedict, M. I., Paine, L. L., Paine, L. A., Brandt, D., & Stallings, R. (1999). The association of childhood sexual abuse with depressive symptoms during pregnancy, and selected pregnancy outcomes. *Child Abuse & Neglect, 23*(7), 659–670. https://doi.org/10.1016/s0145-2134(99)00040-x

Biaggi, A., Conroy, S., Pawlby, S., & Pariante, C. M. (2016). Identifying the women at risk of antenatal anxiety and depression: A systematic review. *Journal of Affective Disorders, 191,* 62–77. http://dx.doi.org/10.1016/j.jad.2015.11.014

Brunton, R., Woods, T., & Dryer, R. (2020). Child abuse, pregnancy-related anxiety and the mediating role of resilience and social support. *Journal of Health Psychology,* 1-11. https://doi.org/10.1177/1359105320968140

Brunton, R. J., & Dryer, R. (2021). Child sexual abuse and pregnancy: A systematic review of the literature. *Child Abuse & Neglect, 11,* 104802 https://doi.org/10.1016/j.chiabu.2020.104802

Brunton, R. J., Dryer, R., Saliba, A., & Kohlhoff, J. (2015). Pregnancy anxiety: A systematic review of current scales. *Journal of Affective Disorders, 176,* 24–34. https://doi.org/10.1016/j.jad.2015.01.039

Classen, C. C., Palesh, O. G., & Aggarwal, R. (2005). Sexual revictimization: A review of the empirical literature. *Trauma, Violence, & Abuse, 6*(2), 103–129. https://doi.org/10.1177%2F1524838005275087

Cloitre, M., Tardiff, K., Marzuk, P., Leon, A., & Portera, L. (1996). Childhood abuse and subsequent sexual assault among female inpatients. *Journal of Traumatic Stress, 9,* 473–482. https://doi.org/10.1007/BF02103659

Collin-Vézina, D., De La Sablonnière-Griffin, M., Palmer, A. M., & Milne, L. (2015). A preliminary mapping of individual, relational, and social factors that impede disclosure of childhood sexual abuse. *Child Abuse & Neglect, 43,* 123–134. https://doi.org/10.1016/j.chiabu.2015.03.010

Eide, J., Hovengen, R., & Nordhagen, R. (2010). Childhood abuse and later worries about the baby's health in pregnancy. *Acta Obstetricia et Gynecologica Scandinavica, 89*(12), 1523–1531. https://doi.org/10.3109/00016349.2010.526180

Finkelhor, D. (1994). Current information on the scope and nature of child sexual abuse. *The Future of Children,* 31–53.

Grimstad, H., & Schei, B. (1999). Pregnancy and delivery for women with a history of child sexual abuse. *Child Abuse & Neglect, 23*(1), 81–90. https://doi.org/10.1016/s0145-2134(98)00113-6

Heimstad, R., Dahloe, R., Laache, I., Skogvoll, E., & Schei, B. (2006). Fear of childbirth and history of abuse: Implications for pregnancy and delivery. *Acta Obstetricia et Gynecologica Scandinavica, 85*(4), 435–440. https://doi.org/10.1080/00016340500432507

Horan, D. L., Hill, L. D., & Schulkin, J. (2000). Childhood sexual abuse and preterm labor in adulthood: An endocrinological hypothesis. *Women's Health Issues, 10*(1), 27–33. https://doi.org/10.1016/S1049-3867(99)00038-9

Hoyer, J., Wieder, G., Höfler, M., Krause, L., Wittchen, H.-U., & Martini, J. (2020). Do lifetime anxiety disorders (anxiety liability) and pregnancy-related anxiety predict complications during pregnancy and delivery? *Early Human Development, 144,* 105022. https://doi.org//10.1016/j.earlhumdev.2020.105022

Hulme, P. A. (2000). Symptomatology and health care utilization of women primary care patients who experienced childhood sexual. *Child Abuse & Neglect, 24*(11), 1471-1484. https://doi.org//10.1016/S0145-2134(00)00200-3

Hulme, P. A. (2004). Retrospective measurement of childhood sexual abuse: A review of instruments. *Child Maltreatment, 9*(2), 201–217. https://doi.org/10.1177/1077559504264264

Jacobs, J. L. (1992). Child sexual abuse victimization and later sequelae during pregnancy and childbirth. *Journal of Child Sexual Abuse, 1*(1), 103–112. https://doi.org/10.1300/J070v01n01_07

Keegan, J., Parva, M., Finnegan, M., Gerson, A., & Belden, M. (2010). Addiction in Pregnancy. *Journal of Addictive Diseases, 29*(2), 175–191. https://doi.org/10.1080/10550881003684723

Kitzinger, J. V. (1992). Counteracting, not reenacting, the violation of women's bodies: The challenge for perinatal caregivers. *Birth, 19*(4), 219–220.

Koss, M. P., & Dinero, T. E. (1989). Discriminant analysis of risk factors for sexual victimization among a national sample of college women. *Journal of Consulting and Clinical Psychology, 57*(2), 242.

Lara, M., Navarrete, L., Nieto, L., & Le, H.-N. (2015). Childhood abuse increases the risk of depressive and anxiety symptoms and history of suicidal behavior in Mexican pregnant women. *Revista Brasileira de Psiquiatria, 37*(3), 203–210. https://doi.org/10.1590/1516-4446-2014-1479

Leeners, B., Görres, G., Block, E., & Hengartner, M. P. (2016). Birth experiences in adult women with a history of childhood sexual abuse. *Journal of Psychosomatic Research, 83*, 27–32. https://doi.org/10.1016/j.jpsychores.2016.02.006

Leeners, B., Neumaier-Wagner, P., Quarg, A. F., & Rath, W. (2006a). Childhood sexual abuse (CSA) experiences: An underestimated factor in perinatal care. *Acta Obstetricia et Gynecologica Scandinavica, 85*(8), 971–976. https://doi.org/10.1080/00016340600626917

Leeners, B., Rath, W., Block, E., Görres, G., & Tschudin, S. (2014). Risk factors for unfavorable pregnancy outcome in women with adverse childhood experiences. *Journal of Perinatal Medicine, 42*(2), 171–178. https://doi.org/10.1515/jpm-2013-0003

Leeners, B., Richter-Appelt, H., Imthurn, B., & Rath, W. (2006b). Influence of childhood sexual abuse on pregnancy, delivery, and the early postpartum period in adult women. *Journal of Psychosomatic Research, 61*(2), 139–151. https://doi.org/10.1016/j.jpsychores.2005.11.006

Leeners, B., Stiller, R., Block, E., Görres, G., Imthurn, B., & Rath, W. (2007). Effect of childhood sexual abuse on gynecologic care as an adult. *Psychosomatics, 48*(5), 385-393. https://doi.org/10.1176/appi.psy.48.5.385

Leeners, B., Stiller, R., Block, E., Görres, G., & Rath, W. (2010). Pregnancy complications in women with childhood sexual abuse experiences. *Journal of Psychosomatic Research, 69*(5), 503–510. https://doi.org/10.1016/j.jpsychores.2010.04.017

Leeners, B., Stiller, R., Block, E., Görres, G., Rath, W., & Tschudin, S. (2013). Prenatal care in adult women exposed to childhood sexual abuse. *Journal of Perinatal Medicine, 41*(4), 365–374. https://doi.org/10.1515/jpm-2011-0086

Lev-Wiesel, R., Chen, R., Daphna-Tekoah, S., & Hod, M. (2009). Past traumatic events: Are they a risk factor for high-risk pregnancy, delivery complications, and postpartum posttraumatic symptoms? *Journal of Women's Health, 18*(1), 119–125. https://doi.org/10.1089/jwh.2008.0774

Liapi, C. A., Tsakalia, D. E., Panitsa-Faflia, C. C., Antsaklis, A. I., Aravantinos, D. I., & Batrinos, M. L. (1996). Corticotropin-releasing-hormone levels in pregnancy-induced hypertension. *European Journal of Obstetrics & Gynecology & Reproductive Biology, 68*, 109–114. https://doi.org/10.1016/0301-2115(96)02508-0

Livingston, G. (2015). *Childlessness falls, family size grows among highly educated women.* Pew Research Center. www.pewresearch.org/social-trends/2015/05/07/childlessness-falls-family-size-grows-among-highly-educated-women/

LoGiudice, J. A. (2016). A systematic literature review of the childbearing cycle as experienced by survivors of sexual abuse. *Nursing for Women's Health, 20*(6), 582-594. https://doi.org//10.1016/j.nwh.2016.10.008

Lukasse, M., Schei, B., Vangen, S., & Øian, P. (2009). Childhood abuse and common complaints in pregnancy. *Birth, 36*(3), 190–199. https://doi.org/10.1111/j.1523-536X.2009.00323.x

Maniglio, R. (2009). The impact of child sexual abuse on health: A systematic review of reviews. *Clinical Psychology Review, 29*(7), 647–657. https://doi.org/10.1016/j.cpr.2009.08.003

Martini, J., Petzoldt, J., Einsle, F., Beesdo-Baum, K., Hofler, M., & Wittchen, H.-U. (2015). Risk factors and course patterns of anxiety and depressive disorders during pregnancy and after delivery: A prospective-longitudinal study. *Journal of Affective Disorders*, *175*, 385–395. https://doi.org/10.1016/j.jad.2015.01.012

Masten, A. S., & Cicchetti, D. (2010). Developmental cascades. *Development and Psychopathology*, *22*(3), 491–495. https://doi.org/10.1017/S0954579410000222

Mastorakos, G., & Ilias, I. (2003). Maternal and fetal hypothalamic – pituitary – adrenal axes during pregnancy and postpartum. *Annals of the New York Academy of Sciences*, *997*(1), 136–149. https://doi.org/10.1196/annals.1290.016

McElvaney, R. (2015). Disclosure of child sexual abuse: Delays, non-disclosure and partial disclosure. What the research tells us and implications for practice. *Child Abuse Review*, *24*(3), 159–169. https://doi.org/10.1002/car.2280

Mezey, G., Bacchus, L., Bewley, S., & White, S. (2005). Domestic violence, lifetime trauma and psychological health of childbearing women. *BJOG: An International Journal of Obstetrics & Gynaecology*, *112*(2), 197–204. https://doi.org/10.1111/j.1471-0528.2004.00307.x

Mohammadi, M. R., Zarafshan, H., & Khaleghi, A. (2014). Child abuse in Iran: A systematic review and meta-analysis. *Iranian Journal of Psychiatry*, *9*(3), 118–124.

Montgomery, E., Pope, C., & Rogers, J. (2015). The re-enactment of childhood sexual abuse in maternity care: A qualitative study. *BMC Pregnancy and Childbirth*, *15*(1), 194. https://doi.org/10.1186/s12884-015-0626-9

Moody, G., Cannings-John, R., Hood, K. Kemp, A., & Robling, M. (2018). Establishing the international prevalence of self-reported child maltreatment: A systematic review by maltreatment type and gender. *BMC Public Health*, *18*, 1164. https://doi.org/10.1186/s12889-018-6044-y

NICE. (2008). *Antenatal care: NICE clinical guideline 62*. National Institute for Health and Clinical Excellence (NICE).

Noll, J. G., Schulkin, J., Trickett, P. K., Susman, E. J., Breech, L., & Putnam, F. W. (2007). Differential pathways to preterm delivery for sexually abused and comparison women. *Journal of Pediatric Psychology*, *32*(10), 1238–1248. https://doi.org/10.1093/jpepsy/jsm046

Oliveira, A., Reichenheim, M., Moraes, C., Howard, L., & Lobato, G. (2017). Childhood sexual abuse, intimate partner violence during pregnancy, and posttraumatic stress symptoms following childbirth: A path analysis. *Archives of Women's Mental Health*, *20*(2), 297–309. https://doi.org/10.1007/s00737-016-0705-6

Pereda, N., Guilera, G., Forns, M., & Gómez-Benito, J. (2009). The international epidemiology of child sexual abuse: A continuation of Finkelhor (1994). *Child Abuse & Neglect*, *33*(6), 331–342. https://doi.org/10.1016/j.chiabu.2008.07.007

Plant, D., Barker, E. D., Waters, C., Pawlby, S., & Pariante, C. (2013). Intergenerational transmission of maltreatment and psychopathology: The role of antenatal depression. *Psychological Medicine*, *43*(3), 519–528. https://doi.org/10.1017/S0033291712001298

Putnam, F. W. (2003). Ten-year research update review: Child sexual abuse. *Journal of the American Academy of Child & Adolescent Psychiatry*, *42*(3), 269–278. https://doi.org//10.1097/00004583-200303000-00006

Robertson-Blackmore, E., Putnam, F. W., Rubinow, D. R., Matthieu, M., Hunn, J. E., Putnam, K. T., Moynihan, J. A., & O'Connor, T. G. (2013). Antecedent trauma exposure and risk of depression in the perinatal period. *The Journal of Clinical Psychiatry*, *74*(10), e942–948. https://doi.org/10.4088/jcp.13m08364

Roesch, S. C., Dunkel-Schetter, C., Woo, G., & Hobel, C. J. (2004). Modeling the types and timing of stress in pregnancy. *Anxiety, Stress & Coping, 17*(1), 87–102. https://doi.org/10.1080/1061580031000123667

Rollans, M., Schmied, V., Kemp, L., & Meade, T. (2013). 'We just ask some questions. . .' the process of antenatal psychosocial assessment by midwives. *Midwifery, 29*(8), 935–942. https://doi.org//10.1016/j.midw.2012.11.013

Romero, R., Dey, S. K., & Fisher, S. J. (2014). Preterm labor: One syndrome, many causes. *Science, 345*(6198), 760–765. https://doi.org/10.1126/science.1251816

Sandall, J., Soltani, H., Gates, S., Shennan, A., & Devane, D. (2016). Midwife-led continuity models versus other models of care for childbearing women. *Cochrane Database of Systematic Reviews, 8*. https://doi.org/10.1002/14651858.CD00 4667.pub3

Stevens, N. R., Tirone, V., Lillis, T. A., Holmgreen, L., Chen-McCracken, A., & Hobfoll, S. E. (2017). Posttraumatic stress and depression may undermine abuse survivors' self-efficacy in the obstetric care setting. *Journal of Psychosomatic Obstetrics & Gynecology, 38*(2), 103–110. https://doi.org/10.1080/0167482X.2016. 1266480

Tanaka, M., Suzuki, Y. E., Aoyama, I., Takaoka, K., & Macmillan, H. L. (2017). Child sexual abuse in Japan: A systematic review and future directions. *Child Abuse & Neglect, 66*, 31–40. https://doi.org/10.1016/j.chiabu.2017.02.041

The American College of Obstetricians and Gynecologists. (2011). *Adult manifestations of childhood sexual abuse.* Committee Opinion No. 498.

Wadhwa, P. D., Sandman, C. A., Porto, M., Dunlosky, J., & Garite, T. J. (1993). The association between prenatal stress and infant birth weight and gestational age at birth: A prospective investigation. *American Journal of Obstetrics & Gynecology, 169*(4), 858–865. https://doi.org/10.1016/0002-9378(93)90016-c

Wilson, D. R. (2010). Health consequences of childhood sexual abuse. *Perspectives in Psychiatric Care, 46*(1), 56–64. https://doi.org/10.1111/j.1744-6163.2009.00238.x

World Health Organization [WHO]. (2003). Guidelines for medico-legal care for victims of sexual violence. In *Child sexual abuse.* WHO.

World Health Organization [WHO]. (2011). Intimate partner violence during pregnancy. In *Department of reproductive health and research.* WHO.

World Health Organization [WHO]. (2015). *The world's women 2015: Trends and statistics.* WHO. https://unstats.un.org/unsd/gender/downloads/WorldsWomen 2015_chapter6_t.pdf

World Health Organization [WHO]. (2017). *Responding to children and adolescents who have been sexually abused: WHO clinical guidelines.* WHO.

Wosu, A. C., Gelaye, B., & Williams, M. A. (2015). Childhood sexual abuse and posttraumatic stress disorder among pregnant and postpartum women: Review of the literature. *Archives of Women's Mental Health, 18*(1), 61-72. https://doi. org/10.1007/s00737-014-0482-z

Yampolsky, L., Lev-Wiesel, R., & Ben-Zion, I. Z. (2010). Child sexual abuse: Is it a risk factor for pregnancy? *Journal of Advanced Nursing, 66*(9), 2025–2037. https://doi.org/10.1111/j.1365-2648.2010.05387.x

Zambaldi, C. F., Cantilino, A., Farias, J. A., Moraes, G. P., & Botelho Sougey, E. (2011). Dissociative experience during childbirth. *Journal of Psychosomatic Obstetrics & Gynecology, 32*(4), 204–209. https://doi.org/10.3109/0167482X.2011. 626092

13 Psychosocial functioning, body image, and pregnancy-related anxiety

Rachel Dryer

Psychosocial functioning, body image, and pregnancy-related anxiety

The main aim of this chapter is to provide an overview of the research that has been conducted on the association between body dissatisfaction and psychological distress during pregnancy, in particular pregnancy-related anxiety. As detailed in earlier chapters of this book, pregnancy-related anxiety is regarded as a condition that affects up to 14.4% of pregnant women (Poikkeus et al., 2006), and is regarded as a possible risk factor for postnatal depression (Austin et al., 2007; Heron et al., 2004; Milgrom et al., 2008; Sutter-Dallay et al., 2004). Moreover, worries, fears, and concerns about body image have long been recognized as one of the cognitive dimensions of pregnancy-related anxiety (Bayrampour et al., 2016), and this is reflected in the available measures that have been developed specifically for this form of anxiety. For example, one of the three core subscales of the Pregnancy-Related Anxiety Questionnaire Revised-2 (PRAQ-R2, Huizink et al., 2016) measures concern about one's own appearance and includes items such as "I am worried about the fact that I shall not regain my figure after delivery" and "I am concerned about my unattractive appearance." Similarly, a core subscale of the Pregnancy-related Anxiety Scale (PrAS, Brunton et al., 2018) measures body image concerns of pregnant women with items such as "I don't feel good with the way I look," "I feel scared that I will never regain my figure," and "I worry that my partner doesn't find me attractive."

However, while there have been numerous studies on pregnancy-related anxiety aimed at understanding its nature and the contributing factors and outcomes for the mother and infant (DiPietro et al., 2006; Hedegaard et al., 1993), the research specifically aimed at understanding the association between body dissatisfaction and pregnancy-related anxiety has only emerged relatively recently. An early example of research examining this association includes the study conducted by Goodwin et al. (2000) who examined whether there were differences in psychological well-being and body image between pregnant women who exercised and non-exercising pregnant women. In this study, the General Health Questionnaire (GHQ) was used as the measure for psychological well-being. While the results pertaining to the anxiety and insomnia subscale was reported in a table,

DOI: 10.4324/9781003014003-17

the focus of the results were primarily on GHQ total scores as a measure of overall psychological well-being. Most of the studies that have examined the association between body dissatisfaction and psychological distress have primarily focused on depression (Meireles et al., 2015; Skouteris et al., 2005). Only recently have more studies on the correlates of body dissatisfaction included other indicators of distress such as disordered eating and state and/or general anxiety (Chan et al., 2018, 2020). Given this situation, this chapter has adopted a broad coverage approach to examining the association between psychosocial functioning and body image during pregnancy by examining the findings in relation to depression, eating disorder, symptomatology, as well as anxiety.

Body image and body dissatisfaction

Body image refers to the individual's internal representation of their outer appearance. This broad multidimensional construct is comprised of attitudinal, behavioral, and perceptual components (Grogan, 2008; Jarry & Ip, 2005). The attitudinal dimension of body image includes the individual's beliefs and evaluations of their own appearance and the appearance of others. The perceptual dimension refers to the accuracy of an individual's judgments of their own body size. The behavioral aspects of body image include appearance-related behaviors aimed at controlling or changing one's appearance and an individual's avoidance of situations that may result in scrutiny or evaluation from others (Grogan, 2008). Body dissatisfaction often manifests as extreme dissatisfaction with one's appearance, body shape and/or weight, excessive appearance management behaviors, frequent appearance checking, and avoidance of situations that may result in appearance-related judgment (Jarry & Ip, 2005). These body image disturbances have been consistently associated with mental health problems, including depression, disordered eating behavior, and lowered self-esteem in both women and men (Barnes et al., 2020; Paxton et al., 2006; Sharpe et al., 2018; Stice & Shaw, 2002).

   Body dissatisfaction, which is recognized to be prevalent and widespread especially among women (Fiske et al., 2014), often occurs when a woman's beliefs about her appearance do not align with a desired or idealized body shape or size (Grogan, 2008; Tiggemann, 2004). Body dissatisfaction has been attributed to societal pressures to meet the thin-ideal beauty standards that continue to be prominent in most Western, industrialized countries (Loth et al., 2011). Notably, the participants in these previous studies have reported that their body dissatisfaction stems from their perceptions of being heavier than their ideal. More recently, high levels of body dissatisfaction have also been reported for pregnant women across many countries and cultures (Chan et al., 2020; Roomruangwong et al., 2017; Skouteris, 2011; Skouteris et al., 2005; Tsuchiya et al., 2019).

Appearance-related sociocultural pressures during pregnancy

During pregnancy women are faced with considerable physical, physiological, and psychological changes. The rapid changes in the woman's body shape and size are the most visible signs of the changes in the body's role and function. While most women adapt well to these physical changes (Clark et al., 2009), others may find the rapid changes challenging as they reevaluate their appearance-related beliefs (Skouteris, 2011). For this latter group, pregnancy can be a period of immense body dissatisfaction, especially if they continue to define their appearance based on pre-pregnancy body shape and weight and have concerns about being able to meet societal beauty ideals post-birth (Clark et al., 2009; Johnson et al., 2004). During pregnancy, women continue to experience societal pressure to maintain their appearance and to limit weight gain during pregnancy (Orbach & Rubin, 2014). Studies examining media representation of celebrities' pregnancy in popular media have reported that pregnancy weight is frequently portrayed negatively, whereas weight loss after birth is portrayed positively (Gow et al., 2012; Roth et al., 2012), with an emphasis on rapid weight loss postpartum (Roth et al., 2012). In other words, the thin-ideal beauty standard expected of non-pregnant women is applied to women in the early postpartum period (Roth et al., 2012).

A relatively recent investigation into the content of pregnancy magazines found that over a third of advertisements in these magazines promoted appearance-related products that fostered the idea that the physical changes associated with pregnancy needed to be rectified or fixed (e.g., belly wraps that fit around the stomach to help shrink the belly, or clothes to minimize the size of the stomach). Ten percent of these products were aimed at body shaping and toning, and quick weight loss after birth (Boepple & Thompson, 2017). These appearance pressures reinforce the "Yummy Mummy" identity of motherhood promoted in popular media. While the label "Yummy Mummy" originally embodied female choice, self-sufficiency, autonomy, and aesthetic perfection (Allen & Osgood, 2009), it has largely been used to celebrate and promote women who are slender and who either quickly "bounce back" to their pre-pregnancy body shape or who obtain a body shape that is "better" than before (O'Brien Hallstein, 2011). Being a "good mother" has been equated to women who ensure that their bodies are slim, toned, and "sexy." In contrast, "fatness" is associated with personal failure, lack of self-discipline, and control, and therefore constitutes being a "bad mother" (Malatzky, 2017). These media-generated appearance pressures and the internalization of these pressures are regarded as contributing to body dissatisfaction during pregnancy and postpartum (Lovering et al., 2018). Therefore, it is not surprising that, similar to non-pregnant women, pregnant women's body dissatisfaction arises from perceptions of being larger than their ideal even when these women were of normal weight or even below normal weight before conceiving (Tsuchiya et al., 2019).

Body dissatisfaction during pregnancy

Quantitative studies that have examined body dissatisfaction in pregnant women have produced inconsistent findings. While some studies have reported that body image remains relatively stable throughout pregnancy (e.g., Duncombe et al., 2008) or improves relative to pre-pregnancy body satisfaction levels (e.g., Clark & Ogden, 1999; Loth et al., 2011), other studies have suggested that levels of body dissatisfaction increase during pregnancy (e.g., Goodwin et al., 2000; Skouteris et al., 2005), peaking during the postpartum period (Gjerdingen et al., 2009; Rallis et al., 2008). These inconsistent findings are likely to be partly due to methodological variations in the study design (i.e., cross-sectional vs. longitudinal), different instruments used to measure body dissatisfaction (e.g., use of figure rating scales vs. questionnaire items assessing level of satisfaction with specific parts of the body), previous experience of pregnancy (i.e., nulliparous vs. multiparous women), and trimester of pregnancy. The gestational time point in which measures of body dissatisfaction have been taken has been found to influence the nature of body shape and weight concerns of pregnant women. For example, the early stages of pregnancy before the body is recognizably pregnant can be challenging for some women due to concerns that the extra weight may be perceived as being "fat" rather than being "pregnant" (Nash, 2012). Whereas the body concerns experienced by women in the mid to late pregnancy are likely more related to concerns of how the body will look after pregnancy and/or gaining too much weight (Bergbom et al., 2017). However, these inconsistent findings also suggest that the nature of body dissatisfaction and appearance-related identity during pregnancy is complex and not fully captured by existing body dissatisfaction instruments and/or study methodology.

Qualitative investigations on this issue have shed light on the nature of this complexity. A systematic review, conducted by Watson and colleagues (2015), of the qualitative studies on body image experiences during pregnancy found that (a) body image ideals change during pregnancy as women adjust to their role as a mother, (b) both body dissatisfaction and satisfaction are experienced at different times during pregnancy, (c) certain body parts like the stomach and breast have prominent influence on women's body satisfaction, and (d) there is perceived pressure to not only limit weight gain during pregnancy but also to quickly regain pre-pregnancy body shape and size postpartum. This review also highlighted that women can have unrealistic expectations about what is acceptable or normal weight gain during pregnancy, as well as unrealistic notions about the pregnant body shape/size (Watson et al., 2015). These sociocultural pressures to attain unrealistic body shape/size have been demonstrated to persist into the post-pregnancy period, contributing to significant body image concerns (Lovering et al., 2018).

The contributing role of sociocultural pressure on body dissatisfaction was further explored in a study conducted by Hicks and Brown (2016). In this cross-sectional study involving 269 pregnant women, the association between social media use (i.e., Facebook engagement) and body dissatisfaction was examined. A significant relationship was found between having a Facebook account and higher levels of body dissatisfaction, particularly in regard to concerns about body shape and size postpartum. This study also highlighted the key role self-comparison played in defining body image in that over half of these women (56.5%) reported that they frequently compared their pregnant body to other pregnant women. While this study was not able to establish the causal link between social media use, self-comparison, and body dissatisfaction, the findings are consistent with the Tripartite Influence Model of body dissatisfaction (Thompson et al., 1999).

The Tripartite Influence Model (Thompson et al., 1999) proposes that three key sociocultural pressures influence the development of psychological distress (e.g., problematic eating behaviors and depression). These sociocultural pressures include pressure from popular media as well as interpersonal sources of pressure from peers, and family members that include other women and partners, to meet societal ideals of appearance. This interpersonal pressure may come in the form of appearance-related teasing or encouragement to lose weight. The model also posits that the constructs of internalization of societal beauty standards and social comparison both mediate the relationship between sociocultural pressures and body dissatisfaction. In addition to the thin-ideal, pregnant women may also encounter other standards in regard to obtaining the "perfect bump," which is where weight gain is restricted to the belly with little weight gain elsewhere (Hicks & Brown, 2016). Other pregnancy ideals may not be related to the woman's body shape and weight but rather to other beauty standards such as clear and glowing skin and having shiny hair. For postpartum women, the body shape/weight ideals may have a particular emphasis on muscle tone (or muscularity) as indicators of being able to successfully regain their pre-pregnancy body shape.

The applicability of this model to postpartum mothers has recently been suggested using structural equation modeling in a large sample of postpartum women (N = 474) who had given birth within the last 12 months of the study (Lovering et al., 2018). While few differences in model fit were observed when comparing women who had given birth within the last 6 months with women who had given birth within 7–12 months, the model accounted for more variance in body dissatisfaction, thin-ideal internalization, drive for muscularity, depression and self-esteem in women within the later stages of the postpartum period. This finding suggests that women in the later stages of the postpartum period are more vulnerable to appearance-related sociocultural pressures. Moreover, a large proportion of the women in this study were actively trying to lose weight with reported weight goals that were lower than their pre-pregnancy weight. These findings are consistent with the "Yummy Mummy" ideals promoted in popular media that women should not only quickly regain their pre-pregnancy bodies but also obtain a body that is "better" (i.e., thinner and/or more toned) than before (O'Brien Hallstein, 2011), and that women experience increasing appearance-related pressures (and therefore higher levels of body dissatisfaction), particularly during the postpartum period (Gjerdingen et al., 2009; Rallis et al., 2008).

Note that at the time of writing this chapter, the applicability of the Tripartite Influence Model in explaining the appearance-related pressures and experiences of pregnant women had not been specifically tested. However, there are a number of studies that have examined the association between sociocultural pressure, body dissatisfaction, and psychological distress such as anxiety, depression, and disordered eating during pregnancy.

The association between body dissatisfaction and psychological distress

Some of the key correlates of body dissatisfaction in pregnant women were summarized in a systematic review conducted by Fuller-Tyszkiewicz and colleagues (2012). In this review of 22 cross-sectional and prospective studies on body dissatisfaction during pregnancy, the researchers identified a consistent, small-to-moderate association between sociocultural pressures (e.g., appearance-related teasing and pressure to meet the thin-ideal) and body dissatisfaction in pregnant women. In addition, a weak but robust association between body dissatisfaction and depression was identified, with this association being observed across different methods of measuring body dissatisfaction, which range from global estimates of body dissatisfaction, dissatisfaction with specific body parts and/or weight, to perceptions of unattractiveness.

However, there is contention in the literature in regard to the direction of the relationship between these two constructs. The findings from some prospective studies suggest that depression predicts body dissatisfaction during pregnancy and postpartum. For example, a prospective study (N = 230) conducted by Downs et al. (2008) found that depressive symptomatology in the first trimester predicted body dissatisfaction in subsequent trimesters, as well as depressive symptomatology and body dissatisfaction in the second trimester. These findings are consistent with those reported by Clark et al. (2009) who conducted a prospective study involving 116 women, who were asked to provide retrospective recall of pre-pregnancy levels of depression and body dissatisfaction and were also assessed during pregnancy and 12 months postpartum. These researchers reported that their data best supported a model of depressive symptomatology (in the later stages of pregnancy) predicting body dissatisfaction at 6 weeks postpartum, as well as perceptions of fatness throughout the postpartum period. In contrast, the findings from more recent studies suggest the opposite causal relationship (i.e., body dissatisfaction contributing to depression during pregnancy and postpartum). For example, in Rauff and Down's (2011) study involving 151 women who were assessed at each trimester, body dissatisfaction at trimesters 1 and 2 predicted depression at trimesters 2 and 3, respectively. Similarly, Riquin and her colleagues (2019) recently demonstrated, in a longitudinal study involving 457 women, that the risk of depression during pregnancy was four times higher in women with poor body image. Based on this finding, Riquin et al. recommended screening for body dissatisfaction during pregnancy to prevent perinatal depression. Further evidence to support the proposition that body dissatisfaction leads to depression comes from a recent prospective longitudinal study conducted by Chan et al. (2020). In this study, 1,371 women were assessed on measures of body dissatisfaction, anxiety (Hospital Anxiety and Depression Scale, Anxiety Subscale – HADS-A), and depression at each trimester of pregnancy and up to 6 weeks postpartum. These women were also asked to provide retrospective recall (i.e., 6 months prior to pregnancy) on both variables. After controlling for identified risk factors, body dissatisfaction before and during pregnancy were positively associated with higher levels of depressive and general anxiety symptomatology during pregnancy and 6 weeks postpartum. More specifically, pre-pregnancy body dissatisfaction significantly and independently predicted depression and anxiety in all three trimesters of pregnancy. While these more recent prospective and longitudinal studies indicate that body dissatisfaction leads to perinatal depression and anxiety, it is possible that there is a bidirectional relationship between body dissatisfaction and distress (i.e., depression and anxiety), which may explain the seemingly contradictory findings on this issue.

While most of the past research has focused on understanding the relationship between body dissatisfaction and depression, more recent studies have also included other indicators of psychological distress such as problematic eating behaviors and anxiety. For example, Chan and colleagues in an earlier related study (i.e., Chan et al., 2018) examined the prevalence and levels of eating disorders during pregnancy in a study involving 1,470 pregnant women. As in their 2020 study, women were assessed at five time points from the first trimester to 6 months postpartum, and at the first time point, they were asked to provide retrospective self-report (6 months prior to pregnancy) of disordered eating, anxiety, and depression. They reported that while problematic eating behaviors decreased from pre-pregnancy to pregnancy, these behaviors increased from pregnancy to the postpartum period. Moreover, after controlling for problematic eating behaviors before pregnancy, anxiety and depressive symptoms were independently associated with eating disorder symptomatology (i.e., binge-eating disorders and bulimia nervosa) across the three trimesters of pregnancy, with variations in anxiety and depressive symptoms accounting for variations in disordered eating behavior during pregnancy. These researchers concluded that both anxiety and depression in pregnancy are potential risk factors for disordered eating during pregnancy, and that food may be used by women as a way to regulate anxiety and depressive symptoms.

The association between body dissatisfaction, depression, and anxiety during pregnancy and postpartum has also been reported in a cross-sectional study involving 126 pregnant women from Thailand who were assessed in the third trimester of pregnancy and at two time points postpartum (i.e., 2–3 days and 4–6 weeks after birth) (Roomruangwong et al., 2017). Greater body dissatisfaction was associated with both higher state and trait anxiety during pregnancy and lifetime history of bulimia. Moreover, greater body dissatisfaction was associated with higher depressive symptomatology.

The few studies that have examined the association between body dissatisfaction and anxiety during pregnancy have primarily focused on general state anxiety as measured by instruments like the State Trait Anxiety Inventory (STAI) or the HADS-A. Only one study has so far used a measure specifically designed for pregnancy-related anxiety. This recent study by Dryer et al. (2020) supports the key roles sociocultural pressure and social comparison play in body dissatisfaction and psychological distress in pregnant women. In this cross-sectional study of 408 pregnant women, appearance-related sociocultural pressure (from peers, family, and media) significantly predicted pregnancy-related anxiety as well as eating disorder symptomatology and depression. Fat Talk (a form of conversation that involves self-derogatory body talk that can encourage body shape/weight comparison with other women) partially mediated the relationship between sociocultural pressure and pregnancy-related anxiety, and between sociocultural pressure and eating disorder symptomatology. Interestingly, Fat Talk fully mediated the relationship between sociocultural pressure and depression. In addition, body dissatisfaction was found to have direct significant relationships with measures of psychological distress (i.e., pregnancy-related anxiety, depression, and eating disorders), with Fat Talk partially mediating these relationships when these distress variables were examined individually in separate mediation models. These findings are consistent with the findings of previous studies that indicate that pregnant women continue to face sociocultural pressure to meet beauty standards despite the body's new role of reproduction, and also add further evidence to support the association between body dissatisfaction and psychological distress (i.e., depression, eating disorder symptoms, and pregnancy-related anxiety). Moreover, the findings suggest that engaging in appearance-focused conversation (such as Fat Talk) heighten these levels of distress. Note that these findings need to be confirmed in subsequent studies, and the exact nature of the association between body dissatisfaction, eating disorder symptomatology, and pregnancy-related anxiety needs to be established. In other words, the causal direction between sociocultural pressures, body dissatisfaction, eating disorder symptomatology, and pregnancy-related anxiety needs to be clarified during pregnancy and postpartum. One could propose that current appearance-related standards that place excessive importance on the thin-ideal may result in greater body dissatisfaction in expectant mothers, which contributes to eating disorder symptomatology and pregnancy-related anxiety. However, this needs to be confirmed in a prospective and/or longitudinal study where all the relevant constructs are measured.

Gaps and limitations in the current literature

There are a number of limitations in much of the research conducted on this issue. First, most of the studies conducted so far have been cross-sectional in nature with samples comprised of women in different trimesters of pregnancy – thus, making it difficult to assess the direction of causality between body dissatisfaction and the indicators of psychological distress. It is only relatively recently that more prospective and longitudinal studies have emerged that allow for changes in these psychological constructs to be measured and examined in relation to whether body dissatisfaction predicts prenatal and postpartum depression, disordered eating, and anxiety. However, due to the methodological design, these studies have high attrition rates, especially postpartum. Women who already face demands on their time, energy, and psychological well-being are likely to feel less able to participate in these studies, which limits the validity and generalizability of the findings. Second, none of the studies reviewed in this chapter have specifically examined the role of parity (i.e., nulliparous vs. multiparous women) on the relationship between body dissatisfaction and psychological distress/well-being. More specifically, there is limited understanding around whether previous experiences of pregnancy and birth influence women's body image and appearance-related identity, and whether nulliparous women are more susceptible to sociocultural pressures and consequently experience greater body dissatisfaction and potentially higher levels of distress, especially during the postpartum period when women are expected to regain their pre-pregnancy body shape and size. Third, another limitation in the research conducted so far is the reliance on self-report measures of body dissatisfaction and psychological distress or well-being. The self-reported ratings on these measures are likely to be influenced by whether the women are having a "good day" versus a "bad day" at the time of assessment. Moreover, the women's ratings may also be influenced by other variables in the immediate context not measured by the researchers.

The application of ecological momentary assessment methodology in future studies holds promise in further exploration of the exact nature of the association between body dissatisfaction and pregnancy-related anxiety as this methodology allows for real-time emotional precursors and consequences of body dissatisfaction across pregnancy. Finally, the measurement of body dissatisfaction during pregnancy has been a contentious issue with most studies employing measures designed for non-pregnant women given that they potentially influence the validity of the reported findings (Fuller-Tyszkiewicz et al., 2012). This limitation has now been addressed by Watson et al. (2017) with the development of the Body Image in Pregnancy Scale (BIPS). The development of this 36-item scale has been informed by the findings of qualitative studies that have examined women's body image experiences across pregnancy. Initial psychometric evaluations of this scale indicate that the BIPS is comprised of seven dimensions (i.e., preoccupation with appearance, dissatisfaction with strength, dissatisfaction with facial features, sexual attractiveness, prioritizing appearance, behavioral avoidance, and dissatisfaction with body parts), with good to excellent internal consistency reliabilities (0.78–0.95) and acceptable test-retest reliabilities for five of the seven subscales. Examination of the concurrent validity of the BIPS indicated that the subscales correlated with measures of global self-esteem (i.e., Rosenberg Self-Esteem Scale) and body image (i.e., Body Attitudes Questionnaire-Short Form). While this scale is an important advancement in the measurement of body image during pregnancy, further evaluation of its psychometric properties, particularly other forms of validity and its applicability to women from other cultures, is still needed.

Future directions

As identified in the previous paragraph, there is a need to conduct further studies using either prospective, longitudinal design or ecological momentary assessment methods in order to fully understand the nature of the relationship between sociocultural pressures, body dissatisfaction, and psychological distress. For example, the applicability of the Tripartite Influence Model to account for the image-related experiences and body dissatisfaction needs to be explicitly tested, with measures of all the key components of this model included in one sample of pregnant women, similar to Lovering et al.'s (2018) study of postpartum women. There is also a need for more studies that examine the association between pregnancy-related anxiety and psychosocial functioning, especially given that this form of anxiety has been identified as a risk factor for postnatal depression (Austin et al., 2007; Heron et al., 2004; Milgrom et al., 2008; Sutter-Dallay et al., 2004). These studies also need to examine factors that may influence a woman's body image and therefore body dissatisfaction. For example, there is a need to better understand whether parity plays a significant role in body dissatisfaction and psychological distress (e.g., pregnancy-related anxiety) and whether first time expectant mothers need additional support. Similarly, there is a need to examine the variables that may moderate and/or mediate the relationship between sociocultural pressure and body dissatisfaction during pregnancy. Self-compassion, which refers to kindness and understanding of one's own personal struggles and imperfections, has been reported to be positively associated with body appreciation, and was a moderating variable in the relationship between body-related threats (e.g., body comparison, media beauty ideals) and body appreciation (Homan & Tylka, 2015). This finding suggests that self-compassion can help protect women's positive body image. However, there has been little research exploring the role self-compassion plays in body image dissatisfaction for pregnant and postpartum women.

Summary and conclusion

There is sufficient evidence from both qualitative and quantitative studies that both pregnant and postpartum women face sociocultural pressures to meet the thin-ideal, and that this appearance-related pressure is negatively associated with women's psychosocial functioning (Fuller-Tyszkiewicz et al., 2012; Watson et al., 2015), especially when women engage in self-comparison behaviors (e.g., Dryer et al., 2020; Hicks & Brown, 2016). More recent prospective and longitudinal studies have resulted in greater clarification of the nature of the association between body dissatisfaction and psychological distress, with some researchers identifying the need for body image screening during pregnancy in order to facilitate earlier intervention for anxiety, depression, and eating disorder symptomatology (e.g., Chan et al., 2018, 2020; Lovering et al., 2018; Riquin et al., 2019). However, there is currently limited research on pregnancy-related anxiety. Therefore, more research is needed, using a range of methodologies, in order to better understand the relationship between body dissatisfaction and pregnancy-related anxiety, especially in regard to possible moderating (e.g., parity) and mediating factors (e.g., self-compassion). This information will not only inform public education programs but also interventions aimed at preventing psychological distress in pregnant and postpartum women.

References

Allen, K., & Osgood, J. (2009). Young women negotiating maternal subjectivities: The significance of social class. *Studies in the Maternal*, *1*(2), 1–17. https://doi.org/10.16995/sim.104

Austin, M., Tully, L., & Parker, G. (2007). Examining the relationship between antenatal anxiety and postnatal depression. *Journal of Affective Disorders*, *101*(1–3), 169–174, https://doi.org/10.1016/j.jad.2006.11.015

Barnes, M., Abhyankar, P., Dimova, E., & Best, C. (2020). Associations between body dissatisfaction and self-reported anxiety and depression in otherwise healthy men: A systematic review and meta-analysis. *PLoS One*, *15*(2), e0229268. https://doi.org/10.1371/journal.pone.0229268.

Bayrampour, H., Ali, E., Mcneil, D. A., Benzies, K., Macqueen, G., & Tough, S. (2016). Pregnancy-related anxiety: A concept analysis. *International Journal of Nursing Studies*, *55*, 115–130. https://doi.org/10.1016/j.ijnurstu.2015.10.023

Bergbom, I., Modh, C., Lundgren, I., & Lindwall, L. (2017). First-time pregnant women's experiences of their body in early pregnancy. *Scandinavian Journal of Caring Sciences*, *31*(3), 579–586. https://doi.org/10.1111/scs.12372

Boepple, L., & Thompson, J. K. (2017). An exploration of appearance and health messages present in pregnancy magazines. *Journal of Health Psychology*, *22*(14), 1862–1868. https://doi.org/10.1177/1359105316639435.

Brunton, R. J., Dryer, R., Krägeloh, C., Saliba, A., Kohlhoff, J., & Medvedev, O. (2018). The pregnancy-related anxiety scale: A validity examination using Rasch analysis. *Journal of Affective Disorders*, *236*, 127–135. https://doi.org/10.1016/j.jad.2018.04.116

Chan, C. Y., Lee, A. M., Koh, Y. W., Lam, S. K., Lee, C. P., Leung, K. Y., & Tang, C. S. K. (2018). Course, risk factors, and adverse outcomes of disordered eating in pregnancy. *International Journal of Eating Disorders*, *52*, 652–658. https://doi.org/10.1002/eat.23065

Chan, C. Y., Lee, A. M., Koh, Y. W., Lam, S. K., Lee, C. P., Leung, K. Y., & Tang, C. S. K. (2020). Associations of body dissatisfaction with anxiety and depression in the pregnancy and postpartum periods: A longitudinal study. *Journal of Affective Disorders*, *263*, 582–592. https://doi.org/10.1016/j.jad.2019.11.032

Clark, A., Skouteris, H., Wertheim, E. H., Paxton, S. J., & Milgrom, J. (2009). My baby body: A qualitative insight into women's body-related experiences and mood during pregnancy and the postpartum. *Journal of Reproductive and Infant Psychology*, *27*(4), 330–345. https://doi.org/10.1080/02646830903190904.

Clark, M., & Ogden, J. (1999). The impact of pregnancy on eating behaviour and aspects of weight concern. *International Journal of Obesity*, *23*, 18–24. https://doi.org/10.1038/sj.ijo.0800747.

DiPietro, J. A., Novak, M. F. S. X., Costigan, K. A., Atella, L. D., & Reusing, S. P. (2006). Maternal psychological distress during pregnancy in relation to child development at age two. *Child Development*, *77*(3), 573–587. https://doi.org/10.1111/j.1467-8624.2006.00891.x

Downs, D. S., DiNallo, J. M., & Kirner, T. L. (2008). Determinants of pregnancy and postpartum depression: Prospective influences of depressive symptoms, body image satisfaction, and exercise behavior. *Annals of Behavioral Medicine*, *36*(1), 54–63. https://doi.org/10.1007/s12160-008-9044-9.

Dryer, R., von der Schulenburg, I. G., & Brunton, R. (2020). Body dissatisfaction and fat talk during pregnancy: Predictors of distress. *Journal of Affective Disorders*, *267*, 289-296. https://doi.org/10.1016/j.jad.2020.02.031

Duncombe, D., Wertheim, E. H., Skouteris, H., Paxton, S. J., & Kelly, L. (2008). How well do women adapt to changes in their body size and shape across the course of pregnancy? *Journal of Health Psychology*, *13*(4), 503–515. https://doi.org/10.1177/1359105308088521

Fiske, L., Fallon, E. A., Blissmer, B., & Redding, C. A. (2014). Prevalence of body dissatisfaction among United States adults: Review and recommendations for future research. *Eating Behaviors*, *15*(3), 357–365. https://doi.org/10.1016/j.eatbeh.2014.04.010.

Fuller-Tyszkiewicz, M., Skouteris, H., Watson, B. E., & Hill, B. (2012). Body dissatisfaction during pregnancy: A systematic review of cross-sectional and prospective correlates. *Journal of Health Psychology*, *18*(11), 1411–1421. https://doi.org/10.1177/1359105312462437

Gjerdingen, D., Fontaine, P., Crow, S., McGovern, P., Center, B., & Miner, M. (2009). Predictors of mothers' postpartum body dissatisfaction. *Women & Health*, *49*(6), 491-504. https://doi.org/10.1080/03630240903423998

Goodwin, A., Astbury, J., & McMeeken, J. (2000). Body image and psychological well-being in pregnancy. A comparison of exercisers and non-exercisers. *Australian and New Zealand Journal of Obstetrics and Gynaecology*, *40*(4), 442–447. https://doi.org/10.1111/j.1479-828x.2000.tb01178.x.

Gow, R. W., Lydecker, J. A., Lamanna, J. D., & Mazzeo, S. E. (2012). Representations of celebrities' weight and shape during pregnancy and postpartum: A content analysis of three entertainment magazine websites. *Body Image*, *9*(1), 172–175. https://doi.org/10.1016/j.bodyim.2011.07.003

Grogan, S. (2008). *Body image: Understanding body dissatisfaction in men, women and children* (2nd ed.). Routledge/Taylor & Francis Group.

Hedegaard, M., Henriksen, T. B., Sabroe, S., & Secher, N. J. (1993). Psychological distress in pregnancy and preterm delivery. *BMJ*, *307*(6898), 234–239. https://doi.org/10.1136/bmj.307.6898.234.

Heron, J., O'Connor, T. G., Evans, J., Golding, J., Glover, V., & ALSPAC Study Team. (2004). The course of anxiety and depression through pregnancy and the postpartum in a community sample. *Journal of Affective Disorders*, *80*(1), 65–73. https://doi.org/10.1016/j.jad.2003.08.004

Hicks, S., & Brown, A. (2016). Higher Facebook use predicts greater body image dissatisfaction during pregnancy: The role of self-comparison. *Midwifery*, *40*, 132-140. https://doi.org/10.1016/j.midw.2016.06.018

Homan, K. J., & Tylka, T. L. (2015). Self-compassion moderates body comparison and appearance self-worth's inverse relationships with body appreciation. *Body Image*, *15*, 1–7. https://doi.org/10.1016/j.bodyim.2015.04.007

Huizink, A. C., Delforterie, M. J., Scheinin, N. M., Tolvanen, M., Karlsson, L., & Karlsson, H. (2016). Adaption of pregnancy anxiety questionnaire – revised for all pregnant women regardless of parity: PRAQ-R2. *Archives of Women's Mental Health*, *19*(1), 125–132. https://doi.org/10.1007/s00737-015-0531-2

Jarry, J., & Ip, K. (2005). The effectiveness of stand-alone cognitive-behavioural therapy for body image: A meta-analysis. *Body Image*, *2*(4), 317–331. https://doi.org/10.1016/j.bodyim.2005.10.001.

Johnson, S., Burrows, A., & Williamson, I. (2004). 'Does my bump look big in this?' The meaning of bodily changes for first-time mothers-to-be. *Journal of Health Psychology, 9*(3), 361-374. https://doi.org/10.1177/1359105304042346.

Loth, K. A., Bauer, K. W., Wall, M., Berge, J., & Neumark-Sztainer, D. (2011). Body satisfaction during pregnancy. *Body Image, 8*(3), 297–300. https://doi.org/10.1016/j.bodyim.2011.03.002

Lovering, M. E., Rodgers, R. F., George, J. E., & Franko, D. L. (2018). Exploring the Tripartite Influence Model of body dissatisfaction in postpartum women. *Body Image, 24*, 44-54. https://doi.org/10.1016/j.bodyim.2017.12.001.

Malatzky, C. A. (2017). Australian women's complex engagement with the yummy mummy discourse and the bodily ideals of good motherhood. *Women's Studies International Forum, 62*, 25–33. https://doi.org/10.1016/j.wsif.2017.02.006.

Meireles, J. F., Neves, C. M., de Carvalho, P. H., & Ferreira, M. E. (2015). Body dissatisfaction among pregnant women: An integrative review of the literature. *Cien Saude Colet, 20*(7), 2091–2103. https://doi.org/10.1590/1413-81232 015207.05502014.

Milgrom, J., Gemmill, A. W., Bilszta, J. L., Hayes, B., Barnett, B., Brooks, J., & Buist, A. (2008). Antenatal risk factors for postnatal depression: A large prospective study. *Journal of Affective Disorders, 108*, 147–157. https://doi.org/10.1016/j.jad.2007.10.014.

Nash, M. (2012). *Making 'postmodern' mothers: Pregnant embodiment, baby bumps and body image.* Palgrave Macmillan. https://doi.org/10.1057/9781137292155

O'Brien Hallstein, D. (2011). She gives birth, she's wearing a bikini: Mobilizing the post-pregnant celebrity mom body to manage the post-second wave crisis in femininity. *Women's Studies in Communication, 34*(2), 111–138. https://doi.org/10.1 080/07491409.2011.619471.

Orbach, S., & Rubin, H. (2014). *Two for the price of one: The impact of body image during pregnancy and after birth.* Department for Culture, Media and Sport and Government Equalities Office.

Paxton, S. J., Neumark-Sztainer, D., Hannan, P. J., & Eisenberg, M. E. (2006). Body dissatisfaction prospectively predicts depressive mood and low self-esteem in adolescent girls and boys. *Journal of Clinical Child & Adolescent Psychology, 35*(4), 539–549. https://doi.org/10.1207/s15374424jccp3504_5.

Poikkeus, P., Saisto, T., Unkila-Kallio, L., Punamaki, R. L., Repokari, L., Vilska, S., . . . Tulppala, M. (2006). Fear of childbirth and pregnancy-related anxiety in women conceiving with assisted reproduction. *Obstetrics and Gynecology, 108*, 70–76. https://doi.org/10.1097/01.AOG.0000222902.37120.2f

Rallis, S., Skourteris, H., Wertheim, E., & Paxton, S. (2008). Predictors of body image during the first year postpartum: A prospective study. *Women & Health, 45*(1), 87-104. https://doi.org/10.1300/J013v45n01_06

Rauff, E. L., & Downs, D. S. (2011). Mediating effects of body image satisfaction on exercise behavior, depressive symptoms, and gestational weight gain in pregnancy. *Annals of Behavioral Medicine, 42*(3), 381–390. https://doi.org/10.1007/s12160-011-9300-2.

Riquin, E., Lamas, C., Nicolas, I., Dugre Lebigre, C., Curt, F., Cohen, H., Legendre, G., Corcos, M., & Godart, N. (2019). A key for perinatal depression early diagnosis: The body dissatisfaction. *Journal of Affective Disorders, 245*, 340–347. https://doi.org/10.1016/j.jad.2018.11.032.

Roomruangwong, C., Kanchanatawan, B., Sirivichayakul, S., & Maes, M. (2017). High incidence of body image dissatisfaction in pregnancy and the postnatal period: Associations with depression, anxiety, body mass index and weight gain during pregnancy. *Sexual & Reproductive Healthcare*, *13*, 103–109. https://doi.org/10.1016/j.srhc.2017.08.002

Roth, H., Homer, C., & Fenwick, J. (2012). "Bouncing back": How Australia's leading women's magazines portray the postpartum body. *Women and Birth*, *25*(3), 128–134. https://doi.org/10.1016/j.wombi.2011.08.004

Sharpe, H., Griffiths, S., Choo, T., Eisenberg, M. E., Mitchison, D., Wall, M., & Neumark-Sztainer, D. (2018). The relative importance of dissatisfaction, overvaluation and preoccupation with weight and shape for predicting onset of disordered eating behaviors and depressive symptoms over 15 years. *International Journal of Eating Disorders*, *51*(10), 1168–1175. https://doi.org/10.1002/eat.22936

Skouteris, H. (2011). Body image issues in obstetrics and gynecology. In T. F. Cash & L. Smolak (Eds.), *Body image: A handbook of science, practice, and prevention* (pp. 342–349). Guilford Press.

Skouteris, H., Carr, R., Wertheim, E. H., Paxton, S. J., & Duncombe, D. (2005). A prospective study of factors that lead to body dissatisfaction during pregnancy. *Body Image*, *2*(4), 347–361. https://doi.org/10.1016/j.bodyim.2005.09.002

Stice, E., & Shaw, H. E. (2002). Role of body dissatisfaction in the onset and maintenance of eating pathology: A synthesis of research findings. *Journal of Psychosomatic Research*, *53*(5), 985–993. https://doi.org/10.1016/s0022-3999(02)00488-9.

Sutter-Dallay, A. L., Giaconne-Marcesche, V., Glatigny-Dallay, E., & Verdoux, H. (2004). Women with anxiety disorders during pregnancy are at increased risk of intense postnatal depressive symptoms: A prospective survey of the MATQUID cohort. *European Psychiatry*, *19*(8), 459–463. https://doi.org/10.1016/j.eurpsy.2004.09.025.

Thompson, J. K., Coovert, M. D., & Stormer, S. M. (1999). Body image, social comparison, and eating disturbance: A covariance structure modelling investigation. *International Journal of Eating Disorders*, *26*(1), 43–51. https://doi.org/10.1002/(SICI)1098-108X(199907)26:1<43::AID-EAT6>3.0.CO;2-R.

Tiggemann, M. (2004). Body image across the adult life span: Stability and change. *Body Image*, *1*(1), 29–41. https://doi.org/10.1016/S1740-1445(03)00002-0.

Tsuchiya, S., Yasui, M., & Ohashi, K. (2019). Assessing body dissatisfaction in Japanese women during the second trimester of pregnancy using a new figure rating scale. *Nursing & Health Sciences*, *21*(3), 367–374. https://doi.org/10.1111/nhs.12608

Watson, B., Fuller-Tyszkiewicz, M., Broadbent, J., & Skouteris, H. (2015). The meaning of body image experiences during the perinatal period: A systematic review of the qualitative literature. *Body Image*, *14*, 102–113. http://dx.doi.org/10.1016/j.bodyim.2015.04.005

Watson, B., Fuller-Tyszkiewicz, M., Broadbent, J., & Skouteris, H. (2017). Development and validation of a tailored measure of body image for pregnant women. *Psychological Assessment*, *29*(11), 1363. https://doi.org/10.1037/pas0000441

Conclusion

Robyn Brunton and Rachel Dryer

In 1956 Norman Pleshette, Stuart Asch, and Janet Chase sought to "examine the nature of anxieties present in primiparas" (p. 436). Many have credited Pleshette and his colleagues as conducting the earliest study into pregnancy-related anxiety (e.g., Guardino & Dunkel-Schetter, 2014). Some 65 years later, research aimed at understanding this form of anxiety continues. This book, being the culmination of the work of dedicated researchers in this area, is a testament to that seminal work by Pleshette and his colleagues.

Pleshette et al. (1956) pointed out that "anxiety of one kind or another is always present within pregnant women" (p. 455). This statement reminds us that in seeking to understand the manifestation of any phenomena that may occur as part of a normative human process, we risk pathologizing that normative process. But, as has been shown in this book, the immutable changes that occur as part of pregnancy, may make a woman more susceptible to anxieties at that time, and indeed it is the presence of impairment that determines pathology. Nadelson (1973) sought to delineate this as the "normal" and "special" aspects of pregnancy.

As presented in Part I of this book (*Understanding pregnancy-related anxiety*), pregnancy-related anxiety is a particular or unique form of anxiety, which is clinically distinctive and has unique antecedents or risk factors. Another aspect that sets this anxiety apart from other anxieties is its contextualization by pregnancy and the maternal and neonatal outcomes that appear to be more closely associated with pregnancy-related anxiety in comparison to other forms of anxiety. Research in this area is compelling with many advancements in recent years.

The application of research can arguably be said to be more important than the research itself. Bridging the research-application gap is an important aspect of our scientific endeavors and for pregnancy-related anxiety (given the implications for both mother and child) this is a critical component. While pregnancy-related anxiety is contextualized by the pregnancy itself, it does more than describe the content of the woman's worries and fears and this, as O'Connor et al. point out (Chapter 3), is what gives this anxiety scientific and clinical impact. Pleshette's original work in quantifying this anxiety was diagnostic in nature and he applied his findings to the clinical setting behooving us toward making great effort toward this goal. Many of his items exist in current scales in a similar form (e.g., *Are you*

DOI: 10.4324/9781003014003-18

afraid the pain may be bad? Are you afraid your baby will not be normal?) and many do not (e.g., *Did the doctor frighten you about getting too fat? Do you want a boy?*) demonstrating advances that have been made in the ensuing decades.

As shown in Part II, *Implications for Practice*, our current diagnostic practices that are not specific to pregnancy-related anxiety may still capture this unique anxiety. While this affords a level of assuredness that women may not necessarily be misdiagnosed or miss being diagnosed, there are consistent calls for more specific screening, which will require the availability of psychometrically sound screening scales. Much work has already been done in this respect, although the accuracy of some of these scales in detecting pregnancy-related anxiety still need to be evaluated against some form of diagnostic gold-standard and/or biochemical markers of distress. Naturally, screening is linked to treatment and while there is emerging evidence of the efficacy of some psychological and psychosocial treatments, it is clear that further research is needed in this area.

Part III considered – *where to next* – examining future directions for pregnancy-related anxiety research. The chapters in this part all considered emerging research and while they lacked a depth of research to draw on, as the work in this areas is still evolving, the insights and foresights (i.e., where we should direct our research attention) should prove invaluable to future researchers. The chapter on cross-cultural perspectives demonstrated that while pregnancy-related anxiety may be a universal phenomenon, it is less universal in its presentation. This was further extrapolated in the chapter on acculturation and the challenges faced by migrant women. The final two chapters each examined specific areas, both integral to the presentation and treatment of this anxiety, namely, childhood experiences of sexual abuse and body dissatisfaction during pregnancy. As explored in their respective chapters, these two issues present as potential areas where women may need specific support and education to reduce the possibility of them developing psychological distress during pregnancy and postpartum.

As illustrated in the breath of research reported in the various chapters of this book, we have come a long way since Pleshette, Asch, and Chase first investigated anxieties in primiparas. However, as Christine Dunkel-Schetter reminds us – *there is still much to do.*

References

Guardino, C. M., & Dunkel-Schetter, C. (2014). Understanding pregnancy anxiety. *Zero to Three, 34*(4), 12–21. www.zerotothree.org

Nadelson, C. (1973). "Normal" and "special" aspects of pregnancy. *Obstetrics and Gynecology, 41*(4), 611–620.

Pleshette, N., Asch, S. S., & Chase, J. (1956). A study of anxieties during pregnancy, labor, the early and late puerperium. *Bulletin of New York Academic Medicine, 32*(6), 436–455. https://pubmed.ncbi.nlm.nih.gov/13316338/

Index

Index

pregnancy concerns 5, 7, 8, 10
pregnancy distress 5
pregnancy-related anxiety 9, 40,
41, 62–63, 117, 158, 189, 203;
acculturation and 163, 164; affective
disorders and 42–44, 46; age and
12; antecedents 53, 134; assessment
108, 109; behavioral mechanisms
14; biological mechanisms 13–14,
46, 47; birth outcomes 10, 12,
32, 33, 61, 63, 64, 68–69; body
dissatisfaction and 189, 190, 197;
child brain development and 84;
child development and 75; child
motor development and 83–84;
child psychopathology and 82;
child sexual abuse and 180, 181,
182; chronic stress and 8; cognitive
development and 83; cognitive
dimensions 145, 151; concerning
the health of the child 46, 65,
181–182; concerns about labor and
delivery 75; contextual factors 146;
cortisol and 33–34, 85; cross-cultural
cognitive dimensions 147, 149–151;
cultural expectations and 7; cultural
factors 14–15, 145–147, 150–152;
cultural variations 143–144;
definition 5, 6–7; demographic
factors 56; depression and 56;
developmental cascade theories 181;
diagnosing 99–100; and DSM-V
classification 100; education and
12–13; ethnophysiological factors
146; ethnopsychological factors
146; fetal programming and 74–75;
first-time pregnancy and 25; future
research issues 66–69; generalised
anxiety disorder (GAD) and 6–7,
27–28; in high-income countries
144; in high-risk pregnancies 7;
history of pre-pregnancy loss and
42–43, 55, 89; history of research
on 6; and hypothalamic pituitary
axis (HPA) regulation 13, 84–85,
89; ICD-10 and 101; impairments
42; infant/child negative affectivity
and 81–82; inflammatory processes
and 13–14; internal stigma and
150–151; interventions 47, 57,
89, 123–124; IVF treatment and
55; in Latinas 14–15, 87; length of
gestation and 9, 10, 13, 64, 66, 68;

low birth weight and 64; in low- to
middle-income countries 144–145;
and maternal cortisol levels 32;
measurement of 75, 81, 110–112;
mechanistic studies 69; versus other
types of prenatal distress 85–86;
parenting stress and 33; physiological
mechanisms 32; predictive validity
of 31–33; predictors of 12–13, 15,
44, 46; pregnancy concerns and 7,
8; pre-pregnancy origins 46; preterm
birth and 10, 63, 64, 65, 182;
prevalence rates 41, 62, 109–110,
143; psychological factors 56, 65;
psychological interventions 16; recent
studies on birth outcomes 65–66;
risk factors 55; screening tools 16,
57; self-reported 109; sex differences
in fetal vulnerability 86–87; social
and contextual factors 88; state
anxiety and 29–30; substance abuse
and 14; symptoms 99, 100, 147;
timing of fetal exposure to 86;
tokophobia and 110, 132, 181–182;
trait anxiety and 29–30, 44; *see also*
antecedents of pregnancy-related
anxiety; antenatal anxiety; birth
outcomes; interventions; migrant
women; psychological interventions
Pregnancy-Related Anxiety
Questionnaire (PRAQ) 6, 65, 75, 82,
83, 110
Pregnancy-Related Anxiety
Questionnaire-Revised (PRAQ-R) 28
Pregnancy-related Anxiety Scale (PrAS)
75, 88, 113–114
Pregnancy-Related Thoughts (PRT)
scale 116
pregnancy-specific anxiety 5, 7, 9, 10,
14; length of gestation and 13–14;
preterm birth and 66
Pregnancy-Specific Anxiety Scale (PSAS)
117
prenatal anxiety: birth outcomes 62–63;
preterm birth and 62
prenatal depression 25; low birth weight
and 12
prenatal general anxiety 8, 9, 61
prenatal stress 8, 10, 12, 27, 88
pre-pregnancy loss, pregnancy-related
anxiety and 42–43, 55, 89
pre-pregnancy origins, pregnancy-
related anxiety 46

For Product Safety Concerns and Information please contact our EU
representative GPSR@taylorandfrancis.com
Taylor & Francis Verlag GmbH, Kaufingerstraße 24, 80331 München, Germany

www.ingramcontent.com/pod-product-compliance
Lightning Source LLC
Chambersburg PA
CBHW060255220326
41598CB00027B/4112